An Introduction to
HUMAN MOVEMENT
and BIOMECHANICS

An Introduction to

HUMAN MOVEMENT
and BIOMECHANICS

SEVENTH EDITION

EDITED BY

Andy Kerr, PhD, MSC, MCSP
Lecturer, Biomedical Engineering,
University of Strathclyde, Glasgow,
UK

and

Philip Rowe, PhD
Professor of Rehabilitation Science,
Biomedical Engineering,
University of Strathclyde, Glasgow,
UK

ELSEVIER

Edinburgh London New York Oxford Philadelphia St Louis Sydney 2019

ISBN: 978-0-7020-6236-0

Content Strategist: Serena Castelnovo/Poppy Garraway Smith
Content Development Specialist: Veronika Watkins
Content Coordinator: Susan Janson
Project Manager: Karthikeyan Murthy
Designer: Bridget Hoette
Illustration Manager: Muthukumaran Thangaraj

Printed in China

Last digit is the print number: 9 8 7 6 5 4 3 2 1

 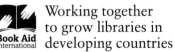

Working together
to grow libraries in
developing countries

www.elsevier.com • www.bookaid.org

ELSEVIER

*We dedicate this book to Professor John Paul for his pioneering work
in the measurement of human movement.*

CONTENTS

SECTION II   Human Movement

PREFACE

This is the seventh edition of *The Human Movement* book. The first edition, *Human Movement: An Introductory Text for Physiotherapy Students,* was published in 1981 and quickly became a major part of physiotherapy undergraduate study. It put the understanding of human movement at the very centre of the physiotherapy profession. After all the hard work in anatomy and physiology this was the book that started the journey into movement analysis and thinking like a therapist. The fact that it has continued for almost 40 years speaks volumes for its appeal and the importance of the area. As new editors we have not only tried to put our own mark on the book, but also retained most of the content and the friendly style. A strength of previous editions has been the recognition that students come from diverse academic backgrounds. With qualifications and experience in physiotherapy (Kerr) and biomedical engineering (Rowe) we understand this diversity very well and have hopefully kept the universal appeal of its plain English delivery, its use of figures and the generally accessible way the content is presented.

After saying all that, this version of the book does differ in tone and content from previous versions. We have removed the anatomical text (this is well covered in many other textbooks that you may already own) and the sociological aspects of previous editions (which are better given their full prominence in a dedicated textbook). We have done this to make room in this book for a more detailed chapter on motor control, as well as new chapters on motor learning and physical activity. We have also spent more time on the biomechanical sections. Too often these concepts are presented with lots of unexplained engineering terms and principles which hinder understanding. In this edition of the book we have taken our time deciphering this information so that it is more easily digested and applied for practical understanding. Finally, we have added a whole chapter of case studies, which will introduce you to movements such as walking, sit to stand, reaching and rowing. The case studies all include real data from either athletes or patients; we hope you enjoy this new section and that it helps inspire your practice. There will also be a supporting website (http://evolve.elsevier.com/Kerr/movement/) where we will add new case studies as well as online quizzes.

Although the book is historically rooted in physiotherapy, understanding human movement is, of course, a key part of many professions, such as podiatry, occupational therapy, biomedical engineering, medicine and sports coaches/therapists. We have tried to bear this in mind by using a broad range of examples from both the clinical and sport worlds. Understanding human movement is a multidisciplinary affair.

Enjoy the book!
Andy and Philip (2019)

Andy and Philip

We have been lucky to get contributions from a range of movement experts across the globe. Movement scientists, physiotherapists, engineers, rehabilitation doctors, podiatrists, orthotists and sports scientists have all contributed, and we are grateful for their enthusiasm and willingness to share their expertise. Their details are listed on the next page. As editors we consider that for understanding human movement our own backgrounds in both medical engineering and physiotherapy has been complementary. We would always advocate a multidisciplinary approach to human movement analysis, combining the engineering principles of objective measurement and the application of physics and maths with the physiotherapist's understanding of how the body works and how the person thinks both in health and illness. Our collaborative research over 30 years is a testimony to the benefits of a multidisciplinary partnership with publications across a range of orthopaedic and neurological movement disorders, as well as developing the movement analysis technology with which to study them. We hope this book will lead some of you to further explore and perhaps even contribute to the understanding of human movement. This has been and continues to be our passion, and we hope you will share it.

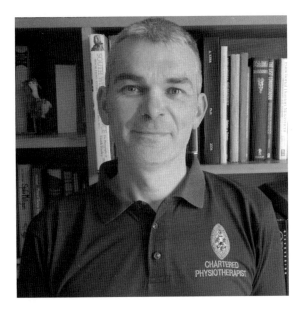

Andy Kerr

After qualifying in 1988 Andy practised as a physiotherapist in the National Health Service for 10 years before undertaking a PhD at the University of Nottingham and then Glasgow Caledonian University, where he also worked as a lecturer teaching biomechanics, exercise therapy and paediatrics. In 2010 he joined the Biomedical Engineering Department at Strathclyde University to conduct clinical research in the area of stroke rehabilitation, and has been awarded several grants in the area of technology-enhanced rehabilitation. His primary motivation in research is the understanding of impaired human movement and its recovery. He is the author of more than 60 scientific papers as well as the undergraduate textbook *Introductory Biomechanics* (Elsevier). He is a Member of the Chartered Society of Physiotherapy and past Chair of the Physiotherapy Research Society.

Recent publications are available from:
http://www.strath.ac.uk/staff/kerrandydr/
https://www.researchgate.net/profile/Andy_Kerr

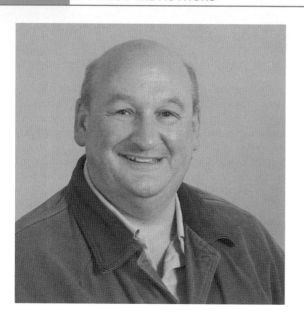

Philip Rowe

Professor Rowe obtained a BSc Hons in Mechanical Engineering from the University of Birmingham (1982) followed by a PhD in Bioengineering from the University of Strathclyde (1990). For his PhD work he was awarded the European Society of Biomechanics, Clinical Biomechanics Award in 1987. After completing his PhD, he held various academic appointments at Queen Margaret University, Edinburgh, UK, where he pursued his own research and was responsible for research development within the School of Health Sciences. He rejoined the Biomedical Engineering Department at Strathclyde in September 2005 as a Professor of Rehabilitation Sciences and is currently the Research Director. Professor Philip Rowe's main research areas lie in clinical movement analysis, functional analysis, biomechanics of the human body in motion, rehabilitation engineering, rehabilitation technology, rehabilitation robotics and robotic surgery especially applied in orthopaedics and stroke.

CONTRIBUTORS

The editor(s) would like to acknowledge and offer grateful thanks for the input of all contributors of previous editions, without whom this new edition would not have been possible.

Seda Bilaloglu, MS
New York University School of
    Medicine,
New York, USA

Roy Bowers, HDip Prosthetics and Orthotics
Principal Teaching Fellow,
National Centre for Prosthetics and
    Orthotics,
Department of Biomedical
    Engineering,
University of Strathclyde,
Glasgow, UK

Bruce Carse, PhD, MEng, MIPEM
Clinical Scientist,
West of Scotland Mobility and
    Rehabilitation Centre,
NHS Scotland,
Glasgow, UK

Megan Caughey
New York Institute of Technology,
Old Westbury,
New York, USA

Philippa Coales, PhD, MSc, PGDip, Health Ergonomics, PGCE
Lecturer in Physiotherapy,
School of Healthcare Sciences,
Cardiff University,
Cardiff, UK

Madeleine A. Grealy, PhD, MPhil, BSc (Hons)
Professor of Psychology,
School of Psychological Sciences and
    Health,
University of Strathclyde,
Glasgow, UK

Kristen Hollands, PhD, MSc, BSc (Hons)
Senior Research Fellow,
School of Health and Society,
University of Salford,
Manchester, UK

Konstantinos Kaliarntas, PhD, MSc, MCSP
Lecturer in Biomechanics,
Sport, Exercise and Health Science,
Edinburgh Napier University,
Edinburgh, UK

Clare Kell, EdD, MSc, MCSP
Director,
Centre for the Enhancement of
    Learning and Teaching,
University of South Wales,
Pontypridd, UK

Andy Kerr, PhD, MSc, MCSP
Lecturer,
Biomedical Engineering,
University of Strathclyde,
Glasgow, UK

Jennifer Muhaidat, PhD
Assistant Professor,
Department of Physiotherapy,
The University of Jordan,
Amman, JOR

Andrew Murphy, PhD, MRes, BSc (Hons)
Senior Lecturer Sport and Exercise
    Biomechanics,
Sport and Exercise,
Birmingham City University,
Birmingham, UK

Daniel Rafferty, HND
Lecturer,
Institute for Applied Health Research,
Glasgow Caledonian University,
Glasgow, UK

Preeti Raghavan, MD
Associate Professor,
Rehabilitation Medicine,
New York University School of
    Medicine,
New York, USA

Philip Rowe, PhD
Professor of Rehabilitation Science,
Biomedical Engineering,
University of Strathclyde,
Glasgow, UK

Tim Sharp, MSc, BSc (Hons), MCSP
Senior Lecturer,
Physiotherapy,
Cardiff University,
Cardiff, UK

Jennifer Stone, MD
New York University School of
    Medicine,
New York, USA

Alvin Tang, BS
New York University School of
    Medicine,
New York, USA

ACKNOWLEDGEMENTS

We would like to acknowledge the contribution from all the previous editors and authors involved in this title. Their work has provided us with a strong platform to deliver the current edition. We would also like to acknowledge the photography of Andy Kerr (senior) in the biomechanics chapters. The book is intended for students of human movement, so we would like to acknowledge the contribution from our previous and current students at the Universities of Strathclyde, Nottingham, Queen Margaret and Glasgow Caledonian for providing us with the motivation and critical feedback that shaped the way we taught biomechanics and human movement. Finally, we acknowledge the many participants in our research without whom we would know very little about human movement.

Introduction

Andy Kerr and Philip Rowe

MOVEMENT

Volitional movement separates animals from plants; from ants to humans, we all move. Every part of us is designed with movement in mind. Science fiction writers like to entertain us with visions of motionless human bodies linked to huge computers running simulations of life. Besides putting physiotherapists out of business, the idea that we can live a motionless life is fundamentally flawed, ignoring the millions of years of evolution that have put us together. Quite simply we are designed to move, and if we do not move, our bodies (skin/bones/muscles/joints/lungs/heart etc.) weaken, our brain loses perception and acuity and our sensory organs become dull. Being deprived of the rich and varying stimuli of actual real movement diminishes our health and well-being and reduces our ability to move. We will always move because we were designed to do this from the very beginning and our very existence depends on it.

UNDERSTANDING MOVEMENT

This book has the sole aim of helping you understand how humans move. You could be a physiotherapy student, a sports science student or even a mad scientist trying to reanimate a long-dead human. The main thing is that you need to understand human movement for whatever your reasons, rehabilitation or terrifying the village down the valley. We have assumed your prior knowledge to be minimal, but we have also assumed your interest and desire to learn. The best way to consolidate knowledge is to apply it immediately to real problems; in the case of human movement this is quite straight forward. You will need to spend time observing lots of people moving, playing sport, acting, walking, limping, standing at the bus stop or slouched at the table next to you as you read this.

Understanding human movement combines five main scientific areas:

1. **Anatomy:** The muscles, bones, joints and motor centres involved in movement. Although we will not go into a lot of anatomic detail (best left to anatomy books), we will make reference to anatomy throughout the book.
2. **Biomechanics:** Using mechanical principles to understand how biologic systems (e.g. human bone, cells, bird feathers, anything that is, or was, alive) move and respond to forces in the physical world.
3. **Physiology:** Understanding the functioning of living systems (e.g. how muscles contract, how the neurons in the brain connect to each other to initiate and control movement, how connective tissue repairs itself).
4. **Psychology:** How movement is learnt, from the early steps taken by toddlers to refining a squash serve. This will include motor learning theories as well as motivation to move.

5. **Metrology:** Understanding any physical phenomenon requires measurement. Measuring human movement involves many levels, from how much a single joint moves to how a person moves around their local community.

Of course understanding human movement is not a new thing. In prehistorical times we probably studied the motor skill of a hunter to emulate them and kill prey. Perhaps the cave paintings found in northern Spain/France were early motion analysis studies of animals so we could be more effective hunters or perhaps just because it was interesting. The first person to put down a record of these movement observations was Aristotle, who wrote *On the motion of Animals* 2500 years ago; you can still buy his book on Amazon (and probably other book vendors). Aristotle, like his contemporary Greek philosophers, began his explorations with observations which felt more like questions. Such as:

> *The movements of animals, quadruped and multiped, are crosswise, or in diagonals, and their equilibrium in standing posture is maintained crosswise; and it is always the limb on the right-hand side that is the first to move.*

This is always a good starting point to understanding movement, making an observation and posing a question. Why is that man keeping his knee straight when he walks? Why is that woman going down the stairs sideways? Why does that runner strike the ground with the outside of his foot?

Try Activity Box 1.1.

These days we have a lot of technology to throw at movement analysis, so we can do a much better job than the ancient Greeks. Video, three-dimensional (3D) motion analysis, accelerometers, gyroscopes etc. can all contribute hugely to movement analysis, and we will cover all these in Chapter 12, but at its heart, movement analysis is still based on making observations (using technology or our eyes) and asking the question *why*. In Chapter 9 we will dip our toe in the world of motor control which will attempt to address this question. In our final Chapter 17, we will consider the altered and abnormal movement patterns presented by patients and athletes.

As we have already said, humans are programmed to move, but that does not mean we know how to move from birth. We do have some basic moves in our early days, called primitive reflexes (see Chapter 10), but these are gradually overridden by more mature movements that we learn through imitation, repetition and feedback. This is a process called motor learning, which we will read about in Chapter 15.

Understanding human movement was given a huge boost in the 19th century with the development of the camera, which provided the means to look at movement systematically and scientifically, applying Newton's principles of mechanics

---

ACTIVITY BOX 1.1 Why Do Quadrupeds Stand and Move Their Limbs in Diagonals?

Ok, let's tackle Aristotle's observation that quadrupeds (think of a dog) position their limbs 'crosswise' or in a diagonal when standing or when they walk. The first thing to bear in mind is that animals (including humans) move in a certain way because it is beneficial, it gives them some kind of an advantage. As Aristotle said himself, 'Nature creates nothing without a purpose.'

What do you think a dog gains from placing its paws in the following position? Think of its balance/stability (which we will cover in Chapter 8); is it better in this position? Is Aristotle's observation true of all quadrupeds?

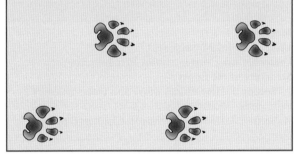

(mass, momentum, force, acceleration) to understand how a human moves. Chapters 2 to 5 will take us through some of this biomechanical understanding. A lot of our knowledge in this area was driven initially by our desire to design replacement joints. Subsequently we attempted to understand the way a child with cerebral palsy walks; this led to groundbreaking surgery and possibly more importantly to a robust approach to understanding human gait (see Case Study one for more information on gait analysis in cerebral palsy). We are now in a new era where we will see motion analysis become ubiquitous in movement training and rehabilitation.

UNDERSTANDING MOVEMENT FOR REHABILITATION

At some point after an injury or illness the body will try to resume normal service. This might be a simple case of regaining movement in your back through gentle stretches after it was injured, or it might be a long process of rehabilitation to recover walking ability after a stroke. For many parts of the body, restoration of movement is absolutely critical to repair and recover, for example:

- Lacking a decent blood supply, the cells that make up the specialised cartilage tissue on the joint surface are nourished through the movement of the joint.

- Collagen fibres laid down during the repair process following a tendon injury are guided by the movements that the tissue is experiencing. No movement will result in a haphazard arrangement, compromising strength and flexibility.
- The way the brain rewires itself after injury (e.g. stroke or traumatic head injury) is influenced by what it experiences. Repetitive movement is a major factor in recovery of functions in the motor cortex (part of brain where movement is initiated and controlled).

Helping an individual recover his or her movement ability (or athletic performance) requires a sound understanding of why that person is moving the way he or she is, including: the way the brain is controlling the movement (see Chapter 9), the way the muscle is contracting (see Chapter 6) and the way the joint is moving (see Chapter 7). But of course we also need to understand the wider picture about movement: why older people are less physically active (see Chapters 10 and 14), the pathologies that stem from not moving very much and perhaps even understanding the shift in our movement behaviour because of the way we now work and travel. Therefore we need to understand three levels of movement: (1) how injury/damage to specific *structures* affects movement, (2) the effect this may have on their ability to perform functional *activities* and (3) the impact a reduction in functional ability might have on an individual's ability to *participate* in their life roles. Structures, activity and participation need to be measured in different ways, and this is considered in Chapter 13. This is important so that we have a rich understanding of movement and not one limited to joint motion or muscle contraction.

For a first attempt at studying human movement, try Activity Boxes 1.2 and 1.3.

> **ACTIVITY BOX 1.2 Classifying Movement**
>
> Wait until you are somewhere with lots of people (a library, a street, the kitchen in your flat, a shopping centre). Find a comfortable place to sit down and, without looking too conspicuous (cutting eye holes in a newspaper does not work), look at the people move around you for at least 20 min. Can you classify their movement? Suggested categories are:
> 1. *Mobility:* They are getting from one place to another.
> 2. *Activity of daily living:* Things they may routinely do to keep healthy and happy (e.g. eating, washing, brushing hair/teeth, getting dressed).
> 3. *Occupation:* For example, paid work, caring for a dependent, studying human movement.
> 4. *Leisure:* Reading, playing sport, hobbies etc.
> 5. *Communication:* We do not just talk with our mouth. Posture and arm/hand movements are also used to communicate.

> **ACTIVITY BOX 1.3 Classifying Movement, Part Two**
>
> From Activity Box 1.2 choose one movement (brushing teeth, making a cup of coffee, walking up stairs etc.) and try the following questions:
> 1. Which joint moves the most?
> 2. Which plane does most of the movement occur in?
> 3. Is there a repetitive cycle in the movement; if so, can you identify the cycle start and finish?

STRUCTURE OF THE BOOK

The book is organised into four very broad sections.

Section 1: How Things Move and Flow: Chapters 2 to 5

In Section 1 will consider biomechanics. This is the application of mechanical principles to better understand all living things (compared with trains or planets); in this book we are chiefly concerned with how these principles apply to movement, human movement in particular. We will look at the relationship between force and movement, how forces (like a muscle pull) can be combined, how bodies become stable and unstable and the energy flow during movement. We will not just look at solid bodies but also fluids; we will look at the way fluids (like blood) move and also the way materials such as skin and tendon behave (a little like fluids) when forces are applied to them.

Section 2: Human Movement: Chapters 6 to 10

In Section 2 we will look closely at the way the human body creates and controls the forces required for movement. We will look at joint mechanics and how this limits or enables movement. The way the central nervous system initiates and controls movement, posture and balance is a hugely complex area, which we will introduce in Section 2. Finally, we will look at how movement develops during early life and then declines with age.

Section 3: Measurement of Movement: Chapters 11 to 14

In Section 3 we will look at how to measure human movement. We will cover the basic principles of measurement (metrology) before going into more details around measurement of movement in a laboratory and clinical environment, the technology available and the biomechanical measures used. We will consider all aspects of movement using the World Health Organisation (WHO) classification of mobility and function (body structure and function, activity and participation). Looking at how the joints move to create gait would be a reflection of body function, how may steps we do in a day would be a reflection of our activity and where, with whom and for what would be a reflection of our participation. In medicine and health care we have tended to look only at body function and assume if we restore this then activity and participation will naturally return. This is increasingly recognised not to be the case, and we must take active steps to encourage/rehabilitate activity and participation as well as function. The final chapter of this section will therefore explore in detail the activity and participation aspects of human movement by looking at physical activity in life and how it is measured.

Section 4: Restoring and Optimising Human Movement: Chapters 15 to 17

In this final section we will consider aspects of movement recovery. Although some of this information has already been raised in previous sections (e.g. restoring flexibility in Chapter 7), in this section we will consider how movement is learned (and relearned) and we will look at aspects of how movement and posture interact with our environment; after all, recovery needs to be made in the context of our working and living environment. In the final chapter we will look at five case studies of movements covering upper limb (reach to grasp), lower limb (sit to stand, gait and use of ankle foot orthoses) and a sports activity (rowing). This last chapter of the book, we hope, will consolidate your understanding of movement and set you on the road to understanding clinical and sports related movement problems, hopefully so that you can do something about them.

All the chapters begin with four or five learning outcomes and end with some self-assessment exercises. These have been included so that you know from the start what we expect you to learn from the chapter and then to check if you have indeed gained this knowledge and understanding. Our advice is to try the questions; even if it is a thought experiment and you do not actually do the exercise, this will help you to monitor progress and focus your attention on the weaker parts of your understanding. We will also provide a longer list of self-assessment activities on the partner website (http://evolve.elsevier.com/Kerr/movement/).

NOTICE ABOUT MATHS AND PHYSICS

Knowledge of physics and maths is NOT EXPECTED, but if you have a strong background in physics do not let this put you off this book. You will find your knowledge helpful in the biomechanics chapters (see Section 1), and this will give you more time to explore the physiology and psychology aspects of movement and look more carefully at the case studies in the final chapter.

For those of you with less confidence in maths and physics and who may be suffering from biomechanophobia (not a recognised phobia, yet), please be patient and give yourself time to absorb the material slowly, try all the activities and self-assessments and most importantly apply your knowledge to the real world. We hope that you can easily follow our explanations in this book and by the end of it you might consider yourself a biomechanists or movement scientist.

ABOUT THE SUPPORTING INFORMATION

There is a supporting website which will contain additional multiple choice questionnaires to test your knowledge. We will also add more case studies and other electronic resources so that you can continue to learn from real cases. So once you have finished the book, log on to the website and carry on learning.

How Things Move and Flow

2

Force

Andy Kerr and Philip Rowe

LEARNING OUTCOMES

After reading this chapter, you will be able to:
1. Define what a mechanical force is.
2. Explain a moment of force.
3. List the four characteristics of force.
4. Explain how forces can be combined and resolved.
5. Demonstrate how trigonometry can be used to analyse force.
6. Describe how you could measure force.

INTRODUCTION

In this first section of the book we will introduce you to biomechanics. Biomechanics is the study of forces acting on living bodies. It is all about applying the laws of mechanics to understand how living things (as opposed to things like steel and bricks) move and take shape. We could simply call it the 'the mechanics of humans' because the bodies, in our case, are human, although we will be drawing comparisons with other animals, such as penguins and turkeys. Understanding how force can produce movement, lead to injury or aid rehabilitation is a central component of many undergraduate and postgraduate courses in health and sport. Biomechanics, like many subjects, can be difficult to grasp but can also be surprisingly easy if you stick to understanding the basic principles and apply your knowledge to the real world.

Force causes movement, so we must begin our exploration of human movement by looking at force. This first chapter in this section will be dedicated entirely to understanding force: what it is, how you describe it, what it does and some principles of analysis. Let's start with some basics: what force is, what it does and the conventions of describing a force.

WHAT IS FORCE?

It is difficult to encapsulate all that the word force means because it is so elemental to our physical world. It is easier, perhaps, to think of its effect on bodies (this does not necessarily mean the human body). It really means any rigid block of mass. This could be a steel box, a wooden door or a human femur; anything providing it has mass and keeps its shape. Simply put, **force changes the motion of bodies.**

There are many different types of force (e.g. electromagnetic force, nuclear force and even spiritual force). In this book, we will be talking about **mechanical force**, which you can think of as a **push** or **pull** (e.g. the push on a wheelchair to set it in motion or the pull on a rope during a tug of war).

WHAT DOES A MECHANICAL FORCE DO?

Mechanical force is an interaction (or exchange) between bodies that results in a change in motion of the interacting bodies. This could be a change in the speed of the body (e.g. resting to moving or moving slowly to moving fast), or it could mean a change in the direction of the body. If this sounds a little abstract, too 'sciency', think about the collision between the white ball and a group of coloured balls in a game of pool; the PUSH from the white ball at impact causes the coloured balls (as well as the white itself) to move off in all kinds of directions and velocities.

Force can also cause a change the shape of a body; like a cushion being squashed when you sit on it or a bone being crushed from the impact of a car crash, we will consider this deforming effect of forces in Chapter 5; for now let's just think of force as something that changes motion.

Take a simple activity, like walking or throwing a ball; behind each change in speed or direction of each part of your body lies a force. Understanding force is clearly important if training (or retraining) movement is one of your objectives. It is pretty relevant then to those of you interested in studying human movement for rehabilitation purposes, so let's begin this understanding with some important information on force.

To improve readability we will refer to mechanical force as simply force for the rest of this chapter and indeed book.

SCALAR OR VECTOR?

To describe a physical **quantity** (length, weight, temperature, speed etc.), typically you just state its magnitude (the **amount** of stuff it has). For example, you might say that a fluid has 200 m³ of volume or that the wind has a speed of 15 miles/h; temperature could also be described in terms of a quantity (e.g. 50°C), and I am sure you can think of many others.

If you need ONLY magnitude to describe something then the thing you are describing is what we call a **scalar**, such as temperature and volume. To describe a **vector**, on the other hand, we need to know details of the direction of the quantity. Force is a vector because we need to say that it is applied in a particular direction (up/down, east/west). Vector is one of those universal words, used in lots of different situations by different people often to mean slightly different things. Pilots will say they are flying along a specific vector,

which is simply the line in the sky they are following, whereas a meteorologist might describe a wind vector (you are probably familiar with the weather maps with all the little wind arrows) (Fig. 2.1). When we talk about force, it is important to remember that it is a vector and so must have a stated direction, we don't you try Activity Box 2.1.

Some terms that describe movement can seem similar, synonymous even, for example, speed/velocity and distance/displacement. These terms appear to mean the same thing, and many people do regard them as the same, which is ok

ACTIVITY BOX 2.1
In the following list, identify the quantities that are scalar and those that are vectors (i.e. need a direction).

Speed	Depth	Circumference	Displacement
Length	Force	Luminosity (brightness of light)	Distance
Mass	Heat	Velocity	Acceleration
Wind	Snowfall	Weight	Time

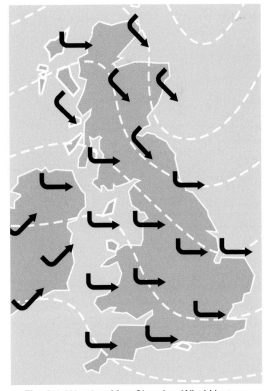

Fig. 2.1 Weather Map Showing Wind Vectors.

unless you need precision in your language. For example, distance is actually a scalar because you need only to state the amount (e.g. 10 miles or 15 km). On the other hand, displacement is a vector, which requires a statement on direction (e.g. 10 miles in a north-westerly direction). An illustration might help:

*If you drive from Aberdeen to Birmingham then back to Aberdeen, you will have travelled a **distance** of 846 miles or 1364 km, unless of course you live in the United States, in which case you will have travelled 2612 miles (Aberdeen, South Dakota, to Birmingham, Alabama). Regardless of the country, **displacement** will be zero because there has been no change in position and therefore no direction.*

It is not only important to know if something is a vector or a scalar; we need to use the same units to describe a quantity. Otherwise we would constantly be making errors. In this book, we will be using the International Systems of Units (SI units). Table 2.1 provides some of the typical SI units used in biomechanics and some equivalent units, mainly

TABLE 2.1 Quantities Used in Biomechanics With Their International Systems of Units and Some Equivalents.

BASE UNITS			
Quantity	**Name**	**SI Unit Abbreviation**	**Equivalent**
Mass	Kilogram	kg	Imperial mass 1 kg = 2.2 pounds
Distance	Metre	m	Imperial distance 1 m = 3.28 feet
Time	Second	s	Nautical time 1 Bell = 1800 s
Temperature	Kelvin	K	Celsius 1 K = −273.15°
Derived Values			
Velocity	Metre per second	m/s	Imperial speed 1 m/s = 2.24 mph
Acceleration	Metre per second per second	m/s^2	Gravity 1 m/s^2 = 0.101 G
Area	Square metre	m^2	Imperial area 1 m^2 =10.76 square feet
Volume	Cubic metre	m^3	Imperial volume 1 m^3 = 220 gallons
Density	Kilogram per cubic metre	kg/m^3	Imperial density 1 kg/m^3 = 0.16 ounce per gallon
Special Units			
Force	Newton	N	Imperial 0.22 pounds of force
Pressure or Stress	Pascal	Pa	N/m^2
Energy, work	Joule	J	1 J = 0.24 calories
Angle	Radians	r	1 r = 57.3 degrees
Power	Watt (J/s)	W	1 W = 0.0013 horsepower
Derived Values From Special Units			
Moment of force	Newton metre	Nm	1 Nm = 0.74 pound feet
Specific energy	Joule per kilogram	J/kg	1 J/kg = 0.0024 kilocalories per kg

SI, International Systems of Units.

from the imperial system used, predominantly, in the United Kingdom and United States of America.

Scalar quantities are easy to add or subtract (provided they have the same units), but vectors are a little trickier. However, because they have a direction, you represent them as arrows and then add them together—a bit like flight navigators (flight path) across the sky (see Fig. 2.2), or meteorologists drawing wind arrow over maps of different countries.

DRAWING VECTORS

To draw a vector, you first need a reference frame. This is just a defined space like the Cartesian graph with X and Y axes that you are probably familiar with from geography and mathematics classes at school—the X axis being the horizontal (bottom line) with positive values going toward the right and the Y axis being the vertical (up) with values increasing as you go up (Fig. 2.3). These axes are perpendicular to each other (i.e. they cross each other at a right angle [90 degrees]). In biomechanics this is sometimes referred to

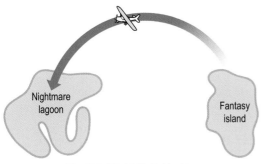

Fig. 2.2 Flight Path Vector.

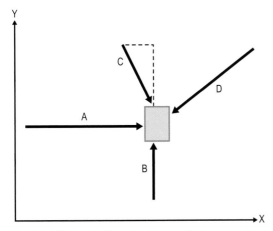

Fig. 2.3 XY Graph Showing Forces Acting on a Box.

as **orthogonal,** which is simply a fancy way of saying they are at right angles to each other.

This frame defines the space within which the force vector is acting. The direction of the vector is defined by the arrowhead at its end. This will tell you whether the vector is positive or negative. For example, force A (see Fig. 2.3) is positive horizontally because it is acting in the same direction as the horizontal (X) axis. If the arrowhead were pointing in the opposite direction, it would be negative.

The magnitude (amount) of force is represented in a force vector diagram by the length of the arrow, so first you need to decide on an appropriate way to translate the force magnitude value into a length value. A scaling factor if you like. For example, 10 N could equal 1 cm, so a force with a magnitude of 35 N would be represented by a line 3.5 cm long. The angle of the force is defined using one of the axes (X or Y) for reference, so it may be 0 degrees to the X axis (which would be same as 90 degrees to the Y axis) or it could be 30 degrees to the X axis. In Fig. 2.3, force A has a magnitude of 50 N, so the arrow length (using our scaling factor) is 5 cm. The force is positive along the X axis (arrow pointing in same direction as X) and is orientated parallel (0 degrees) to the X axis.

Can you translate force B in the same way (assuming the same scaling factor of 10 N = 1 cm)? (Clue: you will need a ruler for magnitude.)

This is easy for straight vectors like A and B, but what if the force is being applied at an angle, for example C? For this you will also need a protractor to measure the angle, as well as a ruler. Therefore force C has a magnitude of 35 N and is acting down to the right at an angle of 30 degrees to the vertical axis (Y). Can you now do the same for force D (40 N)? (Answer is at end of chapter.)

Some of you may have noticed that we live in three dimensions, four if you consider time, but let's not get carried away. The point is that force also exists in three dimensions, so we need to add in another dimension. If we have X and Y, then we must have Z. Like the X axis, the Z axis is horizontal (parallel to ground) and 90 degrees to the other two axes. If you have studied anatomy, this would be synonymous with the mediolateral direction. If you have not studied anatomy, think of it as side-to-side direction as opposed to forward and back (X) and up and down (Y). You can use the right-hand rule to understand this relationship. Put your right hand out as if you were going to shake someone's hand (thumb point up). Now close your ring finger and pinkie, and point your middle finger to the left. The Y is your thumb (positive values in direction thumb is pointing), the X your index finger (positive values in direction finger pointing) and the middle finger is the Z axis (positive values in direction finger pointing) (Fig. 2.4). This is known as the right hand rule and is the convention in biomechanics,

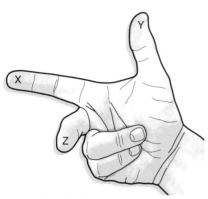

Fig. 2.4 Right-Hand Rule.

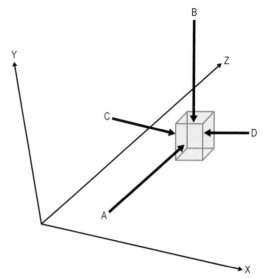

Fig. 2.6 XYZ Graph Showing Forces Acting on a Box.

ACTIVITY BOX 2.2

Get a piece of blank paper and mark two axes, X and Y (see Fig. 2.5). Now get your pencil (sharpened) and push it through the point where they cross (the origin). You now have the three axes: X, Y on the paper and your pencil is the Z axis.

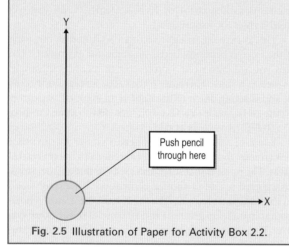

Fig. 2.5 Illustration of Paper for Activity Box 2.2.

---

although some countries use a different combination of XYZ to denote the three axes, a typical alternative being to have the Z as your thumb (vertical), Y as your index (forward and back) and X as your middle finger (side to side). If you are still confused, then try Activity Box 2.2.

The important thing is to avoid confusion by knowing which convention the textbook, scientific journal or movement laboratory is using. In this textbook we will be using the one shown in Fig. 2.4.

As we have said, forces acting in the same direction as the axes will have a positive value; however, forces acting in the opposite direction will have negative values, but this does not mean the push or pull of force is less than zero—it is simply acting in the opposite direction.

Force B in Fig. 2.6 is a vertical force of −60 N because it is acting in the opposite direction to the Y axis (i.e. downward). Force A has a magnitude of 50 N in the Z direction.

POINT OF APPLICATION

From what we have talked about so far, we know that force has magnitude (length of arrow), direction (arrowhead) and angle (angle with axes of reference frame), all defined within our XYZ reference frame, but does it matter where on the object (box or bone) the force is actually applied?

Put your pen or pencil on the table in front of you (Fig. 2.7). Now you are going to:
1. Apply a pushing force, more or less at the centre of the pencil.
2. Apply a pushing force (same magnitude as before) at one end of the pencil.

The movement of the pencil is entirely different, depending on where you applied the force. When the force was applied at the middle of the pencil, the whole pencil moved in the direction of the push; however, when the force was applied away from the centre, the pencil rotated. The first force caused a linear motion (straight line), and the second force caused an angular motion (rotation). A force that causes rotation is called a moment, or torque from the Latin

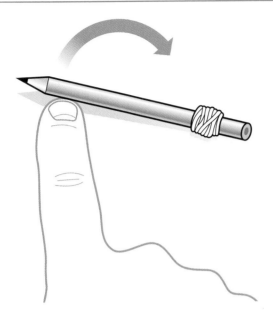

Fig. 2.7 Pencil Being Pushed.

torquere, which means to twist. The point where the force is applied is clearly important to the resulting motion and needs to be stated. This is called the **point of application** and is usually expressed by using a reference frame for the object that is being pushed (i.e. the X, Y, Z coordinates of the box, ball or banana).

FORCE MAGNITUDE AND CHANGE IN MOTION

As we now know, **magnitude** is the quantity, or amount, of push or pull represented by the length of the vector in a vector diagram. When we talk about movement, force magnitude is defined from the **acceleration** that the force produces on a body. Now acceleration needs some clear definition because it does not just mean how fast you are moving. Let's start with velocity (which **is** how fast you are moving and in what direction):

Velocity (V) = Change in displacement divided by time

or:

$$V = \frac{\text{Position}_2 - \text{Position}_1}{\text{Time}}.$$ **Equation 2.1**

So if a ball were rolling down a school corridor from position$_1$ (let's say 3 m along the corridor) to position$_2$ (let's

say 7 m along the corridor) and this took 3 seconds, then the ball had a velocity magnitude of:

$$\frac{7\,\text{m} - 3\,\text{m}}{3} = 1.33\,\text{m/s}.$$

Velocity (unlike speed) is a vector and can be described as positive or negative depending on the direction (which you must state).

Now acceleration is the rate of change of velocity (or the time derivative of velocity) (i.e. how quickly or slowly the velocity of the body is changing, speeding up or slowing down or changing direction). If velocity is constant, then there is no acceleration. The greater the change in velocity, the greater the acceleration; this relationship is formalised in the equation for average acceleration:

$$\text{Acceleration} = \frac{\overset{\text{Change in velocity}}{(\text{Velocity at end} - \text{Velocity at start})}}{\text{Time}}$$

Equation 2.2

Or the magnitude of the acceleration

$$A = \frac{(\text{Velocity}^2 - \text{Velocity}^1)}{\text{Time}}.$$

Let's imagine you went up to the ball, which was still happily rolling down the corridor, and gave it another push (in the same direction that it was rolling). Before you pushed it, the ball had a velocity of 1.33 m/s, and after the push (which lasted 2s), it had a velocity of 2.45 m/s; this would mean there was an acceleration of:

$$\frac{2.45\,\text{m/s} - 1.33\,\text{m/s}}{2} = 0.56\,\text{m/s}^2.$$

During your push, the ball increased its velocity by 0.56 m/s every second.

Acceleration is a vector, like force, and can be described as positive (velocity increasing, i.e. getting faster) or negative (velocity decreasing, i.e. getting slower) which is also known as deceleration. In his ground-breaking book, *Principia Mathematica*, Sir Isaac Newton (1687) laid down the rules that govern how force causes motion. In recognition of his achievement, force magnitude is measured in newtons (N), where 1 N is the amount of force required to accelerate a 1 kg of mass by a 1 kg of mass by 1 meter per second per second (1 m/s^2). We will talk about these laws in more detail in the next chapter; however, for now it is worth remembering that force causes acceleration, or a change in velocity.

If you imagine a 1 kg bag of sugar and apply 1 N to it, then the bag would move (provided we ignore all other forces such as friction and air resistance) in the direction the force is applied, getting faster by 1 m/s, every second for the duration of the push (Fig. 2.8).

Newton described the force of gravity using the analogy of the falling apple. If you knew that an apple was about to fall from a tree and managed to set up a high-speed camera to record the fall, the developed photographs would show the apple falling a greater and greater distance between each photograph (i.e. the velocity of the apple [distance divided by time] was increasing). If, on the other hand, you lived in space with zero gravity (it would be strange to find a productive apple tree in space so, instead, imagine a piece of space debris) and photographed the object falling; there would be the same distance between each snap shot (i.e. it would be moving at the same velocity throughout its 'fall'). We will talk more about falling objects later in the chapter.

Of course, acceleration is not just about gravity, EVERY force has the potential to cause a body to accelerate. We will return to acceleration and Isaac Newton in the next chapter, but for now let's recap on what we know about force.

WHAT YOU NEED TO REMEMBER SO FAR

A mechanical force (force) is basically a **push** or a **pull** that causes a body to **accelerate.** To describe a force accurately you need to remember that it is a **vector** with four characteristics:

1. **Magnitude**; which is measured in newton.
2. **Direction**; which you need to define using a standard reference frame like the XYZ Cartesian frame in Fig. 2.6.
3. **Point of application** on the body, again using standard reference frame.
4. **Angle of application**, in degrees or radians.

THE FORCE OF MUSCLES

Within the human body, force is produced through the contraction of skeletal muscle. This could mean the muscles shortening (known as a concentric contraction), lengthening while tense (known as an eccentric contraction) or being in a state of tension while remaining at the same length (known as a static or isometric contraction). These types of contraction are demonstrated in Fig. 2.9 with the quadriceps muscle group. In the first diagram, the knee is straightening, produced by shortening of the quadriceps. In the second diagram the knee is flexing, this movement is produced by gravity; however, the movement is still controlled by the quadriceps, the muscle is lengthening while producing tension. In the final diagram the knee is being held in the same position, gravity is still trying to pull the leg down but the quadriceps are matching this force with a static

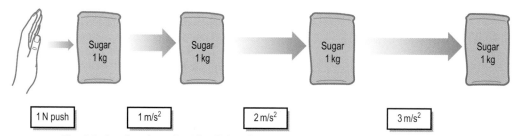

Fig. 2.8 Acceleration of a 1-kg Object From an Application of a 1 N Force (Push).

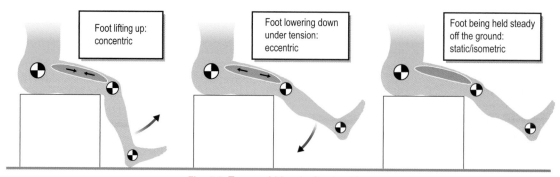

Fig. 2.9 Types of Muscle Contraction.

contraction—no movement. For more detail on muscle contraction, go to Chapter 6.

It is worth noting that, although we can apply pushing **and** pulling forces on an object, our muscles always **pull** on bones, never push, which makes things a little easier to understand. In addition, muscles are not intelligent, they behave very simply, and they can produce only one type of contraction at a time—isometric, concentric or eccentric.

The direction and angle of the muscle **pull** are defined by the anatomy of the muscle, in particular the location of the tendinous attachments on the bone (point of application). The magnitude of the pull corresponds generally to the size of the muscle (i.e. its physiologic cross-sectional area, or how thick it is). However, it is the brain (motor cortex, to be exact) that determines how many muscle fibres are active at any one point, a bit like the conductor in an orchestra pointing to just a couple of cellos when a gentle soft sound is required or the whole ensemble for a crescendo (see chapter 9 for more on how the brain controls movement).

An important mechanical feature of the force generated by most skeletal muscles is that it is applied at a distance from the centre of a joint (Fig. 2.10), like when you pushed the pencil at the end rather than the centre (see Fig. 2.7). This is particularly true of muscles in the body that create motion; these are sometimes referred to as mobiliser muscles.

The importance of this distance between where the force is applied and the joint or fulcrum is best illustrated with a simple experiment.

Walk over to a door, and pull it open.

Where did you apply your pulling force?

I would like to think you all did the same thing there (the handle is a bit of a clue!). The point is, like the mobiliser muscles in your body, you applied your pulling force well away from the joint or in the door's case the hinges. This is the principle of **moments** and is the basis for the simplest (and most efficient) machine known to man: the **lever**, which we will talk about in the next chapter. The turning force (moment or sometimes called torque) is created when a force is applied at a distance away from the turning part (this can be called the pivot, fulcrum, hinge or joint). You know the principle of moments intuitively; otherwise you would sit in the middle of a seesaw!

Of course you know what happens (or rather does not happen) if you sit in the middle of a seesaw, so you can work out what happens if you apply a force at the hinges of a door or if a muscle applies its pulling force at the joint centre. Some muscles are indeed attached so that their pull is close to the joint centre. What function do you think these muscles will perform? They will not rotate the bone, so what do they do? What does your force do when you sit in the middle the seesaw? Can this force serve any purpose?

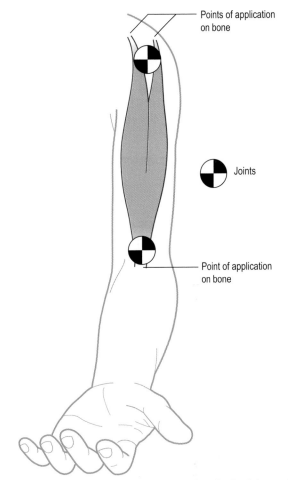

Points of application on bone

Joints

Point of application on bone

Fig. 2.10 Muscle Producing Force Point of application is beyond the joint centre.

In fact, these muscles are critical to movement. They fix (or stabilise if you prefer) a body part to enable motion to occur—a bit like the screws in the door hinge holding the bracket in place or the bolt that secures the seesaw to the ground. These muscles are sometimes called stabiliser muscles, for obvious reasons.

Human movement is generally performed through a series of rotations at joints. Think of the number of body parts that turn when you walk (ankle, knee, hip, pelvis, shoulder, elbow). Each rotation is generated and controlled by muscles. To allow these rotations to occur, the central axis of the body needs to remain stable. A seesaw that moved about on the ground would prove an awkward toy to play with; it has to be fixed to the ground to allow the rotation to occur. The muscles that are attached very close to, or right at, the joint centre act to hold or stabilise the bone.

MAGNITUDE OF MOMENTS

Like the force that causes linear (straight) motion (e.g. the push on a car), moments are also vectors, so we need all the same information as before. Firstly the magnitude: this is the product (multiplication) of the applied force and its perpendicular (at 90 degrees; Fig. 2.11) distance from the fulcrum (this distance is also known as the moment or lever arm).

Moment = Force (N) × Perpendicular distance (m) from pivot.

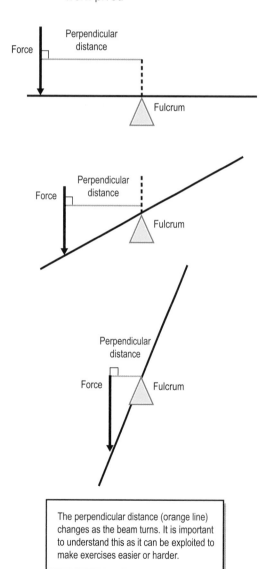

The perpendicular distance (orange line) changes as the beam turns. It is important to understand this as it can be exploited to make exercises easier or harder.

Fig. 2.11 Perpendicular Force.

So, moments are measured in newton metres (Nm) or equivalents, such as pound feet for anyone still using the Imperial system.

Let's say the gastrocnemius muscle (calf) (Fig. 2.12) pulls on the heel with a force of 150 N and this is applied 5 cm (0.05 m) perpendicularly behind the ankle joint. The turning force is therefore 150 N × 0.05 m = 7.5 Nm. If you had a larger calcaneum (heel bone), say one that extended 8 cm (0.08 m) back from the ankle joint, then the turning force will be 12 Nm (150 × 0.08), nearly 40% more for just 3 cm! The point here is that you can change the size of the turning force by changing the distance to the joint, although admittedly changing the size of your calcaneum is a little tricky;

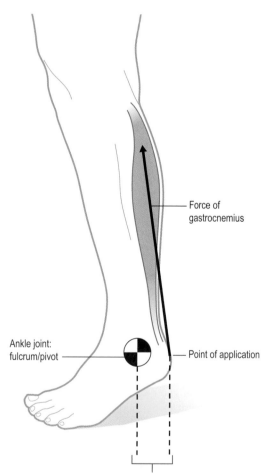

Fig. 2.12 Plantarflexing (Up Onto Toes) Moment Created by a Gastrocnemius (Calf Muscle) Contraction.

ACTIVITY BOX 2.3

Let's imagine you were testing the strength of someone's quadriceps muscle group (muscles on front of thigh that straighten the leg) and you ask the person who is sitting on a plinth to straighten his or her knee while you push against him or her (Fig. 2.13). Where do you place your hand (i.e. your resisting force)?

Of course you place it furthest away from the joint, giving yourself the longest possible moment arm (perpendicular distance between axis of rotation and point where force is applied); your force is at a mechanical advantage compared with the poor old quadriceps, which applied its pull very close to the knee joint.

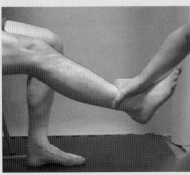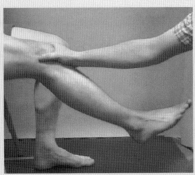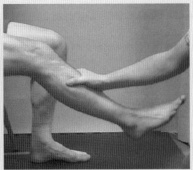

Fig. 2.13 Hand Placement to Resist Knee Extension.

perhaps we will see this kind of *anatomical doping* in future sports events. (Try Activity Box 2.3 [see Fig. 2.13].)

DIRECTION OF MOMENTS

So, the magnitude of a moment is force × distance (Nm). Moments are of course vectors, so we need to state a direction; because rotation is the resulting motion, the convention is to state the moment as positive when it creates a clockwise motion and negative when it creates an anticlockwise movement. When applied to the body, moments can be described in terms of the motion they create about the joint (e.g. a knee flexor moment or a hip abducting moment). The point of application is the same as previously (i.e. the point on the bone [or other object]).

What You Have to Remember About Moments

Moments are turning forces created by a force applied at a distance from a turning point; the magnitude is the product of force and perpendicular distance from joint (Nm). Moments are described as clockwise or anticlockwise. When applied to the human body, they are described according to the anatomical motion they will produce (e.g. a flexion moment or an abducting moment). Forces applied around the centre of a joint help to stabilise it; they do not produce turning motions.

ANALYSING FORCE

Up to now, we have really considered only a single force at a time—one vector, one arrow on the graph. How easy is that! In our body we have around 700 skeletal muscles, each capable of generating individual force vectors—lots and lots of arrows. Some muscles pass over two joints and so are capable of generating more than one moment at a time. Then of course there are the ligaments which change the direction of a muscle's pull (more on this in the next chapter) and we cannot forget all the external forces that act on us (like gravity). Performing daily activities means we have to contend with lots of external forces; this may be the contact forces with the ground or the weight of a handbag on our shoulder. To understand human movement and posture, we need to be able to analyse the action of lots of forces all acting at the same time, some opposing each other, some helping each other. Let's take the first step in this understanding by looking at two forces.

HOW DO FORCES COMBINE?

As you will recall from earlier, the useful thing about forces, being that it is a vector, is that you can draw them as arrows and add them together. Let's take a simple example. Two women are pushing a car (Fig. 2.14). The first woman, Ailsa,

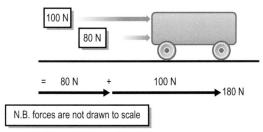

Fig. 2.14 Two Forces Pushing a Car.

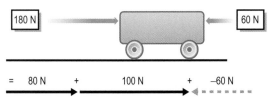

Fig. 2.15 Two Forces Acting in Opposite Directions.

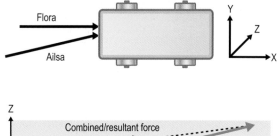

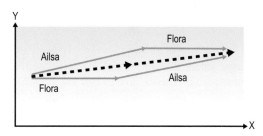

Note that the 'vertical' is Z; this is because we are viewing the car from above, so the vertical axis represents side-to-side movement

Fig. 2.16 Adding Forces at Angles This time you are looking at the car from the air.

pushes in a straight line from left to right with a force of 100 N. The second woman, Flora, pushes with a force of 80 N. To get the combined force (this is also called the resultant), we simply add the two arrows together.

That seems pretty straightforward, and it would be the exactly the same if more people came along. Now, as we know, there is a force acting against Ailsa and Flora (otherwise it would be a pretty easy task); this is the force of friction (which we will talk more about in next chapter), which acts against the two women (Fig. 2.15). Now because it is acting against the two women it has a negative value (remember the reference frames from earlier in the chapter, see Fig. 2.3). If we estimate the magnitude as −60N we can calculate the resultant (combined) force acting on the car as follows:

$$80\,N + 100\,N - 60\,N = 120\,N$$

In the examples so far, we have used forces which are applied at right angles to the object (straight at it), but this is rarely the case either in the physical environment or within our bodies. To understand forces acting at an angle, let's continue with the car pushing.

Ailsa's right hand begins to hurt after pushing for so long, so now she pushes only with her left hand; consequently her force changes direction a little (but still with the same magnitude). Now she is pushing at a 25-degree angle from the horizontal, but Flora continues to push straight. To understand how this affects the resulting force, you can still add the forces together, remembering to maintain the same angles (Fig. 2.16).

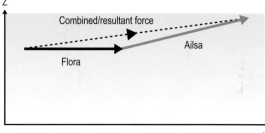

Fig. 2.17 Parallelogram of Forces.

To understand the effect these two pushes have on the car (you could probably guess, but it is good to see how we can calculate the resulting force), we can combine them by adding one to the other (nose to tail). The resultant (dotted line) is the connecting line between starting point and the end of the two combined force vectors.

This is also known as the parallelogram of forces because you can construct a parallelogram (a figure of four sides where the side opposite to each other are parallel) using the two forces for both sides (Fig. 2.17). The resultant then just joins up the start of the first arrows with the end of the second ones.

As well as joining forces together, we can also take them apart. It is just the reverse of combining (I probably did not need to say that). Instead of two people pushing the car, let's say we had one, Barry, who pushes the car at an angle. Now the push Barry creates on the car (dotted arrow in Fig. 2.18, F1) could have been achieved by a number of

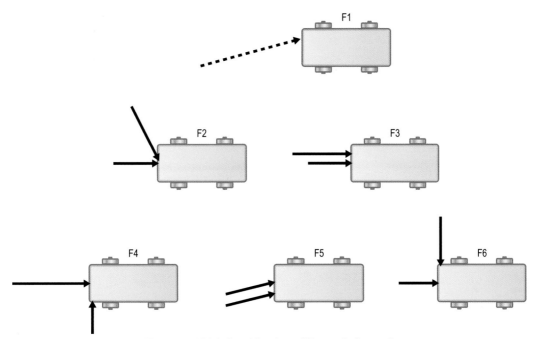

Fig. 2.18 Which Combination of Forces Is Correct?

different combinations. From the following diagrams (see Fig. 2.18), choose the combinations that could provide the same push as Barry (see end of chapter for the answer).

What we are saying here is that we could replace Barry with two smaller forces applied at different angles. For ease of calculation, it is simplest to replace Barry with forces that act at right angles to each other; that way, we can use trigonometry to calculate their size and direction (more of this later).

If you did not understand the car example, let's try something you can do yourself. Go over to a table/chair or anything really that can you can push across the floor (something on wheels would be good; just make sure there is nothing breakable on top before you push). Now push it in the same manner as shown in Fig. 2.19 (i.e. push down and forward).

Because you are pushing the object at an angle, the force you apply could be replaced by a combination of a horizontal/forward push and a vertical/downward push (dotted arrows in Fig. 2.19), depending on the angle of application. You are basically pushing down and forwards. Importantly, these two components of the force will act at right angles to each other. From this breaking down (or resolution) of forces, we can see that only a part of the applied force (the horizontal component) will cause the forward motion of the table/chair and that the vertical part does not contribute toward the forward motion at all. In fact, it will make matters worse

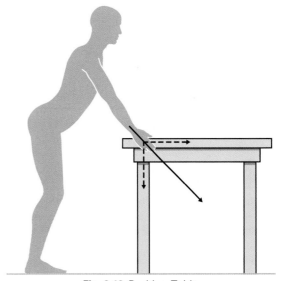

Fig. 2.19 Pushing Table.

because it increases the force of friction acting in the opposite direction (more on this in the next chapter). So, it would be best, of course, to apply the force without any vertical component (Fig. 2.20).

That is enough pushing of things around; let's get back to the human body.

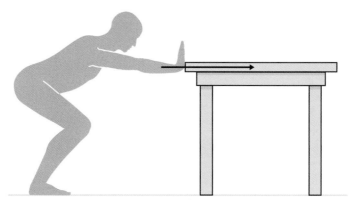

Fig. 2.20 Applying the Force Horizontally.

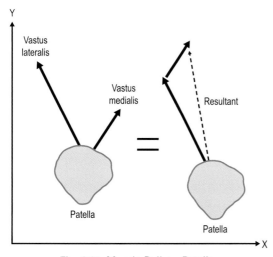

Fig. 2.21 Muscle Pull on Patella.

ANALYSING MUSCLE FORCE APPLICATION

Two thigh muscles pull on the patella (this is the knee cap if you have not covered this in an anatomy class), the vastus medialis and vastus lateralis (there are two other muscles involved, but let's keep it simple, for just now) (Fig. 2.21). We can add the two muscle forces together, just like Ailsa and Flora, (remembering to add nose to tail!) to see the resultant; remember that the length of the arrow represents the size of the muscle's pull, provided, of course, you have kept the same scale throughout (see Fig. 2.21).

You could have probably guessed, just by looking at the arrows, what the resultant force would look like, but this is a useful exercise, particularly when things become more complicated. From these two muscle forces, we get a resultant (or combined) force that acts to pull the patella up and to

the right. This is not a great idea because the patella runs along a kind of groove on the femur (strangely enough this is called the femoral groove). Poor contact between the patella and the femur (from being too far one way) could lead to local inflammation pain, swelling etc., so what can you do to make sure the patella is pulled directly up and not over to one side? (Answer is at end of chapter.)

Q Angle and Knee Pain

In fact, it has been speculated by physiotherapists, podiatrists and sport therapists (among others) that the angle of pull of the quadriceps (Q angle) muscle group is one of the causes of pain around the patella (Fig. 2.22). It has been suggested that a large angle (>15 degrees) to the axis of the long axis of the tibia is a risk factor. Furthermore, it has been suggested that the reason female athletes are more prone to this type of knee problem is from their naturally larger Q angle, due to the female pelvis being broader. It should be noted that this is still disputed because no clear evidence has been produced. Indeed, the notion that females have a broader pelvis (although this may sound intuitively correct) has not been empirically established. What do you think?

There are of course many examples of muscles applying their pull on a bone at an angle. For example, let's look at the pull of gluteus medius (GM) on the femur, which is one of the main muscles that lift your leg out to the side. In Fig. 2.23 the black arrow represents the force vector of GM. (You will notice that the vector has arrows at both ends; really this is just to demonstrate that it can pull in either direction, as all muscles can.) For the moment, just consider the pull is on the femur, look at the angle the vector makes with the femur and think about what we have already talked about regarding breaking forces up into their component parts; you should be able to see that the two thinner lines are the result of this pull on the greater trochanter.

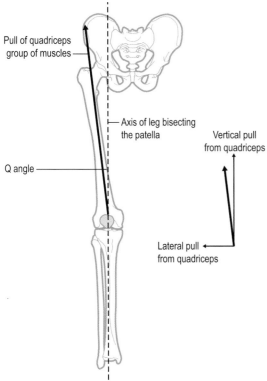

Pull of quadriceps
group of muscles

Axis of leg bisecting
the patella

Vertical pull
from quadriceps

Q angle

Lateral pull
from quadriceps

Fig. 2.22 Q Angle.

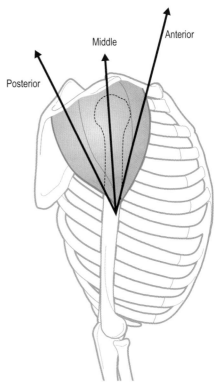

Posterior

Middle

Anterior

Fig. 2.24 Force of Three Parts of Deltoid.

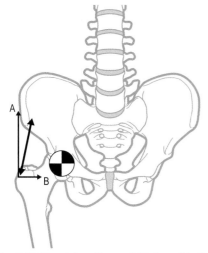

A

B

Fig. 2.23 Resolving Force of Gluteus Medius.

The part of the force (A) pulling directly upward (toward the pelvis) will create the turning force because it is acting at a distance from the joint centre. The other force component (B) is directed inwards toward the joint. The B component may be useful in stabilising the joint but may also lead to injury because it is compressing the joint together. The joint is designed to cope with these compressions (this will be discussed in more detail in Chapter 7); however, over time these compressions can contribute to erosion of the articular surface and ultimately inflammation of the joint (i.e. arthritis).

All our examples so far have been from the lower limb, so let's move up the body. The deltoid muscle wraps around the outside of your shoulder. This muscle is primarily involved in lifting your arm out to the side (abduction); it is usually regarded as a muscle made up of three parts (front, middle and back) that can work separately or altogether. If all three parts (Fig. 2.24) were working what would be the result? Remember that in a vector diagram the length of the arrows represents the relative magnitude of the force.

Can you draw in the resultant? (Answer is at end of chapter.)

We have been looking at the muscle forces that combine (within our body), but how do external forces combine to act on our body?

When you are standing still, you are applying a force down onto the ground (your mass multiplied by the force of gravity—downward-directed arrow in Fig. 2.25), which we have already talked about, and the ground applies a force back onto you (grey upward-directed arrow in Fig. 2.25) of the same magnitude but in the opposite direction (more on this in the next chapter). Now the situation during walking is a bit more complicated; you still apply a force onto the ground, but this time your force (and consequently the ground's reaction force) is applied at an angle. Take the last point of contact with the ground when you walk, which is usually toe off. To understand the effect this force has, we need to break the force down into its component parts (vertical and horizontal). From this breakdown, we can see that some of the reaction force will be directed horizontally forward (which pushed us forward) and vertically up (which lifts our body up).

Have a look at Fig. 2.26 for an idea of the forces applied in the frontal plane at the same point in the gait cycle, and see if you can work out the components of the force based on the resultant vector and what might be the direction of the resulting motion.

Just like linear (straight) forces, we can also add the rotational effect of forces (moments). Moments that create rotation in the same direction (clockwise or anticlockwise) can be added. If they are opposite to each other, they are subtracted. So, for example, imagine two workers using a long lever to help move a boulder (Fig. 2.27). Man A applies

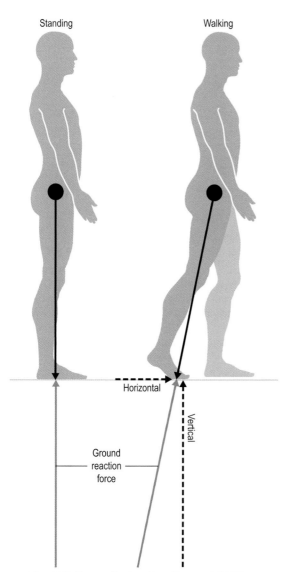

Fig. 2.25 Forces During Standing and Walking.

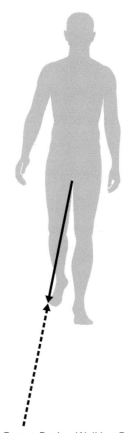

Fig. 2.26 Forces During Walking From Front.

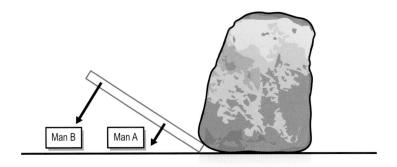

Fig. 2.27 Adding Moments.

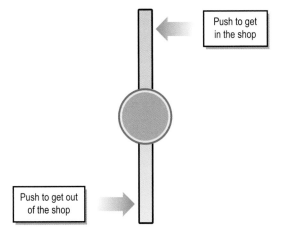

Fig. 2.28 Force Couple: Rotating Doors.

his pull of 90 N 20 cm (0.2 m) from the fulcrum (so a moment of 18 Nm) while man B applies his 75 N at a perpendicular distance of 35 cm (0.35 m) from the fulcrum (so a moment of 26.25 Nm). Because the moments are in the same direction, we simply add them to get the net moment (44.25 Nm). If one of them were pushing rather than pulling, we would subtract the anticlockwise motion form the clockwise.

The moments do not have to be applied on the same side as each other to create the same moment. In a force couple, two (or more) forces are applied in opposite directions and opposite sides of the fulcrum (Fig. 2.28); the result is that they produce the same motion and therefore can be added together. The best illustration of this, from our everyday lives, is the rotating doors that you typically find at the entrance to big shops. To get into the shop, you push one panel of the door, but on the opposite side (trying to get out) is another person pushing on a different panel of the door; the effect is the sum of both your moments. If

you try to push on the same panel (in opposite directions) you will cancel each other out.

There are some examples of these force couples in the human body (e.g. the pull of the different parts of the trapezius muscle on the scapula). Perhaps the easiest to visualise is the complementary action of the hamstring muscles pulling the pelvis down at the back and rectus abdominus muscle (the six-pack muscle on your abdomen) pulling the pelvis up at the front, the combination causing the pelvis to tilt posteriorly (tucking your bottom in).

MEASURING FORCE

One of the tools used in biomechanics to measure force is the forceplate. A forceplate is an example of a transducer. A transducer is a device that changes one type of energy to another (e.g. a solar panel changes light energy into electrical energy and a loudspeaker changes electrical energy into sound). A force transducer therefore transforms (changes) mechanical energy (a push or pull) into an electrical current. After the signal has been calibrated, so we know how much current is created when a force of a certain magnitude is applied, then force can be measured. With careful arrangement of transducers and some mathematics, the other components of force (direction, point and angle of application) can be obtained. Two types of force transducer are common: strain gauges and piezoelectric crystals (Further Information 2.1).

Strain gauges are simple devices used to measure force. They are based on strips of metal (e.g. copper) that change their electrical resistance as they are changed in length (e.g. if they are stretched). Electrogoniometers, for example, are based on strain gauges. Placed across a joint, the electrogoniomter will stretch with movement; this change in length causes a change in electrical current. A calibration process determines how much joint movement will create a certain amount of change in current; this is then converted to degrees.

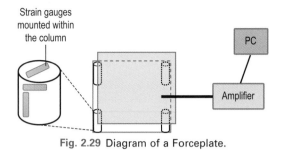

Fig. 2.29 Diagram of a Forceplate.

Force transducers (crystals or strain gauges) are used in force plates to measure the amount, direction and location of an applied force.

The forceplate consists of a rigid metal platform (i.e. the surface that the force will be applied to) which sits on top of four columns located, approximately, in the corners which have force transducers in them. Three transducers are orientated at right angles to each other within these columns. This allows them to pick up force in the different directions (X, Y and Z). The electrical signal is then amplified (volume turned up) and passed onto a personal computer for analysis (Fig. 2.29).

There are four columns in a forceplate so that the location of the force can be calculated. If you stood in the very centre of a square bit of wood that was resting on four weighing scales, the reading on all the scales would be the same. However, if you stood towards the front of the wood, the readings on the front two scales would be higher than the back two. Therefore, if you looked only at the scales, you would know that the person was standing toward the front of the piece of wood. The forceplate works in the same way to calculate what is called the centre of pressure; this is the location (or point of application) of the force on the plate (Fig. 2.30).

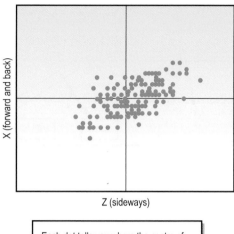

Each dot tells you where the centre of pressure was at a specific moment in time. So if all the dots are close together the person has not wobbled about much.

Fig. 2.30 Centre of Pressure Measured by a Forceplate During Normal Standing.

Basically the forceplate works like a sophisticated bathroom scale. When you stand on bathroom scales you compress small springs; this change in length of the springs is transferred (using levers and cogs) to cause a dial to move, which has been calibrated to show your weight. Because of the way the scales are designed, it does not matter (or should not) where you stand (as long as all your weight is on the plate!), and because it uses springs which are orientated vertically, it can measure only vertical force (which is fine if you are just standing there). The forceplate offers more options; it can locate the exact position of your force on the plate (see Fig. 2.30), and it can calculate the amount of vertical and horizontal force (because the transducers are positioned in different directions, see Fig. 2.29). Finally, the electrical signal from the forceplate can be easily recorded and analysed using a computer. This is quite difficult to do with a bathroom scale because the only 'output' is what you see. The final output from a forceplate has been used to study forces during walking. Have a look at Fig. 2.31, and see if you can interpret the graph. Do not worry if you cannot; there is an explanation in the next paragraph. The graph is the recording of force during a single stance phase of gait (i.e. the bit of walking when your foot is on the ground).

Okay, here is the explanation. Let's consider the vertical force first (the dotted line). The graph begins with initial contact (heel strike usually), so you can see this rapid increase in force as the body crashes down onto the forceplate. This

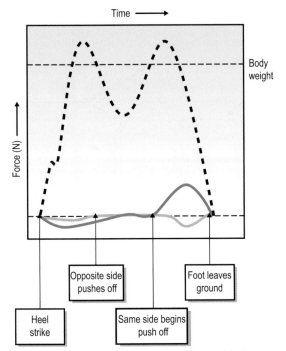

Fig. 2.31 Ground Reaction Forces During Walking.

force will exceed body weight (we will look at the reasons for this in the next chapters). You may notice a little bump in the graph during this increase; this is called the heel strike transient. It represents a brief reduction in force and is caused by shock absorption (hip, knee and ankle movement on impact). Next comes a drop in vertical force. This is primarily due to the action of the opposite side (must not forget we are bipedal), which is accelerating upwards (mainly hip flexion), so there is less force acting on the forceplate (you are moving up!).

Following this dip, the vertical force increases again to the same level achieved previously. This is again due to the action of the lower limb pushing the person up (and forward) but this time by the foot resting on the forceplate.

The horizontal force (black line), although nowhere near as large as the vertical, is still interesting. You will see that the force is immediately negative; this is a braking force. Towards the end, it becomes positive; this is a propulsion force (moving you forward). You might notice that the propulsion force is greater than the braking force, which indicates the individual is probably increasing his walking speed.

How did you get on with that? We will be revisiting force and change in motion in the next chapter, so if you found that difficult to follow, do not worry; the next chapter should help.

USING MATHEMATICS TO RESOLVE FORCE

The graphical method of adding forces is easy to follow (hopefully) with the benefit of being able to see the result. However, it can be quite difficult to be accurate with this method because it involves a lot of measurements, all of which may fall foul of human error. There is another way of adding force that involves trigonometry. There is nothing terribly difficult about it, but it does put some people off, so we will take it easy in this section. If you really hate this kind of thing, just glance through it until the summary at the end; you could always try again later.

The whole principle revolves around some special properties of right-angle triangles that the ancient Greeks worked out 2500 years ago (Further Information 2.2).

Thanks to them, we need only a few bits of information to work out all the dimensions of a right-angled triangle (two of the sides are placed at 90 degrees to each other). For example, let's say side A (Fig. 2.32) has a length of 5 cm and

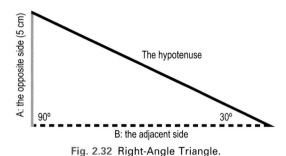

Fig. 2.32 Right-Angle Triangle.

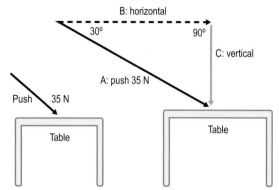

Fig. 2.33 Push on Table Resolved Into Components for Mathematical Analysis.

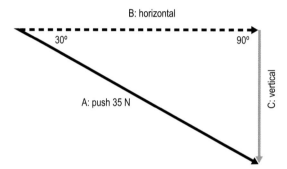

Fig. 2.34 The Push Viewed as a Right-Angle Triangle.

there is an angle of 30 degrees between the adjacent and the hypotenuse. We can work out all the other angles and lengths from these two quantities. We can work out the size of the hypotenuse (sloped line opposite the right angle) because the sine of 30 degrees is equal to the opposite divided by the hypotenuse, that is:

$$\sin 30° = 5/H.$$

Therefore,

$$H = 5/\sin 30° = 5/0.5 = 10.$$

The long sloping side (hypotenuse) is therefore 10 cm long. We could have also used cosine rule, which is the relationship between the hypotenuse and the side adjacent to the known angle (side B in Fig. 2.32).

It states that the cosine of the angle (30 degrees in our case) is equal to the adjacent divided by the hypotenuse (which we know is 10 cm for our triangle):

$$\cos 30 = A/10$$

$$10 \times \cos 30 = \text{Adjacent (side B)} = 8.66 \text{ cm}.$$

So now we know all three sides, but if we only knew two we could calculate the last one using Pythagoras's theorem (see Further Information 2.2).

We have talked quite abstractly so far, so let's get back to force and biomechanics.

Imagine you are pushing a table across a room and the direction of your push is not straight but at an angle (just like Fig. 2.19). Before we just drew the components; this time we will use trigonometry.

The push (black solid line, Fig. 2.33) can be resolved into the two components (at right angles to each other), one acting horizontally (black dashed arrow) and the other acting vertically (grey arrow). This is just as we discussed before; now if we know the size of the hypotenuse, which

in this case we call the resultant and the angle it is applied to the box, then we can work out the other two components exactly.

Let's suggest that the force has a magnitude of 35 N and is applied at the box at an angle of 30 degrees to the horizontal; we can construct a right-sided triangle (Fig. 2.34).

We can now use the sine rule to calculate the size of the opposite length (which in our case is the vertical component):

$$\sin 30° = \text{Opposite/Hypotenuse (35)},$$

therefore:

$$0.5 = \text{Opposite (unknown)}/35,$$

therefore:

$$35 \times 0.5 = \text{Opposite, that is, 17.5 N}.$$

If we know the hypotenuse and we know the opposite, we can calculate the remaining length (horizontal) using Pythagoras's theorem:

Hypotenuse squared = Opposite squared
+ Adjacent squared,

therefore

$$352 = 17.52 + \text{Adjacent}$$
(unknown horizontal component),

therefore

$$352 - 17.52 = \text{Adjacent squared},$$

therefore

$$\text{Adjacent squared} = 918.75,$$

so the adjacent (horizontal) is the square root of this (i.e. 30 N).

So now we know that if we apply a force of 35 N to a box at an angle of 30 degrees to horizontal, that it will result in a vertical component of 17.5 N and a horizontal component of 30.3 N.

The relevance here for the human body is that skeletal muscles apply their forces on moving bones, which will inevitably mean that the force is being applied at an angle. Let's consider the pull of the biceps muscle. If the forearm were positioned at 90 degrees to the upper arm, then the biceps would apply its force completely vertically (i.e. no resolution; Fig. 2.35).

Now if the elbow extends (straightens), even a little, then the angle of pull of the biceps muscle on the radius will change. When it is no longer being applied at 90 degrees the muscle, force is resolved into parallel and perpendicular components. We can use trigonometry again, but we need a few bits of information. The size of the pull, let's say it is 50 N, and the angle of application, let's say 25 degrees, would

be sufficient for us to construct a right-sided triangle and apply the cosine or sine laws (Fig. 2.36).

It does not take a huge leap of imagination to realise that we can apply this analytical method to multiple muscle forces at the same time to work out all the forces involved in a complex problem. This is exactly what bioengineers do by constructing free-body diagrams where some of the forces and some of the angles (e.g. by measuring with a forceplate) are known and the rest can be calculated with Greek mathematics—something for you to look forward to.

SUMMARY PART TWO

What you need to remember from all that.

That was a pretty mathematics-based chapter, so it is probably good to recount the things you have to remember.

Forces are vectors and so can be added nose to tail. Provided the angles and lengths are kept consistent, there is no end to the number of forces that can be analysed in this way. Rotational effects of forces can also be added if you know the motions they will cause. As well as adding forces, forces can be resolved into component parts which act at right angles to each other.

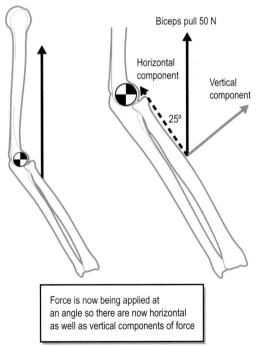

Force is now being applied at an angle so there are now horizontal as well as vertical components of force

Fig. 2.36 Resolution of Muscle Force When Applied at an Angle.

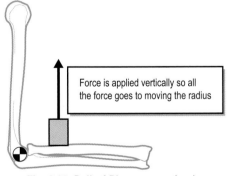

Force is applied vertically so all the force goes to moving the radius

Fig. 2.35 Pull of Biceps at an Angle.

There are different ways of directly measuring force; the forceplate is used for measure different movements, including gait. We examined the outputs from a forceplate; centre of pressure (see Fig. 2.29) and ground reaction force magnitude (see Fig. 2.30), so that will not be new to you next time (it is amazing what you can see in those graphs if you look hard enough!).

Finally, we used mathematics, or more specifically trigonometry, to work out, exactly, what happens when muscle forces are applied at angles.

To conclude this chapter, we thought we could look at an example of force being applied therapeutically, in this case to reduce the symptoms of back pain.

APPLYING A MOBILISATION TECHNIQUE TO THE BACK

The practice of applying force directly to a joint is widely used by many health professionals such as chiropractors, osteopaths and physiotherapists. Let's look at one specific mobilisation technique. A posteroanterior (PA) mobilisation on the spine (or PA for short). This is a downward force applied to the spinous process of a prone patient (lying on their front); the reason for applying this kind of technique might be to improve the range of motion, in the same way that you might wiggle and jiggle a stiff link in a chain or loosen an old door hinge by opening and shutting it. Some therapists perform the technique to create a sedative effect on the painful segment. Whatever the reason, let's look at some of the biomechanical considerations during a typical setup of a therapist applying a PA.

To perform the PA, the therapist stands at the side of the patient who is lying on his or her front on a plinth (firm bed) and applies downward pressure at the stiff segment (Fig. 2.37). The magnitude of this downward force is hard for the therapist to measure exactly, but, using strain gauges, values between 63 and 347 N (quite a difference!) have been recorded (see Fig. 2.3), although it should be said that anything between 100 and 150 N seems to be typical (equivalent to 10 to 15 bags of sugar). The force can be applied through the thumbs of the therapist (surface area approximately 15 cm^2) onto the skin lying over the spinous process; this creates pressure on the skin of around 10 N/cm^2 (150/15), making it quite uncomfortable for the therapist and patient. For this reason, some therapists will use the larger surface area of the hypothenar eminence (pad of soft tissue in the hand just beyond the wrist crease on the little finger side). This compressive stress is applied cyclically (one/off/one/off etc.) at a rate of around two times per second, or 2 Hz.

Although this is quite a lot of pressure, it is unlikely to strain any of the underlying soft tissues (skin, fat, muscle,

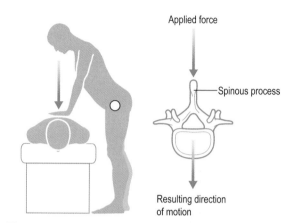

Applied force

Spinous process

Resulting direction of motion

Fig. 2.37 A physiotherapist applying a posteroanterior mobilisation to the lumbar spine, typical direction of applied force.

blood vessels and nerves) beyond their elastic limits (we will cover this in more detail in Chapters 5 ahd 7). This means that when the pressure is released the tissues will quickly reform. If the tissues are only mildly strained and then return to their original shape, what is the point in this mobilising technique? The purpose of repetitive force application may not be to actually change the length/shape of tissues or displace the underlying joint but rather to unstiffen the tissues surrounding the joint(s) by altering their compliance (flexibility). So, it is the repetitive nature of the technique, and not necessarily the magnitude of the force, that is perhaps more important. But what about the underlying bone and joint, which, after all, are the target of the technique, to cause one segment to move on the one next to it (i.e. to move the joint)?

Bone is a much stiffer material, compared with the surrounding soft tissues, which strain. So when the downward force is applied, the bone (and consequently the joint) will hopefully move because it acts like a rigid body (it does not change shape). It is a little like pushing an armchair across a carpet to get a better view of the television (TV); initially your push squashes (compresses) the chair's soft cushioning, but after this your push begins to move the much stiffer frame of the chair over the carpet. However, unlike peripheral joints the segments of the spine are very closely bound together through bony congruency, joint capsules, large discs strong ligaments and multiple layers of muscle. Thus it behaves more like a beam than individual segments (in Chapter 5 we will look in more detail about how beams [like the femur] bend, now try Activity Box 2.4.)

The magnitude of force applied in a PA (100 to 150 N) is unlikely, after it has been reduced by compressing the soft tissues, to cause a great deal of displacement; 2 to 8 mm has been estimated from mathematical models.

Let's change the setup for this mobilising force and see what happens; we will ask the therapist to take a small step backwards. This is an easy alteration to make when applying the technique, but does it change the effect in any way?

Remembering the principles of force resolution, you will know that because this force is being applied at an angle, it resolves into components at right angles to each other (one parallel and one perpendicular). So some of the force will still be directed vertically down (but with a reduced magnitude), producing the same vertically directed motion as before, in this angled position; however, some of the force will be now be directed horizontally along the surface of the body (as indicated in Fig. 2.38).

The effect of this horizontal component would be to generate an anticlockwise moment on the vertebra (as shown in Fig. 2.38) because it is applied at a distance from the fulcrum (which in this case is the centre of mass of the vertebra). However, this moment depends on the tissues overlying the spinous process being rigid enough to

---

ACTIVITY BOX 2.4

You will need a few friends for this activity; five or six should do it. Get your friends to stand up in a line and link arms so that they are holding each other really tightly. Now go up to one of your friends in the middle of this human chain and push them. What happened?

This is similar to what happens to your spine when you push one segment; of course the whole chain moves. This means that the side of the spine/human chain you are pressing on will come close together (compressive strain) and the back of the chain will be opened apart (tensile strain).

ACTIVITY BOX 2.5

Press down on this page with one finger and angle it towards the middle (you may have to hold the book steady) so that the page buckles. Did you find that difficult? Did your finger keep slipping? Now lick the end of your finger and try again. This should prove easier to do because the moisture effectively stuck your finger to the page (increased the coefficient of friction). This time when you pushed the page, (hopefully) it moved but it was probably only the top page. This is because there is not much friction between the layers or pages. The same is true for the layers of tissue under the top surface of skin in your own body.

Find a bit of your skin (e.g. the back of your hand, inside of your elbow), and press directly down on the skin with your finger. Now (without changing the force of your press) turn your finger so it is now pressing on your skin at an angle. You should find that your finger (a) is not pressing down as much and (b) moves over your skin because the layers of soft tissue are sliding on each other. So when applied at an angle, the strain becomes more shear than compressive.

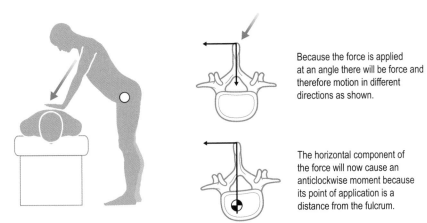

Because the force is applied at an angle there will be force and therefore motion in different directions as shown.

The horizontal component of the force will now cause an anticlockwise moment because its point of application is a distance from the fulcrum.

Fig. 2.38 A physiotherapist applying a posteroanterior mobilisation to the lumbar spine, changing the direction of applied force.

translate the force. To let you understand what I mean, try Activity Box 2.5.

Therefore you can see that a force applied to the spinous process at an angle is a very different proposition from one applied directly down, different direction, different point of application (if the soft tissues slide) and different magnitude. A small step backwards can dramatically change the technique.

In this mobilisation technique, we have considered the direction of the force, the point of application, the effect of overlying soft tissues and the repetitive loading (Further Information 2.3).

Before you proceed to the next chapter, it might be worth looking again at the learning outcomes and then trying the self-assessment exercises.

FURTHER INFORMATION 2.3

In an effort to understand, as well as standardise, spinal mobilisations, simulators are becoming increasingly popular in universities and training institutes. These vary but usually include a mocked-up spine complete with the overlying soft tissues and some way of measuring force such as a strain gauge (see p. 21). The novice practitioner now has the ability to practice their technique while receiving information on direction, rate, frequency, magnitude and point of application of their force. They may for example be able to compare themselves to an experienced practitioner: a good way to refine the technique. Afterall we cannot fit strain gauges to the spines of our patients and clients.

SELF-ASSESSMENT: QUESTIONS

1. Define what we mean by a mechanical force.
2. Which of the following are vectors?
   a. Displacement
   b. Speed
   c. Force
   d. Length
   e. Acceleration
3. From the following list, identify the four characteristics needed to describe a force.
   Distance from pivot, speed, time, magnitude, friction coefficient, point of application, direction, angle of application
4. Is the following statement true or false?
   Velocity is synonymous with speed.
5. Muscles cause joints to rotate because
   a. The joint shape is usually curved.
   b. The muscle is attached at a distance from the joint centre (centre of rotation).
   c. More than two joints work together.
6. If the biceps brachii muscle pulls on the radius with 50 N of force (acting perpendicularly) at a distance of 5 cm from the elbow joint centre, it will create a turning of
   a. 250 Nm.
   b. 10 Nm.
   c. 2.5 Nm.
   d. 25 Nm.
7. If a pulling force (such as a muscle) is applied at an angle, the overall force is
   a. Reduced.
   b. Increased.
   c. Broken down/resolved into horizontal and vertical components.
   d. Unchanged.
8. Provide an example of a force couple (muscular or otherwise).
9. Name the two types of force transducer commonly used in a forceplate.
10. Define a moment of force

ANSWERS TO QUESTIONS POSED IN THE TEXT

Scalars are: speed, depth, circumference, length, distance, luminosity, mass and heat

Vectors are: displacement, force, velocity and acceleration

- Force D vector has a length of 4.76 cm, and therefore a magnitude of 47.6 N; it is applied downwards at an angle of 37 degrees to the horizontal (X) or 53 degrees to the vertical (Y).
- The correct force combination for the car push (see Fig. 2.18) would be F4 and F5; adding the forces in both these combinations would produce the same force vector as Barry (F1).
- To stop the patella moving more towards one side than the other, we need to make sure the resultant is straight. Because we cannot alter the direction of the muscle (we would need the help of an orthopaedic surgeon for that), we can achieve this only by increasing the size of the vastus medialis vector (by strengthening). We could try to reduce the size of vastus lateralis (weaken it), but this would mean resting the muscle, which would also weaken vastus medialis. Therefore we need specific exercises for vastus medialis, which is just what physiotherapists and sports therapists do.
- Simultaneous activation of the three parts of deltoid would result in a combined force similar to the following figure:

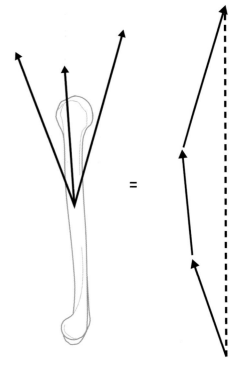

Stability and Balance

Andy Kerr and Philip Rowe

LEARNING OUTCOMES

After reading this chapter, you will be able to:
1. Distinguish between weight and mass.
2. Locate the body's centre of mass (CoM) in quiet standing and describe how it alters with movement and different postures.
3. Define the stability of a body based on its base of support (BoS) and CoM location.
4. Describe how gravity creates moments about the joints.
5. Explain commonly used strategies for remaining balanced.

INTRODUCTION

In this chapter we will look at how the body achieves stability in the context of gravity. We will also look at balance, which, although closely related to stability, is conceptually different with the active involvement of multiple body systems to sense and control the body's position. Balance will be considered in more detail in Chapter 8 but it is worth introducing in this chapter as it follows logically on from our discussions and activities on stability. As always, please try the activities, where possible, and when you have completed the chapter re-read the learning outcomes and try the self-assessment exercises.

GRAVITY: THE ULTIMATE FORCE

The force we have to contend with constantly, and one which has literally shaped our bodies, is **gravity**. Gravity is a pulling force. Theoretically, every piece of mass in the universe pulls other pieces of masses towards it. Before you ask why you are not all sticking together, the strength of the pull depends on the amount of the mass; generally you have to have the same mass as a planet before you create a gravitational (pulling) field worth talking about.

Distance is also a factor with gravity; after all, if gravity was just dependent on mass then all of us would be pulled toward the object with the most mass, which in our case would be the sun, but the sun is too far away to exert that much of a pull on us individually. Gravity becomes stronger the closer you get to the large mass and weaker the further away you are from it. Newton worked this out and called it the Law of Universal Gravitation. Being a mathematician he expressed this law with the formula for calculating the strength of gravity:

$$\text{Gravity} = \frac{G \times (\text{Mass}_1 \times \text{Mass}_2)}{\text{Distance between the two masses squared}}.$$

Note: G is a constant value which is consistent throughout the universe; the inclusion of this value helps make the equation work (probably best to leave it at that).

The large mass closest to us is, of course, our beloved planet, Earth. The mass of the Earth is constantly pulling us towards its centre. The amount it pulls is measured in terms of how much acceleration (see Chapter 2, Fig. 2.8, for a reminder of acceleration) it produces on bodies located on its surface. This has been measured at 9.81 m/s², so every piece of mass on the surface of Earth is pulled towards its centre at a rate of 9.81 m/s², every second. Put it another way, when an object falls to the ground every second it will increase it's speed by 22 miles per hour (mph, which is equivalent to 9.81 m/s²), after 1s it will be traveling at 22mph, after 2s 44mph, after 3s 66mph etc., it wouldn't take long before it gets pretty fast; something to think about before you lean over the side of the Eiffel Tower. We will cover the relationship between force and acceleration in more detail in Chapter 4.

The reason gravity isn't causing you to move while you are sitting there reading this book (it hasn't just given up or been switched off) is that you have hit a hard block, that is the ground or any supporting surface you are sitting/lying/standing on. If you didn't have this hard block under you, for example if you found yourself falling from a bridge or just after you cleared the bar during a pole vault jump, then you would accelerate downward. As Galileo demonstrated in the year 1604, every object accelerates at the same rate on Earth regardless of its weight (Further Information 3.1, see Fig. 3.2). Why not try for yourself; get a coin and a pen and drop them at the same time (Fig. 3.1).

They should have reached the ground at the same time.

They didn't!!

If you dropped them from a small height, you may not have been quick enough to notice much. If you dropped them from a higher point, you may be ready to argue that they don't hit the ground at the same time. They do experience exactly the same accelerating force (gravity); however, the forces that slow them down (decelerating forces) may have been different. This relates to the shape and smoothness of each falling body—we will talk more about this in Chapter 5—but basically the pencil will experience more air resistance than the coin due to its larger surface area in contact with the passing air. Because of this it will slow down more than the coin. If you did the same experiment on the Moon (where there is no air to slow things down) then the objects will definitely hit the ground at the same time, although they will fall slower than on Earth due to the reduced gravity!

Because the Moon is smaller and lighter than Earth it has less gravity (around a sixth that of Earth's). This means that visitors to the Moon, like Buzz Aldrin and Neil Armstrong, felt less of a downward pull when they were walking about on the surface, illustrating the difference between weight and mass. Let me explain; the astronauts had more

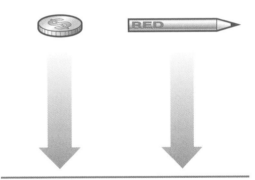

Fig. 3.1 Pen and Coin Dropped Together.

FURTHER INFORMATION 3.1

As an experimental scientist, Galileo Galilei was a bit of a rarity in the 17th century; most scientists of the day preferred thought experiments (useful in some ways but lacking the word evidence that we are so enamoured with in the 21st century). Even at the beginning of his career he was unhappy with the untested, yet widely held, idea that objects of different weight fell at different speeds. I would guess that some people today still believe it to be true, and to be honest it doesn't seem so weird under casual observation. But Galileo was not one for casual observation; he wanted to test it and in Italy there are

some handy leaning towers to help inquisitive scientists. From the leaning tower of Pisa (yes, it was leaning even then), Galileo dropped objects of various mass (but of similar size and shape) at the same time: cannon balls, wooden balls, musket balls and balls made of different metals. When he found that the objects, (more or less) hit the ground at the same time, the accepted wisdom (championed by Aristotle; more on him later) was rejected and Galileo's hypothesis, that every object is subjected to the same acceleration (gravity), was accepted. This is also known as the equivalence principle and was the

Continued

FURTHER INFORMATION 3.1—cont'd

foundation for Newton's Laws of Motion (see Chapter 4). The falling objects are subjected to different amounts of friction and air resistance (depending on their shape) which explains why we perceive heavier objects to fall to the ground faster than light ones (Fig. 3.2).

In fact astronaut David Scott repeated Galileo's experiment on the Moon using a falcon feather and a hammer (it could have been anything really) and found that without air resistance they did indeed fall at the same rate.

Historians still debate whether Galileo actually conducted the experiment, but whether he did or didn't, he was right, as thousands of schoolchildren and the odd astronaut can testify to.

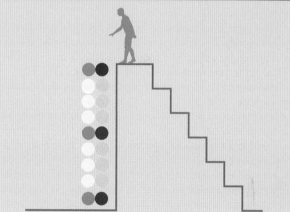

Fig. 3.2 Dropping Objects of Different Size From a Tower.

or less the same amount of mass as they had when on Earth and yet if they stood on a weighing scale on the Moon they would weigh less (around a sixth) than they did on Earth because there is less of a force (gravity) pulling them down. So weight is the amount of mass you have multiplied by the acceleration of gravity (which may vary according to the planet you are living on).

Put another way, weight will vary according to the accelerations the body is experiencing whereas mass is simply the amount of stuff you have contained within the confines of your skin which won't alter (well not easily or quickly). Although both are often confusingly measured in kilograms, weight is really a force, so should be measured in newtons. We will talk a bit more about this later but if you didn't understand that why not try Activity Box 3.1 (see Fig. 3.3; Further Information 3.2).

Let's come back down to Earth and try to understand more about mass, because, as hopefully you will see, it is critical to understanding human movement, as well as space travel.

CENTRE OF MASS

When gravity acts on an object, such as your body, it acts on every particle of mass within that body. This makes analysis very difficult, so to simplify this situation (always desirable) we can think of the force acting about a single average point—the centre of mass (CoM).

The CoM is the average position of all the bits of the body's mass. Consequently it will depend on the density (the concentration of mass) and its distribution within the shape of the body. The CoM of a ball filled with foam would

FURTHER INFORMATION 3.2 The Advantages of the Moon's Atmosphere

Low gravity and lack of air resistance (remember the feather and coin being dropped) are behind proposals to build a Moon base for launching space flights to Mars. In this way the energy cost of lifting a large mass (the shuttle, at lift off, has a total mass of around 109,000 kg) off the surface is much reduced. Also when it comes to landing, the lack of air will not cause the same high temperature that spacecraft can experience on re-entry to Earth's atmosphere (the surface of the shuttle can rise to 816°C!). The Moon would be easier because there is no friction on the vessel's surface from the air but you will need big retro rockets to slow down rather than the parachutes deployed during an Earth landing.

be at its geometric centre, provided the ball is a perfect circle of course and the mass (foam) within it is evenly distributed. If the mass was denser (more packed in) at the top than the bottom, then the CoM would be higher. The CoM simply reflects where the mass is (Fig. 3.4).

Look around at some of the objects in the room you are in just now, chair, filing cabinet, TV, computer, bookcase etc., and try to guess where the CoM is. Don't just pick the centre of the shape; perhaps there are some bits heavier than others, the top of the table for example. There may be empty spaces within the object, for example within a personal computer, which can alter the CoM position. Maybe there are some components that are very dense like the screen of a visual display unit.

ACTIVITY BOX 3.1

This is quite a fun experiment that will demonstrate the difference between mass and weight as well as showing you a really easy and quick way to lose weight. Get a set of analogue weighing scales (ones with a dial, not digital) and go to one of the lifts in your building (if you don't have access to a lift, don't worry; there are alternatives mentioned at the end). Now, making sure you have the lift to yourself, stand on the scales and take a note of your weight. Now press the up button while looking at your dial. What happened? Did your weight momentarily increase? Next time, I want you to press the down button and watch the dial again. This time your weight should drop; although brief, it isn't a long-term alternative to dieting if you want to lose weight.

So why did you lose and gain weight simply from going up and down in a lift? Let's analyse the forces (Fig. 3.3). First when the lift was standing still (Box A): You are applying a force (mass × gravity) down onto the weighing scale and it is pushing you back (otherwise you would

fall), by exactly the same amount. This push up is what is displayed by the dial. Basically the forces are in balance. When you pressed the up button, the bottom (Box B) of the floor started to push up more on your feet (you might even be able to feel your knees buckle a little). This upward acceleration increases your weight. When you pressed down (Box C), the opposite occurred: the increased downward acceleration means you (temporarily) weigh less. You will notice that these changes are brief and that the scales quickly return to normal, even when you are still moving at a constant velocity. This is because although you might still be moving, there are no accelerations.

'The point to remember here is that an acceleration alters your weight'. You can get the same feeling from a rollercoaster, or even driving over hilly country lanes. Even if you bounce up and down on a set of weighing scales your apparent weight changes, even if your actual weight (mass) remains the same, because you are accelerating.

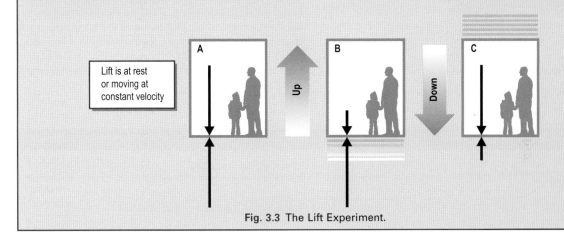

Fig. 3.3 The Lift Experiment.

Calculating the Centre of Mass

Rather than guess the location of the CoM it may be necessary to calculate its exact position; this is critical for engineers designing large structures such as bridges and office blocks and, although arguably less critical, can provide a better understanding of movement performance and injury in sport and rehabilitation. Various methods for calculating the CoM of the human body have been used. In the 17th century, the Italian scientist Borelli used balance boards to estimate the CoM location; this worked because the point about which the body balances is the same as the CoM.

Remember those long boring days at school when, instead of listening to your maths teacher, you were busy trying to balance your pencil on your rubber (you were not alone); well, you were actually doing the same thing as Borelli, finding the pencil's CoM, the balance point on your pencil being the same as its CoM. If there were more pencil mass on one side of the rubber than the other then it would tip in the direction of most mass; there has to be equal amounts of mass on either side for the pencil for it to be balanced, so the rubber must lie at the CoM (Fig. 3.5, Activity Box 3.2 and see Fig. 3.6).

By applying this type of analysis (balancing bodies) to elderly male cadavers, research studies have shown that the

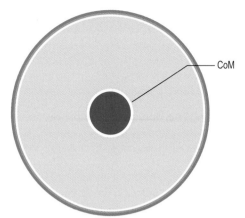

Fig. 3.4 Centre of Mass *(CoM)* of a Ball Filled Evenly With Foam.

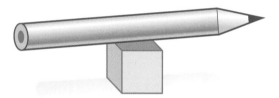

Fig. 3.5 Balancing a Pencil on a Rubber.

overall CoM of the human body, when standing upright with arms by the side, lies within the pelvis. To be more precise, it has been placed at 5 cm anterior to the second sacral tuberosity (Fig. 3.7), the bone at the base of your spine. Sports textbooks sometimes use a value of 55% of height (from feet up), which is approximately the same point (why not measure it on your self and see if it is the same).

The vertical arrow pointing down from the CoM in Fig. 3.7 is the **line of gravity** (LoG) and is a useful way of understanding posture and movement used by rehabilitation workers and sports professionals. It represents the direction of gravity which is acting through (on average) the CoM (see Fig. 3.7). In Chapter 8 we will use the LoG to analyse different postures.

This may or may not be obvious to you, but the CoM does not necessarily have to lie within the mass of the body. The CoM of a doughnut, for example, is in the centre, that is in the hole in the middle. It's just something to bear in mind when you come to analysing body positions.

We have looked at the CoM location in quiet (very quiet in the case of the male cadavers) standing; however we are constantly on the move, changing postures from sitting to lying, standing to walking, standing to swimming etc.; as the CoM represents the location of all the body parts it will change as the body changes. So for example if you move your hands forward, there will be more mass forward than previously, so the overall CoM will have moved forward.

ACTIVITY BOX 3.2

To do this activity you will need a wobble board and a strong plank of wood, but if you don't have these things you can just imagine the activity.

Finding the balance point of a human can be done just as crudely as you balancing the pencil on top of the rubber, by using a wobble board. Do not be confused with the instrument used by Australian aboriginals to replicate the sound of thunder; by wobble board we mean the mini seesaw used to train balance. Get a plank of wood and place it on top of the wobble board so that it is balanced; this will need a bit of adjustment. Now get a piece of chalk or something similar and draw a line from the point on the ground that the fulcrum touches up and over the board (black vertical in Fig. 3.6). Now carefully sit down in the middle of the wobble board (more or less on your chalk line) and slowly lie down. One of three things will happen: either your head end falls down, your feet end falls down or you are balanced. To become balanced will require a little bit of shuffling up or down. Now, when

you finally get balanced, look at the position of the chalk mark (you may need a friend to help); it should now be at your centre of mass. There is just as much of your mass below the chalk line as above it.

From this balanced point, try lifting your hands up. What should happen and what did happen? Can you explain any movement that occurred? Try moving other parts of your body but before you do try to predict what might happen.

Of course we have only really estimated the **height** of your CoM; to get a truly three-dimensional location, you will need to repeat the experiment when standing. I will let you get on with that in your own time. Estimating the height is good enough for me.

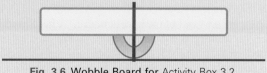

Fig. 3.6 Wobble Board for Activity Box 3.2.

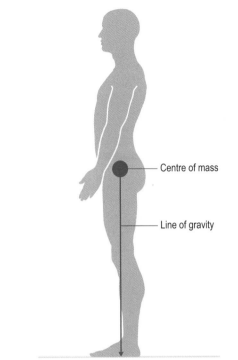

Fig. 3.7 Centre of Mass of a Typical Human in Quiet Standing: 5 Cm in Front of the Second Sacral Tuberosity.

As soon as you stand up your CoM will also rise, because more of your mass is higher up. On the following group of pictures (Fig. 3.8) put your finger where you think the CoM is located. Think where it was in quiet standing (within pelvis) then look at how the body parts are arranged now: is there more mass further forwards or further back than in standing, or is it lower or higher? (Answers at end of chapter.)

We hope you found that a useful exercise and one that you can practice on real people performing sport as well as everyday activities; just be careful not to stare for too long; some people won't understand.

Now of course things are not as simple as looking at a picture, or even videos. We have made a big assumption (assumptions are pretty commonplace in biomechanics; otherwise you would keep getting stuck, but they have to be reasonable) that the mass was evenly distributed within the shape. That there is the same amount of mass within the same area in the legs compared to the trunk is clearly wrong.

Humans are made of different kinds of material, which we will talk about later in Chapter 5, with different amounts of stuff within them. Muscle is one of the most densely packed structures in our bodies and our legs (generally) have the greatest amount of muscle tissue (because of their

constant battle against gravity), so basically there is more mass in our legs than in our trunk, which may look large but contains a lot of spaces (think of the air in your lungs and other organs to a lesser extent). So if we move a leg forward then the CoM will move further forward than if we had moved our arms or bellies by a similar amount.

What Should You Remember About Mass?

Mass is the amount of stuff within a shape. It is measured in kilograms (kg). It is different from weight which is synonymous with your body force. To make life easier, you can represent the whole mass of a body by its CoM. The CoM moves with the body so that it could even be outside the body shape in some circumstances. We will talk more about mass and how it relates to movement in Chapter 4 when we look at Newton's laws of motion.

Moments Created by Mass

Gravity pulls us straight down; we have probably laboured this point already, but it's worth remembering. Our bodies are made up of lots of linked segments; each segment has its own mass and therefore a point that we can call the segmental CoM, as opposed to the overall CoM we have been talking about so far. Now because each segment is linked by a rotational point (joints) this will mean that gravity (which, on average will be applied at the segmental CoM) can create moments, which are (as you will hopefully recall; if not then go back to Chapter 2) the rotational effects of forces, caused by a force being applied about a pivot/hinge/joint. To illustrate this effect of gravity let's try a simple exercise, Activity Box 3.3 (see Fig. 3.9).

Moments created by gravity are a useful way to structure resistance exercises, for example, if you were trying to train a group of muscles. Consider the following problem:

An athlete is recovering from a serious shoulder injury. Following a long period in a sling his muscles are generally very weak. You decide to work first on strengthening his shoulder abductors (muscles that lift your arm out to the side) by getting him to hold a certain position for 5 seconds at a time. Which position would be the easiest?

1. Lying on his side with the weak arm raised toward the ceiling at 90 degrees? (See Fig. 3.10.)
2. Standing up with arm raised out to side (i.e. the same position as Fig. 3.10 but now as standing)? (See Fig. 3.11.)

After a couple of sessions he has improved and you would like to introduce more resistance to the muscles, so how could you alter the position in Fig. 3.10 to create a little bit more resistance to the shoulder abductors?

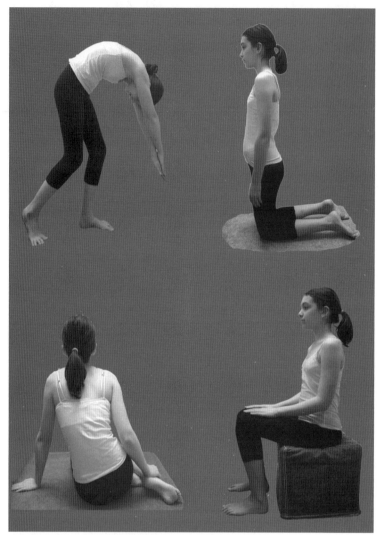

Fig. 3.8 Find the Centre of Mass.

ACTIVITY BOX 3.3

Stand up and move your right arm out to the side (abduction), like you would if you were signalling to turn right on a bike (Fig. 3.9). Hold it there. You should feel the muscles around your shoulder working pretty hard to hold this abducted position. So, what are your muscles working against? Let's analyse the forces at work:

There is a moment caused by gravity acting directly down (I said you would need to remember that) on the mass of your arm. Now, although gravity is acting on every particle of mass in your arm it can be averaged out to act

at the CoM, which is probably around your elbow (depending on how muscular you are), which if I am not mistaken is some distance from your shoulder. The force of gravity acting at the CoM of the arm (represented by the LoG) will therefore cause an adducting moment about your shoulder; that is, it is trying to bring your arm down to your side. The size of this moment depends on the mass of your arm (and anything it is holding, weight or cup of coffee) and where this is centred (i.e. CoM) in relation to the joint centre (see Fig. 3.9). So for example if you were

ACTIVITY BOX 3.3—cont'd

wearing a plaster of Paris cast on your wrist, the CoM would move further down your arm, increasing the distance from the fulcrum (shoulder), as well as increasing the amount of mass and therefore increasing the adducting moment.

Now bring your arm closer to your body (let's say halfway down) and hold it there. Now, does that feel better?

You should have found that holding your arm closer to your body was easier. The reason for this is the reduced distance (moment arm) between the LoG and centre of rotation. This doesn't mean that your arm has shortened

but it has moved through an arc that brings the CoM and centre of rotation closer, reducing the moment. If you continue to move your arm down, the CoM will lie more or less directly underneath the centre of rotation. Therefore no moments will be created, which is why it is easier to walk with your arms by your side than holding them out to the side (just in case you were wondering).

What about if you held your arm out to the side with your elbow bent; how does that change the difficulty? Clue: the CoM of the arm will have moved.

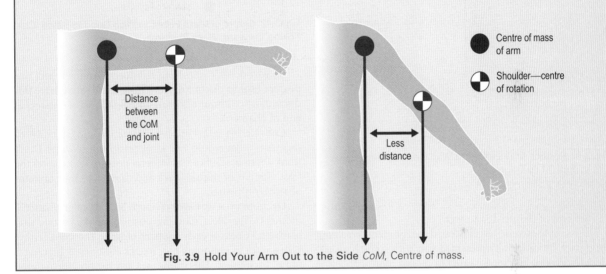

Fig. 3.9 Hold Your Arm Out to the Side *CoM*, Centre of mass.

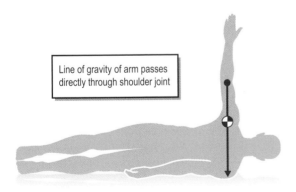

Fig. 3.10 Position a: Lying on Side With the Weak Arm Raised Towards the Ceiling at 90 Degrees.

(Answers to both questions are at end of this chapter.)

Let's try another one: following a hip replacement operation the hip abductor muscles (muscles that move the leg out to the side; predominantly this is gluteus medius) are generally weak due to the damage from the surgery on the lateral side of the hip. You are not sure which exercises to start with so decide on the easiest ones for the hip abductors. Considering the moments caused by gravity (don't forget it pulls things directly down!) place the following positions in order of the difficulty (easiest first).

1. The patient lying on their back moving the operated leg out into abduction (out to side).
2. Standing and moving operated leg out into abduction.
3. Lying on 'good' side and lifting operated leg directly up into abduction.
4. Lying on 'good' side with knee bent and moving leg directly up into abduction.

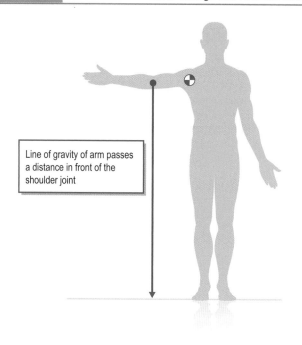

Line of gravity of arm passes a distance in front of the shoulder joint

Fig. 3.11 Position B: Standing Up With the Weak Arm Raised Out to Side at 90 Degrees.

(See end of chapter for answer.)

This simple exercise has illustrated the moments created by gravity and hopefully presented you with some logical ideas for making an exercise easier or indeed more difficult.

MOMENTS AND POSTURE

Of course these gravitational moments are not limited to our limbs. Think about your sitting position at the moment and in particular, your head. If, like in the diagram below (Fig. 3.12), your head is jutting forward on your neck (if it isn't, then just try it for a few moments) then the CoM of the head will be placed relatively forward of the joints in the neck. What does this mean for muscle effort?

The downward force, created by gravity acting on the mass of the head, will be located at the CoM. Poking your head forward moves this CoM (and therefore the force) forward from the joints in the neck thereby creating a turning force which is trying to flex the neck (bring the head down onto the chest). If this is difficult to imagine then try to think what would happen if someone came up to you and pushed down on your head, with it still poking forward; in this position it would flex down. This is exactly what gravity is trying to do.

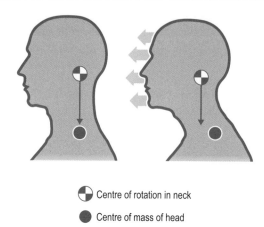

⊕ Centre of rotation in neck

● Centre of mass of head

Fig. 3.12 Centre of Mass Location With Good and Bad (Chin Poking Forward) Neck Postures.

So why doesn't your head fall down? And why will this posture lead to discomfort and how could you relieve this discomfort (without resorting to painkillers)? (Answers at end of chapter.)

Considering gravitational moments and stability of segments what would the ideal posture look like? Don't think about aesthetics but rather a posture that creates the least amount of muscle work and causes the least amount of stress on tissues.

Ok, from what we have previously said about gravitational moments, the ideal standing posture would be one that places the CoM of each segment close to the joint centre. Like a stack of children's play blocks all squarely placed on top of each other. This minimises any turning force in the same way that sitting in the middle of a seesaw means you don't tilt one of the sides down. This will minimise any resulting muscle activity. An ideal standing posture has therefore been suggested to be one where the LoG, from the head down, passes (Fig. 3.13):
1. Through the mastoid process (the bony lump behind the ear).
2. Just in front of the shoulder joint.
3. Just behind the hip joint.
4. Through or just in front of the knee joint.
5. A couple of centimetres in front of the ankle joint.

We will consider this ideal standing posture again in Chapter 8; it is a useful template when considering postural back pain.

STABILITY

Generally when we talk about the stability of a rigid body it refers to its ability (or inability) to return to its original position after experiencing an external force(s), such as a push. If a body was unstable, its position is likely to change when it is pushed; this could result in a fall and injury or, for a sportsman, it could mean being pushed out of an important position, for example a goalkeeper being jostled out of the way during a corner kick in a game of soccer. A more stable body is less likely to fall or be displaced from a push or pull, so how can you improve stability?

The previous section on mass and CoM is very important to understanding a body's stability. We need to know where a body's CoM is located and we also need to know about its base of support (BoS). This is the area of contact a body has with its supporting surface. For example, a box sitting on the ground has a typically large BoS as indicated by the shaded area in Fig. 3.14. We can calculate the BoS simply as the area that is width × length of the contacting surface.

The box is a simple example; what about the BoS for more complex shapes like the human body? While standing with feet apart the BoS of a human is defined by the shaded areas in Fig. 3.15.

As you can see from the footprints in Fig. 3.15 the BoS does not have to be all in contact with the supporting surface; rather it is the area defined by the perimeter round all the points in contact. Think of the 'feet' of the Eiffel Tower; it wouldn't be as much fun if you couldn't walk under the tower but the fact that the actual contact points are relatively small doesn't alter its stability because the area between the points is what matters. Take another example: if we look at

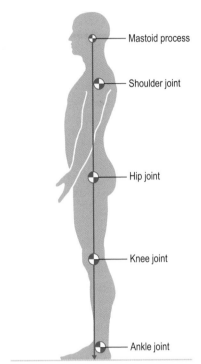

Fig. 3.13 Ideal Standing Posture.

- Mastoid process
- Shoulder joint
- Hip joint
- Knee joint
- Ankle joint

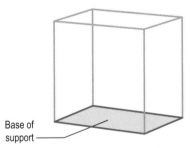

Base of support

Fig. 3.14 Base of Support of a Box.

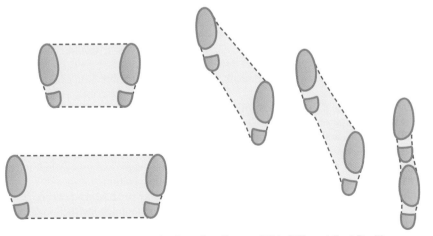

Fig. 3.15 Base of Support of a Standing Human With Different Feet Positions.

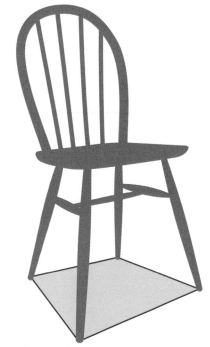

Fig. 3.16 Base of Support of a Chair.

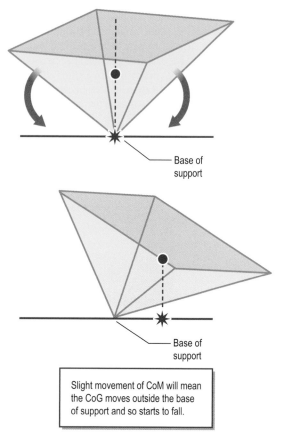

Base of support

Base of support

Slight movement of CoM will mean the CoG moves outside the base of support and so starts to fall.

Fig. 3.18 Inverted Pyramid Showing Centre of Mass *(CoM)*, Centre of Gravity *(CoG)* and Base of Support.

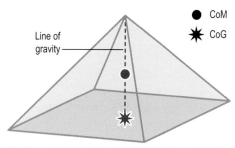

Line of gravity

● CoM

✶ CoG

Fig. 3.17 Pyramid Showing Centre of Mass *(CoM)*, Centre of Gravity *(CoG)* and Base of Support, darker shaded area.

a chair (Fig. 3.16) the points in contact are relatively small; however the BoS is actually quite large.

A body is considered to be stable if its CoM lies within the BoS. Well, actually it's the centre of gravity (CoG) that should lie within the BoS, the CoG is slightly different from CoM and easily confused. If you take a line vertically down from the CoM (if you remember this is called the LoG), then the point where this line meets the ground is the CoG, so the CoG is a point on the ground. A stable body has the CoG within the BoS. Think of the Egyptian pyramids (Fig. 3.17); they are pretty stable structures with the CoG well within the BoS.

What happens if we turn the pyramid upside down? It can still be a stable body but only if we manage to balance the CoM directly above the very small BoS. You can see how this inverted pyramid could easily become unstable, that is, it wouldn't take much for it to topple (Fig. 3.18).

A body's stability (you could also use the word equilibrium) could be described as one of three types.

1. Unstable—if pushed, a body will move and continue to move until it reaches a stable position.
2. Neutral stability—if pushed a body will move to a new position where it will remain.
3. Stable—if pushed a body will move then return to its original position.

Now once you have made a cone (see Further Information 3.3 for simple quick instructions) try to position it in the three types of equilibrium, see Fig. 3.19 (see also Further Information 3.4 and Activity Box 3.4).

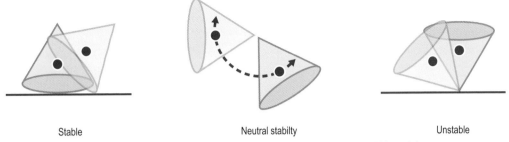

Fig. 3.19 Three Categories of Stability: Stable, Neutral and Unstable.

Stable   Neutral stabilty   Unstable

FURTHER INFORMATION 3.3   How to Make a Paper Cone

Get a piece of A4 paper, a small plate, pencil, sticky tape and scissors.

Use the plate to draw a circle on the paper; the bigger the circle, the bigger the cone. Now carefully cut out the circle, and fold it in half and then half again so you have a pizza slice. Open out your circle so you can see the four triangles and cut one of them out. Now bring the two edges you have cut together and overlap them (the more you overlap the narrower the cone) so that you have a cone. Tape the ends down.

FURTHER INFORMATION 3.4

The Belarussian Aleksandr Bendikov incredibly managed to balance 783 dominoes on top of a single domino, so that it was basically an upside-down pyramid. Unbelievably this structure stood for a couple of days in his apartment before the media came to witness it. It couldn't have been an easy wait and I don't suppose he was very tolerant of anyone slamming the door. Why don't you try to build one for yourself: all you need is 800 or so dominoes, a flat surface, plenty of time to kill and a very steady hand.

ACTIVITY BOX 3.4

Have another look at Fig. 3.8. You have already identified the CoM; now define the base support so that you have some indication of stability. Is the CoG within the BoS? How close is the CoG to the borders of the BoS? Think about how easy it would be for the person to become destabilised and what direction of push would they be most vulnerable to.

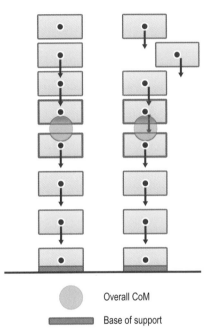

⬤ Overall CoM

▬ Base of support

Fig. 3.20 Intrinsic and Extrinsic Stability *CoM*, Centre of mass.

LOCAL AND GENERAL STABILITY

Because we are made of multiple segments, you could have a situation where there is instability between a couple of segments but overall the body is still stable. The spine gives us a good illustration of this difference, between intrinsic and extrinsic stability. The spine consists of 12 segments (vertebra) stacked on top of each other with their characteristic three curves. Let's look at the spine from the back and consider each segment at a time (Fig. 3.20). The CoM of the top segment is located (more or less) at its centre and lies nicely within the BoS of the supporting surface (i.e. the top surface of the next segment down). At this level the segment is stable, locally or intrinsically stable. In a well-aligned spine this situation carries on all the way down to the bottom segment which in turn rests on the sacrum. The structure of each individual intervertebral segment and the way they are stacked on top of each other confers a great deal of intrinsic stability to the spine; stripped of all its muscles the spine would still be regarded as an intrinsically very stable structure.

Now consider a small lateral shift in one of the segments, the second one down. Although overall (extrinsically) the spine is still stable, because the overall CoM (and therefore the CoG) still lies within the BoS, the second segment down is outwith its BoS and is therefore intrinsically unstable.

Any local instability, even if it does not affect overall stability, still requires a local solution. If you were an engineer and this was a tower you might bolt some plates or extra cables over the local instability; otherwise it could cause the tower to fall because that individual will eventually break because of the stress. In the body, additional muscle work and perhaps some adaptation of other tissues (ligaments and capsule) prevents an individual segment from being further displaced. This additional work can cause local damage and discomfort.

The stability of a body is a fundamental design consideration in the construction of many structures from simple furniture to high-storey buildings. Wheelchairs are no exception. It's pretty important that a wheelchair remains stable despite being pushed back and forward, bumped up/down kerbs, moved up and down slopes and manoeuvred around obstacles. It is also important to know if the stability is affected by changes in the user's body mass (e.g. putting a lot of weight on) or the attachment of a rucksack over the back.

So how are wheelchairs designed for maximal stability? First let's just look at a standard wheelchair and identify the CoM, CoG and BoS. When estimating CoM you should consider the person and wheelchair as a single unit. The BoS is defined by the parts in contact with the ground (i.e. front wheel and back wheel).

As you can see (Fig. 3.21), on a flat surface the wheelchair is stable with the CoG well within the BoS; however what happens if the wheelchair goes up a slope? (See Fig. 3.22.)

This is obviously a precarious situation, with the CoG close to, if not past, the rear boundary of the BoS. What can you do to reduce the risk of the chair (and occupant) tipping backwards?
- Lean forwards?
- Increase the BoS at the back?

Both options can increase stability. Leaning forwards, of course, moves the CoM forward and therefore returns the CoG within the BoS again. Increasing the BoS at the back is achieved with wheelchairs that have their back wheels fixed further back, thereby increasing the BoS (this does however make them a little less manoeuvrable). Many wheelchairs

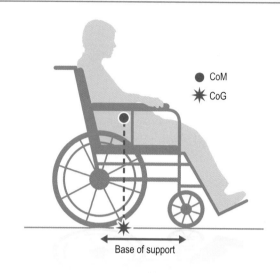

Fig. 3.21 Stability of a Wheelchair User *CoM*, Centre of mass; *CoG*, centre of gravity.

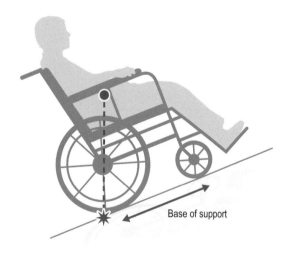

The CoG is now behind the base of support, the wheelchair and occupant are therefore unstable and in danger of tipping backwards

Fig. 3.22 Stability of a Wheelchair User Going Up a Slope *CoG*, Centre of gravity.

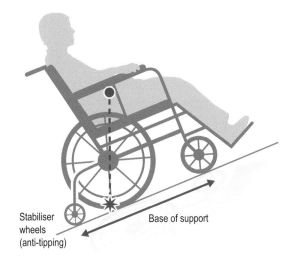

Stabiliser wheels (anti-tipping)

Base of support

Fig. 3.23 Stabiliser Wheels to Prevent Tipping.

have included small stabiliser wheels at the back; these are designed so that they will come in contact with the ground with the slightest posterior tip (Fig. 3.23). This contact moves the BoS backward so that the CoG is again within the BoS, that is it stabilises. This is a bit like moving your foot back to keep balanced when someone pushes you from the front, you change your BoS to accommodate a new CoG position.

Can you think of any other situations when a wheelchair may become unstable?

- What would happen when moving down a slope?
- What about hanging a rucksack on the handles at the back?
- Or how about if the occupant became a lower-limb amputee?

(Answers at end of chapter.)

Of course, we have just looked at wheelchair stability from one perspective, that is forwards and backwards; the wheelchair can also be unstable from side to side as well (Further Information 3.5). The same kind of analysis that we applied for the side view can be applied for the front/back view. How might side-to-side stability of the wheelchair be compromised?

STANDING BALANCE

Being upright has produced some excellent outcomes for humans—seeing over walls, freedom to use your hands and skipping—but it has also made us fairly unstable. When you think about it, since we decided to become bipedal, the

---

FURTHER INFORMATION 3.5

The sports of wheelchair basketball and rugby involve a lot of potentially destabilising collisions and rapid accelerations. To minimise the risk of tipping over (difficult to play when you are rooted to the ground), the wheels in these wheelchairs are angled out to increase the width of the BoS, conferring greater stability on the wheelchair and occupant, particularly from the side.

ACTIVITY BOX 3.5

Stand up and close your eyes (make sure you have a clear space around you and don't try this if you have a problem with your balance) and feel yourself gently sway. It is like a tree swaying in a gentle breeze. But why don't you just stand still?

As a living organism there are systems constantly at work: your lungs expand, your heart beats and blood gushes round your body and there are constant fluctuations in your body mass. These movements cause the body's CoM to move a little, which is counterbalanced by muscle activity, a little contraction here, another there, to dampen any movements of the CoM. Before you know it, you are swaying.

---

human body is quite unstable, one of the reasons we have such a big problem with falls in older adults. After all, you do not see many dogs falling over. Becoming upright has moved our CoM much further away from our BoS; now it can easily (and often does) move outside the BoS. With this arrangement, we have been likened to an upside-down pendulum (like an old-fashioned metronome musicians use to keep rhythm when playing), with our mass swaying back and forward and side to side over a relatively small fixed point (our feet); try Activity Box 3.5.

If we look at the body in a standing position from the side, we can see how this swinging pendulum develops (Fig. 3.24). Imagine if the CoM moved forward a little, for example, you moved both your arms in front of you. With the CoM moving forward, the LoG is further in front of your ankle creating a moment that will bend (dorsiflex) your foot. If left unchecked this moment will mean the whole body will begin rotating forward. Try it if you like. Stand up and put both arms in front of you; you should feel yourself starting to fall forwards. If you can't feel anything you may be too tense; for this to work you have to be pretty relaxed and in tune with your body. If you do start to fall forward you only have a short period of time for your body to respond

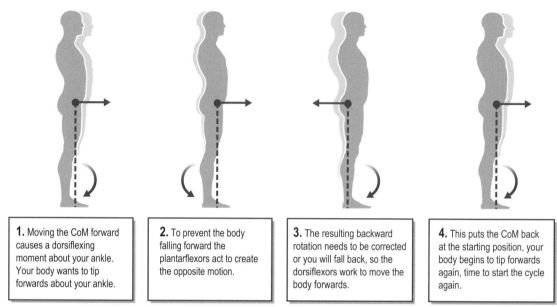

1. Moving the CoM forward causes a dorsiflexing moment about your ankle. Your body wants to tip forwards about your ankle.

2. To prevent the body falling forward the plantarflexors act to create the opposite motion.

3. The resulting backward rotation needs to be corrected or you will fall back, so the dorsiflexors work to move the body forwards.

4. This puts the CoM back at the starting position, your body begins to tip forwards again, time to start the cycle again.

Fig. 3.24 Inverted Pendulum *CoM*, Centre of mass.

because, powered by gravity, it has started to accelerate towards the ground. Of course your body reacts quickly by creating a counter moment to rotate your body backwards. This is achieved through contraction of the ankle plantarflexors (calf muscles) which rotate your leg, and consequently the rest of the body, backwards. Unfortunately this means your CoM is accelerating backwards, and unless there is another muscle action the body will fall backwards. If you don't believe me, why not try it yourself.

Stand up and contract your plantarflexors (press your toes down into the ground so that your heels lift momentarily). You should feel yourself moving backwards. So yet again the body has to produce a corrective force to make you rotate forwards again. How will this be produced? Step forward the heroic tibialis anterior (the muscle that brings your foot towards your lower leg, a movement known as dorsiflexion). Practically single-handedly this muscle pulls the body forward again. Again, try it if you like; stand up and quickly pull your toes (both sides) up in the air (a reasonable distance) so that only your heels are on the ground, then immediately let them drop down again. Following this movement you should start to feel your body move forward. So now we are back at the start again with the CoM rocking forwards, the pendulum starts its swing again. This model of balance was first proposed by David Winter, one of the pioneers of biomechanics.

This back and forward rocking movement about your ankle, controlled by the dorsiflexors and plantarflexors, has been called the ankle strategy. It has been suggested that as

you get older this strategy for controlling balance is not so effective due to a decrease in the speed that your nerves carry information from your brain to your muscles. Basically the muscles are too far away for an older person to use them quickly enough to react to changes in body position. When this happens the muscles about the hip are used to move the body forwards and back; this has been called, unsurprisingly, the hip strategy. The hip strategy is also used if a large shift in the body's CoM is required, for example if you are pushed, with a largish force from the front or back.

Despite our inherent instability humans accomplish some incredible feats of balance; consider one of the most spectacular circus acts, walking along the high wire.

During high-wire balancing acts (Fig. 3.25), the BoS is not only small and narrow (the width of the BoS will be essentially the width of the wire), it also moves; really nasty. Lateral (side-to-side) stability is crucial; the acrobats will need to absolutely limit lateral movement and if it does occur, to respond quickly enough to correct the movement before it's too late. They don't have time for an inverted pendulum because that takes too long. One thing that all tight-rope or high-wire acrobats do is that they all seem to either carry something (usually this is a pole held horizontally but sometimes an umbrella) or hold their arms out to the side. Why is this? Try Activity Box 3.6; it might give you some clues!

Holding the pole means there is more mass distributed away from the pivot point; this creates moments about the central axis (if you imagine a line up from the pivot point

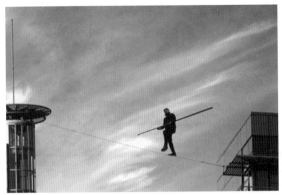

Fig. 3.25 Walking Along the High Wire.

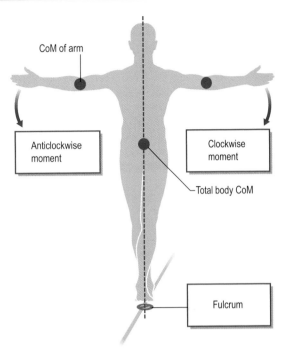

Fig. 3.26 Using Equilibrium of Moments to Perform the High Wire Act *CoM*, Centre of mass.

ACTIVITY BOX 3.6

Why not try this balancing act yourself? No, not on a high wire (we don't want any casualties)! Just imagine (or draw) a line on the floor and attempt to walk along it. First do it with your arms pinned to your side, then try it with your arms out to the side. Finally try it while holding a pole (an unopened umbrella would be fine) level in both hands in front of you. Hopefully you should have felt steadier the second time and even steadier the last time with possibly less muscle work going on around your ankle.

dividing the body; Fig. 3.26) of the body. These moments can be used to quickly create accelerations of the body, correcting any destabilising movement, a quick flick of the pole producing a rapid change in the lateral rotation of the body. There is also a slowing down effect caused by moving mass outwards from the pivot point. This is a bit like making the beam of a seesaw longer so that it takes longer to rotate when a force is applied. We'll talk more about this in Chapter 4.

Some tight-rope artists hold a pole which is bent downwards. Why do you think they do this? (Answer at end of chapter.) (See Further Information 3.6.)

Other primates such as orangutans employ much the same principle when they walk; they deliberately move their arms out to the side so that they can counterbalance lateral momentum. Next chance you get to go to the zoo have a look at any monkey walking on two legs, do you think they could walk if their arms were tied to their sides?

Now that you have thought a bit about gravity, moments and stability, why not have a shot at Activities Box 3.7 and 3.8 (see Figs 3.27 and 3.28). Try to imagine your CoM location throughout the activities.

FURTHER INFORMATION 3.6

In the late 1800s the Great Blondin walked across the Niagara Falls on a tight-rope. Although an amazing accomplishment in itself, he attempted to make the spectacle even more entertaining with theatrical twists including carrying his manager (I wonder who was the most frightened) and stopping halfway across to cook a meal!

Understanding a body's stability by identifying the CoM and BoS (see Activity Box 3.4) is, of course, limited because we are considering static situations, snapshots during a movement. We are constantly moving, changing position, direction and velocity and therefore changing our stability; to illustrate this consider the stability of a sprinter at the beginning of a 100m race. At the start he has a large BoS (defined by the feet, knees and hands—all the points of contact with the ground) and the CoM (or rather CoG) is clearly within this boundary; Fig. 3.29.

As the start gun fires, the sprinter lifts his head and hands simultaneously; this means the BoS rapidly reduces and moves backwards. The CoM (if you imagine it to lie somewhere around the lower abdomen/upper pelvis) and

ACTIVITY BOX 3.7

To remain standing we need a really well-tuned ability to detect our body position (this is also called kinaesthesia). Take a moment to check out your kinaesthetic awareness. Stand up with a bit of space around you so that you are free of objects on the ground and try the following:

1. Close your eyes. Starting at your head think about each body part. Is your head forward on your neck? Is it slightly tilted? Now move down your body, shoulders, arms, hands, pelvis etc., and try to build a three-dimensional map of yourself. This ability to locate all your body parts in space is critical to balance, as you will see.

2. Now take your shoes off and stand up again. This time concentrate on your feet. Can you identify which bit under your feet is being squashed the most by your weight: Heels? Instep? Toes?

3. OK, now that you have located the area of most pressure under your feet, start to move your body around (without moving your feet). First, slowly lean your trunk forwards until you feel the pressure under your feet move forwards to your toes. Think about your legs and try to identify which structures in your body are being stressed. Can you feel any muscles working harder? This is basically the inverted pendulum we talked about before; see Fig. 3.27.

4. Now, go back to normal standing and, without changing anything else, move your arms forwards, starting a little then reaching further forward. How does this change your stability and why?

5. Now remembering to keep your eyes closed, lean your trunk backwards. This time you should feel the centre of pressure move back. Unfortunately, you don't have much BoS in this direction so you can quickly come to the edge of your stability. Before you reach the point when you have to take a step back, move your arms forwards. Like the last experiment, think about the movement of your CoM in relationship to your BoS and why the forward movement of your arms was helpful. Do you think it would matter if you moved your arms forwards slowly or quickly?

Once you have done these experiments, why don't you try to move just a small part of your body, for example, bending your elbow, and see if it changes the position of the pressure under your feet. You will need very good kinaesthetic awareness for this!

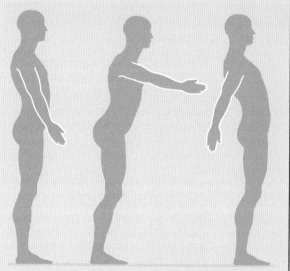

Fig. 3.27 Feeling Your Balance, Activity Box 3.7.

ACTIVITY BOX 3.8

Try this fun activity based around stability and gravitational moments (Fig. 3.28).

Kneel down on the floor and put your hands behind your back. Just as a precaution put a pillow on the ground about a metre in front of you. Now bend down to lightly touch your nose onto the ground just in front of your knees and straighten up, quite easy. Now try to touch the ground further and further away. Sooner or later you will get to a point when you are no longer able to straighten up. Compare your distance with your friends and then try to work out why some people can go further than others. Is there a gender difference?

The first time you did this it was easy (relatively) because your CoM was not creating a very large moment. In fact your CoM was probably directly above the knee joint (which is where the body is pivoting) and just a little in front of your hip (so a small flexor moment was created). The next time your CoM was further forwards, creating a larger hip flexor moment and introducing a knee extensor moment. Basically the weight of your trunk/head/arms was rotating your thigh forwards. To prevent you falling forwards you create a counter moment—hip extensor and knee flexor moment—by contracting your hip extensors (gluteus maximus and hamstrings) and knee flexors (hamstrings).

ACTIVITY BOX 3.8—cont'd

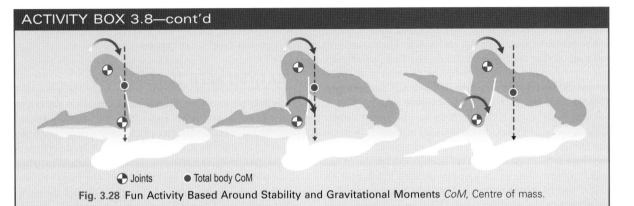

● Joints   ● Total body CoM

Fig. 3.28 Fun Activity Based Around Stability and Gravitational Moments *CoM*, Centre of mass.

If you put your hands on the back of your thigh during the movement, you would feel a lot of muscle work. Now the effect this muscle activity has on your lower leg is to lift it up (knee bends). This is unavoidable and just adds to your problems by moving the CoM further forwards and reducing your BoS. You might say you have reached the tipping point, which is why you need the pillow.

Try the same thing again and this time get someone to hold your feet down; you will find that with a stable fixed point, the moments created by your hip extensors and knee flexors will allow you to reach further forwards.

Right, did you work out why some of your friends managed to do this better than others? It's all to do with how your mass is distributed. Those of you with more mass higher up in your body, for example large muscles in your arms and upper body, will find the task more difficult because when you bend forwards you create a larger flexing moment.

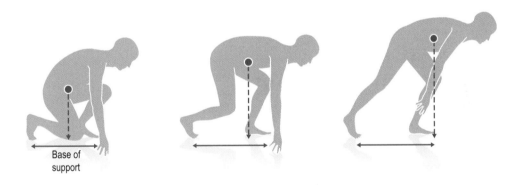

Base of support

Fig. 3.29 Sprint Start.

therefore CoG is now positioned well in front of the BoS. From our discussions and activities on stability, we would expect the athlete to fall flat on his face. Although this would probably be very funny, it doesn't happen. So WHY doesn't the athlete fall?

You may already know the answer but if you don't try this activity.

Stand up from your chair. Sit back down and do it again but this time do it much slower. Difficult? You probably fell back down onto the chair the second time (if you did it slowly enough). When you performed the movement at normal speed there was a theoretical possibility that you might fall (destabilise) because the body travels through an unstable position between the point when you come off the chair until you are upright. However because you performed the movement at speed you were able to able to keep the time spent in this period to a minimum and also the forward momentum counteracted the gravitational moments that are pushing you back down toward the chair.

Try the movement again and attempt to stop at the moment of lift off, look at your BoS and then estimate where (more or less) your CoG is located. The reason you fall back is that the CoG is behind your BoS, which only consists of your feet. Performing the movement at speed means the body gets to the new BoS without destabilising. Is there anything you could do to improve your stability if, for some reason, you had to perform the movement slowly? What about your foot position (BoS), try it yourself; perform the movement slowly with different foot positions.

There is more information on stability during the sit-to-stand movement in the case studies detailed in Chapter 17.

Let's get back to the sprinter. The sit-to-stand experiment should have given you the answer. The sprinter is momentarily unstable as he leaves the blocks, but his speed moves his CoM over the new BoS (his feet) before he has a chance to fall, although his feet have to move pretty quickly to create the new BoS.

Even during normal walking the body will move in and out of unstable positions. Just before you put your foot down to strike the ground, where is your CoM? And where is your BoS? So how would you describe your stability at this point? No wonder walking has been described as a series of falls narrowly avoided; this becomes all the more obvious when you watch a toddler learn this very human skill (see Chapter 10).

So, a body can be theoretically unstable at different points during a movement provided it is moving towards the next BoS quickly enough. There are many other examples when the body is 'theoretically' unstable but the person does not fall. Can you think of any more?

WHAT YOU NEED TO REMEMBER

So, gravity pulls us (speaking as bits of mass) to the centre of the Earth, and it is the main force we have to contend with. The size of this downward force is a product of our mass (the amount of stuff in our body) and the acceleration due to gravity (9.81 m/s); this is what is measured when you stand on bathroom scales. Even if our mass remains constant, our weight could change if we change the vertical accelerations acting on our body, for example, going to the Moon, even bouncing up and down or travelling in an elevator. The CoM is a single point that represents all the mass in a body; in quiet standing it is positioned within the pelvis.

Gravity can be considered to act at the CoM of each body segment; this may cause gravitational moments depending on how the limb is positioned.

The stability of a body is determined by the relationship between the BoS and position of the total body CoM. The body may be technically unstable but not fall provided it is moving towards a stable situation fast enough. We also found out how wheelchairs are designed for stability and why high-wire walkers use umbrellas to balance.

▍ SELF-ASSESSMENT: QUESTIONS

1. Is the following statement true or false?
   The magnitude of the force of gravity is exactly the same wherever you are in the universe.
2. If you have a mass of 75 kg and live on planet Earth how much will you weigh?
   a. 75 kg
   b. 735.75 kg
   c. 7.65 N
   d. 735.75 N
3. Can the centre of mass lie out with the surface of the body?
   a. Yes
   b. No
4. If a body is described as being stable it means that if it is pushed it
   a. Will move momentarily to a new position but then return to its original state.
   b. Will move and continue to move until it reaches a stable position.
   c. Will move to a new position and remain there.
5. What is force measured in?
   a. Kilograms
   b. Newtons
   c. Newton metres
   d. Pounds per square inch
6. What function do the rear stabiliser wheels on a wheelchair perform?
   a. They help with training when someone starts using a wheelchair.
   b. They improve lateral stability.
   c. They prevent the chair tipping forward.
   d. They prevent the chair tipping back.
7. Why would a clown carry an umbrella when walking over a tight rope?
   a. In case it rains
   b. To provide an additional counterbalancing moment
   c. To use as a parachute when she falls
   d. Because it looks good

8. Which of the following muscle groups helps prevent the body swaying backwards while standing?
   a. Ankle dorsiflexors
   b. Ankle plantarflexors
   c. Knee flexors
   d. Ankle evertors
9. The ideal standing posture
   a. Minimises gravitational moments.
   b. Minimises muscle activity.
   c. Has the line of gravity passing close the joint centres.
   d. Has the line of gravity passing just in front of the ankle joint.

10. During movement there are often periods when the body is theoretically unstable; how does the body avoid a fall in these situations?
    a. It moves more slowly to reduce forces.
    b. It moves rapidly to a new stable position.
    c. It keeps the CoM low.

ANSWERS TO QUESTIONS POSED IN THE TEXT

Answer 1

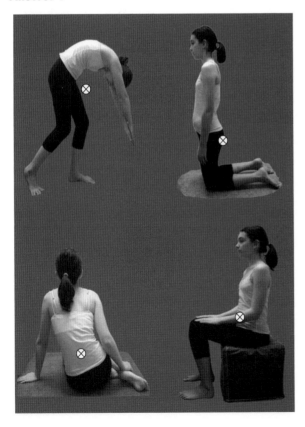

Answer 2

The lying-down position (see Fig. 3.10) would be easiest because the CoM is positioned directly above the joint centre. If you drew a vertical line down from the CoM it would pass through the joint; just like a child sitting in the middle of a seesaw, this produces compression but not a turning force (moment).

Answer 3

If you want to gradually increase resistance from the lying-down position, you could simply move the limb a little out of position, 80 degrees rather than 90 degrees. This would create small moments that the muscles have to resist. Why not try it for yourself: lie on your side and lift your arm directly up so that your fingers are pointing to the ceiling. Feel how much muscle work is required and then move it a little closer to your body; can you feel the moderate difference this makes?

The order of difficulty for the hip abductors would be, from easiest to hardest

1, 2, 4, 3

This is due to the difference in magnitude of the gravitational moment; 2 and 4 are probably quite similar and it would of course depend on the angle achieved.

Answer 4

In Fig. 3.12 the forward location of the CoM on the neck will create a flexor moment (the force is trying to bend the neck forward, chin to chest). To avoid this there must be an opposing extensor moment created by activity of the neck extensors. The further forward the head is placed the greater the flexor moment created by gravity and therefore the counteracting extensor moment from the neck extensors. Increased muscle activity can result in joint compression as well as fatigue and discomfort within the muscles. This is particularly the case if the posture is held for long periods. The solution is straightforward: educate the individual to hold their head in a more retracted position (chin in head back) so that the head CoM is more closely aligned to the neck joint centres.

Answer 5

Moving down a slope will shift your CoG forwards so that it is closer to the forward limit of your BoS. There is a small risk that you could become unstable; however, leaning back into the chair is likely to be all that is required to ensure the CoG is maintained within the BoS. Leaning forwards is not advisable.

- What about hanging a rucksack onto the handlebars at the back?

Hanging a rucksack onto the handlebars at the back of a wheelchair shifts the CoM backwards. This means you are more prone to backward instability, for example when going up a slope or a pavement kerb.

The loss of a lower limb means there is less mass located forwards, a topsy-turvy way of saying your CoM will move backwards, bringing it closer to the limits of your BoS at the back. This, of course, presents a greater possibility of destabilising backwards. To combat this, wheelchairs for amputees are designed with their wheels positioned further back to extend the BoS and ensure stability.

Answer 6

Some tight-rope artists hold a pole which is bent downwards. What do you think is the advantage of this?

The reason for a pole that bends downwards is that as well as improving the lateral stability, it also lowers the CoM, increasing stability (at least by a little bit).

Energy and Movement

Andy Kerr and Philip Rowe

OUTLINE

LEARNING OUTCOMES

After reading this chapter, you will be able to:
1. Define inertia.
2. Explain the relationship between inertia, force and movement (law of inertia).
3. Explain the relationship between momentum and impulse (law of acceleration).
4. Apply the law of action and reaction to everyday movements such as walking.
5. Define work and power.
6. Differentiate between types of levers.
7. Define what energy is and describe the different mechanical forms.
8. Discuss movement strategies designed to optimise efficiency.

INTRODUCTION

Up to now we have dealt with forces in a static kind of way; all the forces were balanced, or in equilibrium if you like. In this chapter we will look more at forces when they are out of balance; this will necessarily feature Isaac Newton's laws of motion. We will consider how movement starts (and stops), how it is controlled and how it is described. We will look at bodies moving in straight lines (linear) and those moving in circular motions (rotation). We will also consider friction and pressure as these are key concepts in understanding force and movement as well as biomechanics in general. From there we will explore the concepts of work and energy as applied to machines and humans.

QUICK REVISION

Let's start with a reminder of what a force does.

The push or pull of a mechanical force does two things to a body:
1. Produces a change in velocity; this could be magnitude and/or direction because velocity is a vector.
2. Changes its shape; for example lengthening, compressing or distorting (we will find about more about this in Chapter 5).

Of course, the chances are that both of these will occur to a greater or lesser extent.

NEWTON'S FIRST LAW (INERTIA)

The way that the motion of a body is affected by a force is enshrined in Newton's three laws of motion which we will get to in a moment. However, it is easier to understand these laws if you consider the body to be rigid so that it won't deform (change shape) when the force is applied.

Let's imagine this rigid body, a brick for example (Fig. 4.1).

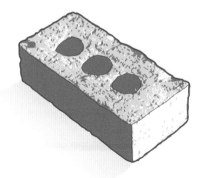

Fig. 4.1 Brick.

The brick is happy where it is and sees no good reason to move. For the brick to move, someone or something is going to have to apply a big enough external force (push or pull). This reluctance to move is a property of all bodies and is called *inertia.* Inertia has been in our scientific knowledge since the experimental work of **Galileo Galilei** almost 400 years ago (Further Information 4.1). In fact inertia comes from the Latin word for laziness and is dependent on the amount of mass a body has; this is a simplification, but the more mass a body has the more reluctant it is to move. Put another way, you need a bigger push to get a big brick moving than a small one.

Inertia is a key principle in biomechanics but it doesn't just apply to objects sitting at rest; the same principle applies to bodies in motion. Let's consider the brick again. Once you apply the push it will move off in the direction of the push; you have changed its velocity. Now that it is moving, it really doesn't want to change again; it's happy moving along at this new velocity, in this direction, forever. Before it was reluctant to move from rest; now it is reluctant to

FURTHER INFORMATION 4.1

As we have already discussed, Galileo was not happy with theory; he wanted to test things. Galileo explored the idea of inertia with a simple, yet elegant experiment. He placed balls on curved tracks of varying gradient. The ball, placed at one end of the slope, would roll down the slope (pulled by the force of gravity) and up the other end (slowed down by the pull of gravity) until it reached its original height, theoretically at least (Fig. 4.2A). In this way the balls behaved very similarly to a pendulum. Galileo made smoother and smoother slopes and balls until he found the balls were very close to achieving the same height. Galileo then reduced the gradient of the slope (see Fig. 4.2B) and found that the ball would move along the slope until it reached the same height, even though it had to travel a greater distance. This continued as the slope was reduced more and more until it became flat (see Fig. 4.2C), at this point, Galileo concluded, the ball would continue to move forever in the same direction. What he demonstrated was inertia. The fact that the ball doesn't continue, no matter how smooth the slopes were made, is evidence of friction.

The experience of being in a rollercoaster is a bit like Galileo's experiment; once you have been pulled up to the first high point you rush down to the bottom, pulled by gravity, and then up to the next top. In the classic (old-fashioned) rollercoaster each top was a little lower than the previous one; why do you think this was?

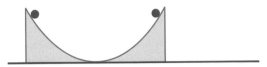

(A) Ball returns to the same height (in a friction-free slope).

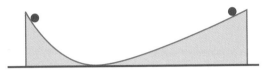

(B) Even if the gradient is altered.

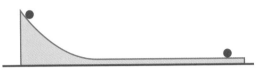

(C) If the gradient were zero (i.e. flat) the ball should continue forever.

Fig. 4.2 (A to C) Galileo's friction-free slopes.

change from a constant velocity; rigid bodies can be pretty stubborn! If we want to change its velocity (stop it, slow it down, increase it or change its direction) we will need to apply yet another force.

In reality we know that the brick, once pushed, does not travel in that direction for very long; when you push a brick it might move a couple of reluctant metres before stopping. It certainly doesn't continue moving at a constant velocity forever. This isn't, however, a contradiction to what I have just said. The reason the brick slows down is that another force is acting on it; *sliding friction* (which we will talk more about later in this chapter) as well as some resistance caused by moving through air (more on this in Chapter 5). These forces are acting in the opposite direction to the brick's motion, eventually making it stop. Everything back in balance again.

What we just talked about is known as the law of inertia; although first described by Galileo, it was Isaac Newton who clearly described its relationship with force. Newton wrote:

Every body perseveres in its state of being at rest or of moving uniformly straight forward, except insofar as it is compelled to change its state by force impressed (Newton and Halley, 1744).

Written in the florid language of the time this is a bit of a mouthful so we can paraphrase to:

A body continues to maintain its state of rest or of uniform motion unless acted upon by an external unbalanced force.

We will continue to talk about inertia in this chapter as it is a really important principle of biomechanics; for simplicity you could just think of it as a reluctance to move or laziness, as Isaac Asimov described it.

One of the important aspects of the law of inertia is that force is **not** required to keep a body in motion (once it has started). You might not think this sounds right, which is what most people thought before Galileo (see Further Information 4.1) and Newton. To understand why this is correct you need to understand all the forces involved when an object moves, **friction** and **air resistance** being the main forces that oppose movement. If we could remove these opposing forces then the force we applied to the brick would indeed cause it to move at a constant velocity (and direction) potentially forever.

MOMENT OF INERTIA

Up to this point we have considered the reluctance of a body to move in a linear direction. Inertia is also an issue if you want to rotate a mass but it's not as simple as how much mass there is. If you want to rotate a lump of mass, such as your leg when walking, then you must overcome its rotational inertia or moment of inertia (a body's resistance to rotation). In a rotating body the distribution of the mass relative to the point about which it is rotating is also a factor. This is called the *moment of inertia*.

The moment of inertia (I) is calculated from the body mass (kg) multiplied by the square of the distance (radius-r) from the point of rotation; for simplicity we can consider the centre of mass (CoM) to be the position of all the bits of mass, which saves us working out the moment of inertia of every particle.

This can summarised as:

$$I = mr^2$$

and is measured in kg.m^2

So, for a point of mass rotating about an origin, the further away it is from the centre the greater its moment of inertia. This is just the principle of moments restated; the further away from the fulcrum, the harder it is to move.

If you had to push a child in a swing and there were two swings free, one with a long chain and one with a short chain, pushing the child in the short swing would require less push from you. This is because there is less resistance to a rotational force because the mass is distributed closer to the pivot. For the same reason it is easier to swing a flexed leg when you walk than a straight one. There is one other major advantage to bending the swinging leg during gait; have a think what this could be. If you try it out it might become obvious.

If you are musical you may have come across the mechanical metronome (that little upside down pendulum that ticks back and forwards to help you keep rhythm). To alter the speed of the metronome you slide the counter (lump of mass) up and down the swinging arm, or in other words, you alter the moment of inertia of the pendulum. We will talk more about metronomes later when we consider conservation of angular momentum.

To recap, inertia is the property of a body that resists changes in motion. This is determined by mass when the motion is in straight lines; for rotating bodies it is the mass and how it is distributed relative to the point of rotation that resists rotation.

LINEAR MOMENTUM

Let's get back to the brick which was happy in its sleepy inertia until another force comes along, a push, for example. The brick will move in the direction of the applied force. Basically the push has changed the brick's velocity; before it had none and now it is moving at a velocity measured in metres per second (m/s). If a body is moving it has **momentum**; this is simply the product (one multiplied by the other) of its mass (in kg) and its velocity (in metres per second) so the units of momentum are kg.m/s.

We can find plenty of examples of the relationship between momentum and force (in fact anything that moves would do). For example, imagine a game of golf. You lift your club up and swing it down to strike the little white ball; the ball (if you managed to hit it which I often don't) instantly changes its momentum and travels in the direction of your applied force. If you got this right, the ball will have horizontal and vertical momentum as it sails towards its target. Of course, as you know, the ball doesn't fly forever, impeded by air resistance and our old friend gravity which oppose horizontal and vertical motion, respectively. The ball hits the ground and continues to move forward because it still has some horizontal momentum; the resistance from the grass and perhaps the friction from the ground reduces this momentum until it reaches zero, the ball has stopped. Friction and air resistance have opposed the ball's motion, just like Galileo's slopes (see Further Information 4.1). One force—the impact of your club—increased the ball's momentum; the opposing forces of gravity, air resistance and friction have conspired to reduce this momentum until the balls stops, close to the pin hopefully.

The point from all this talk about golf balls is that to **change** a body's momentum, for example, stop it, start it, speed it up, slow it down or change direction, requires a force (e.g. your push) applied over a period of time. This is the essence of Newton's second law of motion, the law of acceleration which we'll cover in more detail a little further on.

Momentum is a vector so we need to state a direction, down, up, east, west, etc., using a common reference frame (see Fig. 2.3). Because we live in a three-dimensional world a body may have momentum in three different directions at the same time. Like any other vector (e.g. force, see Chapter 2) you can combine momenta (plural of momentum) vectors and you can resolve them into component parts.

When you are walking you simultaneously have forward, lateral and vertical momentum; behind each direction of momentum is a force. Take the point at the beginning of the swing phase when your trailing leg is about to be brought forward (Fig. 4.3); during this movement your body (represented by the CoM) moves forward, lifts up and moves laterally towards the opposite standing foot. This momentum is generated by the pushing down action of the leg behind you. Well actually it's the reaction force from the ground that pushes you forward but we don't cover action and reaction until later in this chapter, so keep that bit of knowledge to yourself.

Separating the body's momentum into component parts provides a useful method of analysing a movement because it tells us about the forces acting on the body, their direction and magnitude. Think about the motion of your body during the sit-to-stand movement. Fig. 4.4 is reconstructed from a movement analysis study that tracked the motion of the CoM during a sit-to-stand movement. The dark orange line represents horizontal momentum and the light orange line represents vertical. You can therefore see the relationship between the two. Horizontal momentum reaches a peak early in the movement due to the rapid trunk flexion created by the turning force of the trunk muscles while still seated. This momentum then reduces rapidly as vertical momentum increases brought about by large moments about the hip and knee which accelerate the body vertically against gravity; this occurs around about the point when your bottom comes off the seat (seat off).

The reduction in horizontal momentum around seat off is clearly important; otherwise you would fall forwards. Try it: stand up from your chair without stopping your forward motion; your additional step was necessary, otherwise you would become unstable. So you need to create a force in the opposite direction (a braking force) to reduce this forward momentum, in the same way that friction and resistance reduced the horizontal momentum of the golf ball.

From the graph you can see that around seat off there is a change in direction of momentum, from predominantly horizontal to predominantly vertical, so as the horizontal momentum reduces the vertical increases. This period of the movement has been called momentum transfer because this is exactly what is happening. The forward motion of the trunk is transferred to vertical motion of the thigh and lower leg.

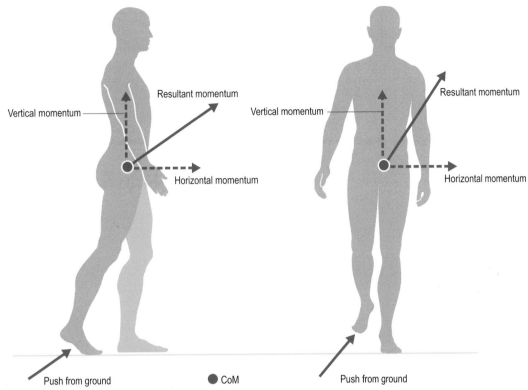

Fig. 4.3 Momentum of Centre of Mass (CoM) During Gait: From Side and Front.

How do you think this transfer occurs? (Answer at end of chapter.)

Again it is worth remembering that each of these momenta and any change in its direction or magnitude is caused by a force acting over a period of time.

ROTATIONAL MOMENTUM

In the previous examples of sit to stand and gait we have considered the body's momentum to be directed in straight lines (linear), acting about the CoM. Of course this total body motion is achieved through rotation of the peripheral joints and trunk, the lower limbs in particular. So we really need to understand the momentum of rotating bodies.

As you will recall from Chapter 2, velocity was the rate of change of displacement, how quickly a body moved in a straight line from A to B. If a body is rotating we can still calculate its velocity but this time we use angular displacement, which can be measured in degrees or radians (Further Information 4.2). Let's look at an example to illustrate this. When sprinting, the knee flexes (bends) by around 110 degrees (depending on how fast you run), and it does this rapidly; let's say the movement takes 0.1 s, so angular velocity

> ### FURTHER INFORMATION 4.2   Radians
>
> A radian is a measure of angular displacement which is equal to 180/π. If you are used to using degrees one radian can be approximated to 57 degrees.

is change in angular displacement (110 degrees) divided by time (0.1) which is 1100 degrees per second (pretty fast!). What we have calculated is the rotational velocity of the whole lower leg; things become more complicated when we consider different points on the rotating body. To demonstrate what we mean try Activity Box 4.1. You will see that the instantaneous linear velocity of the mass furthest away from the centre of rotation will be greater than the mass next to the centre of rotation, which is why photographs of runners tend to have blurred feet.

Now you may have noticed that we have used the word velocity and not momentum in the last paragraph. This was simply so that you can see how angular velocity is calculated. Of course, a rotating body, such as a leg, has mass and therefore momentum.

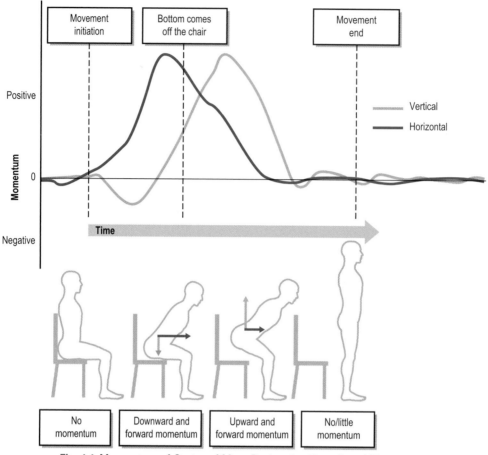

Fig. 4.4 Momentum of Centre of Mass During the Sit-to-Stand Movement.

CENTRIPETAL AND CENTRIFUGAL FORCE

When a body is rotating it is constantly changing direction to keep it turning in a circle. A change in direction can only be achieved by a force. This force has two directions which act at right angles to each other (well really three because we live in three dimension but let's keep it simple). One force causes the forward motion (Fig. 4.6) and the other keeps changing the direction of the body so that it moves in a circle; this force is directed towards the centre (along the string in Activity Box 4.2), and is called **centripetal force**. This combination of forces causes the rubber to move in an arc.

Now we talked previously (Chapter 3) about forces being in balance; therefore the centripetal force needs to have an opposite balancing force; otherwise the rubber would start coming towards you. This force is called **centrifugal** and is the opposite (in direction and magnitude) of centripetal; it pushes things out, away from the centre of rotation.

Everything is now nicely balanced. You can quite easily feel centrifugal force by trying Activity Box 4.3. While the centripetal force changes the direction of the rotating body, the centrifugal force pushes mass outwards.

We calculated the linear momentum of a body as the product of its mass and its velocity. Rotational momentum, though essentially the same, has to consider the distribution of mass so it is calculated from the product of the moment of inertia and 'angular velocity, that is;'

$$\text{Angular momentum} = I \times \omega,$$

where I = moment of inertia and ω = angular velocity (typically stated in radians).

CONSERVATION OF ANGULAR MOMENTUM

You can probably remember when you were a child, lying on your back on a roundabout and stretching your legs in and out causing the roundabout to slow down and speed

ACTIVITY BOX 4.1

Get a pencil with a rubber on the end and a paper clip. Undo one of the twists in the paper clip so that you have a long bit which you pierce through the rubber until it comes out the other end (then pull it back so it doesn't protrude). Place the pencil on your desk. Now, if you hold the paper clip you should be able to rotate the pencil about the fixed point, with the paper clip as the axis. Now, with a pen, mark three dots along the length of your pencil more or less evenly spaced (Fig. 4.5). Imagine these dots represent particles of the pencil so that when you spin the pencil you can see them individually rotate about the origin. You will notice that the dots closest to the centre of rotation move the slowest because they have a smaller circumference to travel through and the ones at the end travel the fastest.

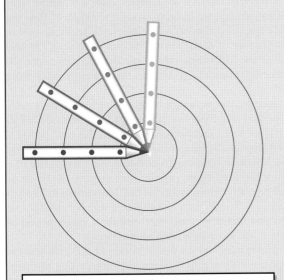

The further away the dot is from the point of rotation, the more movement (greater circumference to its journey) it will experience. Because the pencil is a rigid body, all the dots move at the same time; therefore the velocity of the dots towards the outer end will move the fastest.

Fig. 4.5 Rotational Momentum With a Pencil and Paper Clip.

ACTIVITY BOX 4.2

Get a piece of string (30 cm should do it) and tie your rubber to it. Now go outside to your backyard/garden and twirl the rubber round and round. Now, as we saw in the previous activity, the rubber is going through the same angular displacement as every other point on the string. However, the rubber is travelling through a much bigger distance (greater circumference) so therefore has a greater velocity.

Now let go of the string (being careful to avoid hitting anyone or anything). The rubber moved off in a straight line, right? It didn't continue to move in an arc. This means that the rubber had linear momentum at the time of release, so angular momentum is really just plain old linear momentum. At every moment during the rotation the rubber (mass) has a linear velocity which is directed at right angles to the string. This is well known by discus and hammer throwers who release their projectile at a precise point in the rotation so that the linear velocity is directed up the field. If they get this timing wrong the hammer/discus will move off at an angle which means less distance.

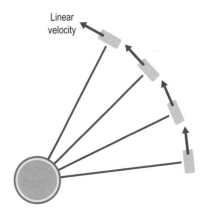

Linear velocity

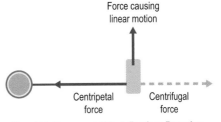

Force causing linear motion

Centripetal force   Centrifugal force

Fig. 4.6 Forces at Work During Rotation.

When you run or jog your arm provides some additional momentum (vertically at least). The CoM of your arm is located somewhere around the elbow so you have to generate sufficient force to overcome its rotational inertia, which comes from the mass multiplied by the distance the CoM is from the shoulder. OK, jog up and down the hall, driveway or wherever and keep your arms straight. Your hands are going through a really big arc of movement compared to your elbows, so there is greater velocity (and of course momentum) at your hands. You may feel more pressure in your hands, which is caused by the centrifugal force (see previous discussion) pushing more blood into your hands as well as stopping blood returning from your hands. You may also feel a little silly.

So what do you do? Of course you bend your elbow. This reduces the moment of inertia so there is less inertia and less muscle to overcome, or if you continue with the same muscle effort your arms will move faster. This is important to keep in time with your leg movement (you may have found this difficult to do with your arms straight).

up. What you were doing was proving that angular (rotational) momentum is conserved. This is a fundamental principle of moving bodies (linear and angular) that is derived from Newton's laws of motion. Quite simply, the total momentum of all the objects (ignoring outside interference) will always be the same.

This is what was happening: the roundabout (including yourself) is a rotating body, whose angular momentum is defined by its velocity and moment of inertia. Now when you stretch out your feet you are increasing the moment of inertia by shifting more mass away from the centre of the roundabout (point of rotation) because angular momentum has to be preserved (energy can't just go away—more on this later); this means that to balance the equation, angular velocity must decrease. In contrast, if you draw your legs back in, the moment of inertia will decrease, meaning angular velocity must increase.

If you can't remember doing this as a child, why not experience it now; it will only serve to consolidate your understanding of biomechanics and it would be fun. The idea can also be replicated with your rubber and string (see Activity Box 4.2) by shortening and lengthening the string. Why not try it, but make sure you have plenty of room and no valuables around; outside might be best.

The conservation of rotational momentum is elegantly demonstrated in figure skating when the skaters do those amazing spins on the spot; the velocity of the spin is controlled by the skater moving their arms and legs inwards and outwards. The skater eventually stops the turn by straightening their arms and leg outwards. There are many other examples of rotational momentum being conserved (e.g. the Dad's favourite Christmas toy, a Newton's cradle).

There are of course lessons for human movement. Shortening your arms and legs while running increases the rotational velocity simply by reducing the moment of inertia, angular momentum being conserved of course.

NEWTON'S SECOND LAW: IMPULSE AND MOMENTUM

Now we know that if you want to change the way a lump of mass is moving (direction or velocity) you need to apply a force and it will accelerate or decelerate in the direction the force was applied, acceleration being the rate of change of velocity; see Chapter 2 for a reminder. This is clear enough we hope; however, the length of time the force is applied also has a bearing on the resulting motion of the lump of mass. This is the nub of Newton's second law of motion which relates impulse to momentum. To understand this let's go back to that stubborn brick from earlier.

As you recall we got the brick moving by giving it a push. Now the force from the push must have been applied to the brick over a certain period of time; this time period is critical to the change in momentum of the brick. As any of you who have been taught how to strike a tennis ball or a golf ball should know, you continue to move the racket or club even after impact with the ball. Instructions like 'follow the swing through' may be familiar to you. For example, we all know that if we push our brick for a longer period of time it will move away with more velocity.

The reason you do this is to extend the time you are applying the force, to continue the racket swing so that it keeps in contact with the ball for longer. Force applied over a time is called *impulse* and this is what causes the change in motion of the body, that is, **impulse causes a change in momentum**. This relationship is a form of Newton's second law, the law of acceleration, and is described neatly by the formula:

$$\text{Impulse (Force} \times \text{Time)} = \text{Change in momentum}$$

or

$$F \times T = \text{Mass} \times \text{Velocity (after the impulse)} - \text{Mass} \times \text{Velocity (before the impulse)}$$

and

$$\text{Force} = \frac{\text{Mass} \times \text{Velocity (after)} - \text{Mass} \times \text{Velocity (before)}}{\text{Time}}.$$

ACTIVITY BOX 4.4   (More of a Thought Experiment Really)

There are three ice pucks resting on the ice rink ready for target practice, pucks A, B and C. They are identical in shape and mass (and distribution of mass; Fig. 4.7).

Johnny the hotshot striker hits puck A with a force of 35 N; this impact lasts 0.1 s (a snap shot!).

He then comes up to puck B and hits it with less venom (25 N) but increases the duration of impact (0.5 s).

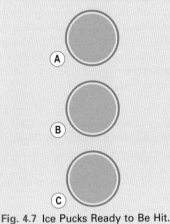

Fig. 4.7 Ice Pucks Ready to Be Hit.

Finally he comes to puck C and decides to wallop it (75 N) and is able to follow through with the stick so that he is in contact for 0.3 s.

Which puck receives the largest impulse and should, therefore, attain the greatest velocity (we can assume the mass doesn't change and there are no other forces acting on it)?

Remember that force × time = change in momentum and that the puck was at rest at the beginning:

For puck A the impulse was 35 N × 0.1 s = 3.5 Ns = $V^2 - V^1$ (zero).

The resulting velocity (V_2) of puck A as it left the hockey stick was 3.5 m/s.

For puck B the impulse was 25 N × 0.5 s = 12.5 Ns = $V^2 - V^1$ (zero).

The resulting velocity of puck B as it left the hockey stick was 12.5 m/s.

Finally for puck C the impulse was 75 N × 0.3 s = 22.5 Ns = $V^2 - V^1$ (zero).

The resulting velocity of puck C as it left the hockey stick was the greatest at 22.5 m/s.

So force × time (or rather impulse) changes momentum and it's exactly the same for decreasing momentum as it is for increasing it.

Because change in velocity divided by time is equal to acceleration, this equation for impulse is the same as the typical presentation of Newton's second law:

$$Force = Mass \times Acceleration.$$

The relationship between impulse and momentum is an important principle so we are going to conduct a small experiment to make sure you understand; try Activity Box 4.4.

Let's try some examples based on human movement:

Imagine a rugby (or an American football) player running for the score line; he is big (let's say 100 kg) and fast (let's say he's running at 8 m/s) so he has a lot of momentum (800 kg.m/s) and he's 15 m from scoring; you are the only player close enough to him to tackle. With every scrap of energy you apply a force of 150 N for 5 s (after which you collapse, beaten), but did you do enough to stop the score? (See Fig. 4.8.)

Let's look at what your impulse (force × time) will do to his momentum:

Force × Time = Change in momentum (Mass × V^2 − Mass × V^1)

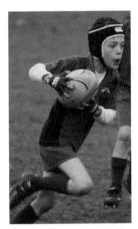

Fig. 4.8 A 100 kg Rugby Player (artistic license) Running for the Try Line.

V^1 is his velocity before your impulse.

V^2 is his velocity after your impulse (this is what we want to find out).

Now the force you apply will be negative as it is against the direction of the other player's motion:

$$-150\,N \times 5\,s \text{ (your impulse)} = (100 \times V^2) - (100 \times 8)$$

$$V^2 = \frac{-750 + 800}{100} = \textbf{0.5 m/s}.$$

After your impulse he is still moving! Although at a much slower velocity (0.5 m/s). Critically at this current velocity and with only 15 m to go he will score in 7.5 s (0.5 m/s × 15 m). Let's hope someone else can get there within this time; otherwise he will score.

What About Trying a Patient Problem?

To get out of a chair, an old lady has to move her body forward at a velocity of 4 m/s. Because she weighs 65 kg this means she has a momentum of 260 kg.m/s. Unfortunately she is a little apprehensive about her balance and so prefers to stop for a moment when she stands up before starting to walk. So she needs to change her momentum from 260 kg.m/s to zero; she can hardly change her mass so she must reduce her velocity. Her muscles contract at the same time to provide a braking force of −80 N (negative, as it is acting in the opposite direction), so how long does it take for her to stop her forward motion?

$$-80\,N \times T\,s = V^2 \times 65\,kg - V^1\,(4\,m/s) \times 65\,kg$$

V^2 is zero (motion stops) so:

$$T = \frac{260\,kg}{80\,N} = \textbf{3.25 s}.$$

This would seem a rather long period of time to decelerate, causing potential problems with stability. What do you think she should do?

Let's end with a rotational problem.

An up and coming javelin thrower has been given a new javelin to throw; it is a little heavier (0.5 kg) than the previous one. If he is to reach his usual distance the javelin must be rotated at a velocity of 2.5 radians per second. The CoM of his arm (including javelin) is 0.5 m from the shoulder and the total mass is 0.7 Kg. How much angular momentum does he need to create? We are going to ignore any existing momentum due to his run up (makes things easier).

So the mass of the rotating body is 7.5 kg and the radius is 0.5 m (we will assume all the mass is located at the CoM). This means the moment of inertia is:

$$Mass \times Radius^2 = 7.5 \times 0.25 = 1.875\,kg.m/s.$$

If he needs to achieve a velocity of 2.5 radians per second, this means he will need an angular momentum of:

$$\begin{aligned} Angular\ momentum &= Moment\ of\ inertia\ (1.875) \\ &\quad \times Angular\ velocity\ (2.5)\ . \\ &= 3.95\,kg.m^2s^{-1} \end{aligned}$$

If we knew how long it takes him to throw the javelin we could also work out how much force he needed but that is probably enough calculations, for now.

NEWTON'S THIRD LAW: ACTION AND REACTION

Implicit in our understanding of force and motion is the principle that every action has an equal and opposite reaction, or put another way, momentum is always conserved. So, for example, the centrifugal force was a reaction to the centripetal action when we talked about rotating bodies, and the ground reaction force is a reaction to the force we apply to the ground (see Chapter 2). Although mentioned before, it is worth making sure you are clear on the law of **action and reaction**.

Newton described this law:

For a force there is always an equal and opposite reaction: or the forces of two bodies on each other are always equal and are directed in opposite directions.

Or more simply:

For every action there will be an equal and opposite reaction.

It's a simple enough law, but like the previous two laws, is absolutely fundamental to our understanding of motion. Let's try a quick experiment; walk over to the wall and put your hands on it with your elbows a little bent, and lean into it as if you are about to do a vertical press-up; now apply a force on the wall by straightening your elbows.

Did the wall move away from you (let's hope not) or change its shape (perhaps imperceptibly)? But you did (or should if you tried hard enough) move a little backwards; this is the reaction force of the wall onto you. You pushed the wall and the wall pushed back on you.

Let's consider another example (this time one that moves): two balls colliding, for example in a game of pool. The four ball and the eight ball crash into each other, and each applies a push to the other and receives a reaction force (at the same instant). The thing to observe is that the interaction between the two balls has resulted in them moving off in opposite directions, but importantly with the same (if we forget friction and air resistance) total momentum. Just like rotating bodies, total momentum in a system (e.g. a group of pool balls) is conserved even after a collision. (See Fig. 4.9.)

We should look at a human movement example of this. Stand on the bottom step of your stairs and jump down onto the floor. When you land you will apply a large force to the ground; simultaneously the ground applies a force back on you. There has been an equal and opposite exchange of momentum between the two bodies, you and the Earth.

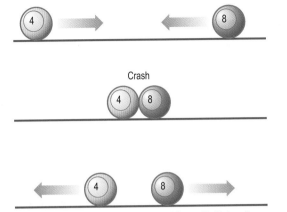

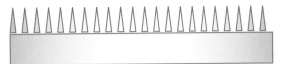

Fig. 4.10 Using Pressure to Explain Bed of Nails.

Fig. 4.9 Conservation of Momentum After a Collision Between Pool Balls.

The size of the reaction force (acting vertically up) from Earth was enough to stop you dead in your tracks (changed the momentum drastically); the size of the action force from you to the Earth was enough to change its orbit, even if it is not observable. The size of your force on the Earth is far too trivial to change its orbit perceptibly, but in theory it did, just a little bit. Perhaps if we all tried a jump at the same time it might be enough to change the Earth's orbit!

SUMMARY OF NEWTON'S LAWS OF MOTION

We have covered a lot in the last few pages so it is probably worth recapping a few important points.

- Bodies prefer to stay at rest or move with unchanging velocity (including direction). For objects moving in a straight line this inertia depends on the amount of mass. For rotating bodies, inertia depends on the amount of mass **and** where it is distributed relative to the point of rotation. This is called the moment of inertia.
- An unbalanced force applied over a period of time (impulse) alters a body's momentum (stop, start, slow down, speed up and change direction).
- During rotation a body has linear velocity which is constantly changing direction due to a force which pulls the body towards the centre of rotation (centripetal force); this force is balanced by a centrifugal force.
- In a rotating body momentum is conserved: if the moment of inertia changes there is a matching change in angular velocity. This principle of conservation also holds true for linear momentum.
- Each time a force is applied (action) there is an equal and opposite reaction force. This means the same as momentum being conserved during an exchange between two (or more) bodies. Although the word reaction implies

some kind of time delay, in fact this occurs instantaneously and might be better regarded as an interaction.

PRESSURE AND FRICTION: BODIES IN CONTACT

When force is applied to a body it is distributed over an area, for example, when you sit on a chair the combined downward force of your head, arms and trunk presses down onto the chair, but not at one point (which would be a little uncomfortable); instead it is spread over an area, your bottom, back of thighs, back and possibly feet.

Close your eyes for a moment and think about all the points that are in contact with the supporting surface (chair, floor, sofa or whatever you are perched on). Unless you are pretty uncomfortable you should have identified a number of areas (shoulders, back, buttocks, etc.) but not any specific points.

What we are talking about is pressure. Pressure is simply the applied force divided by the surface area. So this could be your force (mass × acceleration of gravity gives you the force) divided by the area of contact, for example, the contact surface of your foot on the ground, such that:

$$\text{Pressure} = \text{Force (N)}/\text{Area (m}^2).$$

The units of pressure are Nm^2, otherwise known as pascals, where 1 pascal = 1 Nm^2.

Consider the old Indian trick of lying down on a bed of nails (Fig. 4.10.). If you try to sit on one nail, of course it will hurt (quite a lot probably so don't try it), but if you spread your mass (and therefore your force) over all the nails, the load on each nail is reduced to the point where it can be tolerated. 'The more nails the better because there are more points of contact.'

This principle of increasing the surface area to decrease pressure is exploited across the animal kingdom. Consider the lowly water skater (or strider): by spreading its legs over as much of the surface area of the water as possible the force at any one point is low enough for it not to break the water surface, allowing this delicate insect to glide over the water.

Working in rehabilitation you will come across the effects of pressure on tissue. This could be a life-threatening pressure sore experienced by a bed-bound patient or a blister on your heel from wearing shoes that are too tight. So how does pressure cause such trauma? If you pinch one of your finger nails for a second or two you should see it blanche (go from pink to white). The pressure you applied has pushed the blood away; once you take the pressure off, the blood returns and your nail bed returns to a healthy pink colour. Damage occurs when blood is pushed away from tissue for prolonged periods; ultimately the tissue dies because it has been deprived of the oxygen and nutrients it gets from the blood. The resulting dead tissue can become infected with disastrous results. The remedy is not hard to understand, take the pressure off. Practically, this can be difficult for some patients who cannot move themselves.

How does understanding pressure help the rehabilitation worker or sports therapist? There are numerous examples:
1. Alleviating pressure in the foot by increasing the contact area with a moulded insole.
2. Applying force in a more comfortable manner, for example by using the palm of your hand when moving and handling a patient, rather than your fingers.
3. Modifying furniture to minimise pressure, for example a moulded seat cushion in a wheelchair.

Centre of Pressure

The centre of pressure (CoP) is a term often used by gait analysts, biomechanists and podiatrists, among others. You could consider this as the location of the average point of all the pressure applied to a body (we explored this a little in Activity Box 3.7). Stand up (if you haven't completely relaxed on that bed of nails) and consider where your averaged CoP is.

You are applying a force more or less evenly across the surface area of both your feet, so the averaged point would be somewhere in the middle, roughly at point A in Fig. 4.11. When you are standing nice and quietly then this point will coincide with the centre of gravity (point on the ground from the vertical projection of the CoM). Ok, now press harder down on your right leg (but don't move); you are now pressing the ground more on the right side than the left so the average CoP will move to the right, roughly at point B. What if you pressed your toes down? The CoP would move forward, point C. You can probably guess the rest, but it is important for you to distinguish between CoP

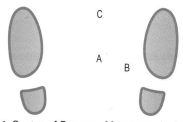

Fig. 4.11 Centre of Pressure Movement in Standing.

and CoM or even centre of gravity. It is easy to get mixed up with all these centres.

Friction

We have already talked quite a bit about friction as an opposing force in this and previous chapters; it's a difficult thing to avoid when you are talking about movement and one that most people have some understanding of, at least superficially. Hopefully this last section of this chapter will give you a greater understanding of friction.

Friction is usually regarded as something we don't really want around. Indeed engineers (and rollercoaster designers) spend a lot of their time trying to reduce it to a minimum. It gets in the way of efficient movement. If friction was invited to a party it would sit (unmoving) in the corner, drink all the expensive beer, eat all the pretzels and bore everyone with stories about how it saved a mountaineer from falling to certain death and stopped an old lady slipping. But these stories are not just some drunk's exaggerations; friction can be a force of good. Let me explain.

Friction is a resisting force. It opposes the movement of one body over another, but that doesn't mean it is not useful; without the friction of a carpet or wooden floor we would find it pretty difficult to stand up, walk or run. We use this resistance to propel ourselves; imagine trying to live on an ice rink all the time, difficult to get anywhere quickly.

There are three types of friction:
1. the friction within fluids (this will be considered in Chapter 5),
2. the friction between sliding surfaces and
3. the friction from an object rolling over a surface.

Sliding friction, as the name suggests, opposes the sliding motion of a body across another surface. There are two factors involved. The first is how much the body is pressed against a surface, for example its weight (mass × gravity). The heavier an object is the greater the sliding friction; this makes sense; a sleeping dog is much easier to push away from the fire than a drunken overweight man. This is only part of the story, however, because the amount of friction is also dependent on the smoothness of the surfaces. From experience you know that the smoother the surface the easier it is to push something across it; this is called the coefficient of friction and is, essentially, a measure of the roughness of surfaces. These two factors cause the relative surfaces to interlock with each other to a greater or lesser extent (try Activity Box 4.5).

So sliding friction can be represented as:

$$F = \mu \times N$$

where F = force of friction; μ = coefficient of friction (roughness of surface) and N = weight of object pressing down onto surface.

ACTIVITY BOX 4.5

Sliding friction is ubiquitous. Put your finger on the top of the table/desk and push it along the surface. Depending on the roughness of your finger and the desk surface you should feel some degree of resistance. Now push down harder (increase the N value) and try the movement again; this should have been much harder because you are squeezing the surfaces together more. You will also experience some heat; this is converted from kinetic energy of the movement and isn't particularly useful, unless you use it to warm your hands up by rubbing them together.

Put a paper tissue on the desk and try to do the same thing with the tissue between your finger and the desk. The movement becomes much easier because the interface between the tissue and desk top has a lower coefficient of friction (metres). I am sure you can think of many other ways to reduce the coefficient of friction of the table top.

Sliding friction is of interest to a range of professionals. Let's look at a couple of illustrations from health care and sport. Nurses need to move dependent patients about their beds. This can be difficult if the patient is large (therefore a large N) and not helped by the sheets which can be ruffled, thereby creating a large coefficient of friction (μ). So what can be done? You can't reduce mass (well not quickly anyway) but you can reduce the coefficient of friction by introducing smoother surfaces such as special sliding sheets (like the tissue in Activity Box 4.5) or simply tightening the sheets to make them smoother. Talcum powder may be another useful option.

There are many examples of sliding friction in the world of sport. In curling, for example, one or two 'sweepers' are employed to brush the ice immediately in front of the sliding stone to reduce sliding friction, preventing the stone from slowing down as much. The action of the sweepers melts the top layer of ice, making it very slippery. On the other hand, reduced friction caused by the sweat of volleyball or basketball players needs to be quickly mopped up to prevent injurious slips. Friction has also created challenges and solutions in the workings of the human body.

To improve efficiency the body has attempted to reduce the effect of friction where it can. The sliding up and down of a tendon, for example, is made easier by wrapping it in a sheath filled with a lubricating fluid which, among other things, reduces the coefficient of friction.

Where sliding friction resists sliding, the other main type of friction, rolling friction, resists rolling motion (you could

have probably guessed that!). Rolling resistance is caused by deformation of a circular surface (such as a wheel) as it moves over a flat surface (such as the ground). This deformation basically means more of the moving object (e.g. the wheel) comes in contact with the ground. There are many factors which affect rolling resistance, for example the shape of the surfaces, the type of material used and the pressure within the material (e.g. in tyres).

Rolling resistance may become a problem for wheelchair users, worn and flat tyres deforming more as the wheelchair rolls over the ground, creating greater resistance. When it comes to movement, however, sliding friction is a greater consideration.

Finally, although a lack of friction on a surface can predispose to a fall, too much friction can also cause injuries; consider the graze from falling on rough ground or a blister from your foot moving up and down in an ill-fitting shoe. Even your nipples don't escape friction; jogger's nipple is quite an uncomfortable experience resulting from the friction of your t-shirt as it slides up and down your body.

Summary of Friction and Pressure

Friction opposes movement. There are three types; in this chapter we considered sliding friction, which was to do with how rough the sliding surfaces were and how much they were squeezed together, and rolling friction, which was about circular surfaces rolling over flatter ones, the resistance, in this case, coming from the amount the surfaces deformed (think of tyres being pressed onto the road).

Pressure is simply force divided by area and is a consideration for parts of the body under prolonged periods of compression. The CoP is the averaged point of all the pressure points.

So far we have talked about the laws that govern how bodies move; in this next section we will look at energy. We will start with the concept of work.

WORK

In mechanics **work** means that energy has been transferred from one body to another through the application of a force. This means, for example, that work is done when you throw a baseball (energy moving from your upper limb to the ball) or lift a child or move a patient's leg. But work is also done if you **catch** a baseball (energy moving from the ball to your upper limb), **lower** a child or **resist** a patient's movement; the principle is that energy has moved from one body to another. Work can be calculated as the size of the force multiplied by the distance the body was moved by that force, that is:

$$\text{Work} = \text{Force} \times \text{Distance}.$$

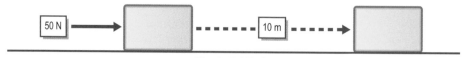

Fig. 4.12 Work.

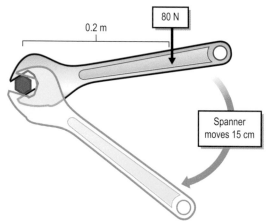

Fig. 4.13 Moment of Force to Turn a Spanner.

This formula would mean the scientific units are newton metres (force × distance), which would cause some confusion with moments which are also newton metres. Instead the convention is to use joules (J; Further Information 4.3), where 1 J is equivalent to 1 N of force acting over 1 m. Work has magnitude only (no direction is required), so work is a scalar quantity.

Example of Work in a Straight Line

Let's consider a simple situation. You want to push a box 10 m along the ground; to achieve this you need to push with a force of 50 N (Fig. 4.12).

This would mean that you have performed 500 J of work (50 N × 10 m).

So, provided you know distance and force, you can calculate work. The same calculation can be made for rotational movement, but we need the rotational equivalents of force and distance. Instead of force we have the rotational effect of a force (moment) and instead of distance we have angular rotation (this is usually measured in radians which are basically a different way of expressing the degrees of an angle, see Further Information 4.2).

Example of Angular Work

Being safety conscious, you decide to tighten up a nut that is holding a table together. You decide to use a spanner (30 cm long) for the job. To turn the spanner you wisely place your hand toward the end of the spanner, let's say 20 cm (0.2 m) from the nut (which will act as the pivot/fulcrum); of course you push down so that the spanner turns in a clockwise (positive) direction (Fig. 4.13). Let's

say that the force you apply with your hand is 80 N and, as we said, it is applied 0.2 m from the nut; this means the moment you apply is 16 Nm (0.2 m × 80 N). You apply this moment of force until the end of the spanner moves 15 cm and the nut tightens.

We can calculate the angle the spanner actually moves through by dividing the angular distance (0.15 m) by radius (0.3 m) which gives us 0.5 radians, a value equivalent to 28.5 degrees.

The work done is 16 Nm × 0.5 radians = 8 J of work.

MUSCLES AT WORK

It's about time we got back to looking at muscles. In rising up from a chair the quadriceps muscle group (muscles on the front of your thigh) pull on the femur (which, in our example, has a length of 53 cm) to rotate it in a clockwise direction (Fig. 4.14). To lift your thigh (along with the mass of your trunk, arms and head) the muscle needs to generate a moment of 200 Nm (perpendicular component of force = 500 N multiplied by the perpendicular distance 0.4 m) and the femur moves through an arc of 0.3 m (an angle of 0.75 [0.3 m/0.4 m] radians or 43 degrees). This would mean that 150 J of work (200 Nm × 0.75) were performed by the quadriceps muscles.

Have a look at the following questions; the first one has been done for you (along with some additional information); then try the other two yourself.

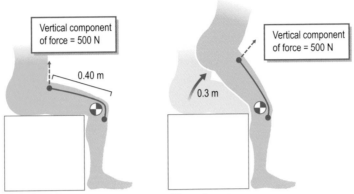

Fig. 4.14 Sit to Stand.

Question 1

A woman is out jogging. For every step she takes her CoM lifts by 0.15 m and moves forward by 0.9 m. She weighs 65 kg.

Calculate the work she does during every step.

Work is performed to move in two directions (there is of course a third direction—side to side—but we will keep it simple for now). To raise her body 0.15 m she must apply a force greater than the downward force (mass [65 kg] × acceleration [9.81 m/s^2] = 637.65 N). We can estimate the magnitude of this force is 700 N (approximately 10% more than body weight; this is an estimate based on literature).

So the work done vertically to lift her body against gravity is 105 J (700 N × 0.15 m).

Let's not forget that she is moving forward, as well as up. To take each forward step, 100 N of force are needed to displace her forwards by one step (0.9 m; again this is an estimate based on literature). So the work done is 100 N × 0.9 = 90 J.

In total then she performs 195 J of work (105 + 90) for each step.

For those of you counting calories, this is equivalent to 0.05 calories so every twenty steps we will expend 1 calorie. Just to put it in perspective, a popular nutty chocolate bar contains around 500 calories = 2000 steps. Of course this is the amount of work she performs (output) but not the amount her body actually consumes (input) because we are inefficient mechanisms; we will talk about this more later in the chapter.

Question 2

Calculate the magnitude of force and amount of work in the following situation:

A hoist is used to lift a disabled customer weighing 105 kg into a swimming pool. How much work does the hoist perform when lifting the man 1.7 m up?

Question 3

An angler catches a fish. The fish pulls hard on the end of the line and the angler begins to turn his reel (the pulley thing at the end of the rod) to bring the fish into shore. He pulls on the handle with 90 N; the handle is 0.064 m from the centre of the reel. The circumference (distance right round reel) of the reel is 40 cm. See Fig. 4.15. The man turns the reel three times to lift the fish. How much work did he perform?

DIRECTION OF WORK

As we have said, work is a scalar quantity because part of its calculation—distance (which could be linear or angular)—is a scalar. This means we do not need to state a direction; however, work can be positive or negative. If the applied force is in same direction as the resulting body movement, as in throwing a baseball, then the work is positive. If, however, the force is applied against the motion (as in catching a baseball) then the work is negative.

In the body, muscles perform positive work when the pulling force they apply to a bone(s) causes joint movement in the same direction as the muscle pull; for example if you straighten your leg while you are sitting there just now, the quadriceps muscle will shorten to pull on your lower leg (via the patella) which obligingly rotates round to straighten the knee. This is positive work or could be described as a concentric contraction (see Chapter 6 for further details).

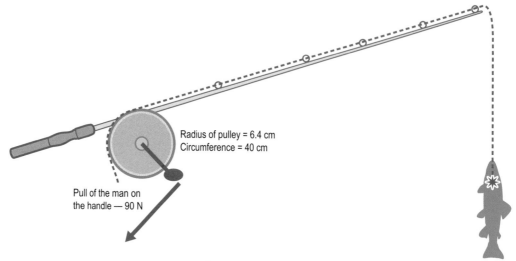

Radius of pulley = 6.4 cm
Circumference = 40 cm

Pull of the man on
the handle — 90 N

Fig. 4.15 Fishing Rod.

The muscle shortens and the bone moves in the same direction.

Negative work is performed when the bone(s) moves in the opposite direction of the muscle pull; for example with your leg straightened out in front, lower it down slowly to the ground. The knee is flexing; however, the quadriceps are working reasonably hard to oppose this motion (or at least control it) which means that the muscle has to lengthen as it continues to pull on the bone. This type of muscle activity is negative work or could also be described as an eccentric contraction.

So, work is performed when a force (like a muscle pull) changes a body's (or body segment's) position. It could be positive or negative.

Vertical jumping provides a good illustration of muscle work. On the way up the muscles that extend the hips, knees and ankles provide a huge amount of positive work (depending on the size of person and how high they want to jump). On landing, this reverses as the same muscles perform a huge amount (similar to the amount of work on the way up) of negative work; the hips, knees and ankles flex while the extensors create tension to slow down the rate of flexion (Further Information 4.4).

USING MACHINES TO DO WORK

The genius of man has been in the development of machines to help them perform work, whether this is a plough to push soil aside or a can opener to…well you know what that does! They have the same purpose; to make it easier to perform work on another body. A machine is simply a device that can help you do work. You put work in

(e.g. muscle work) and you will get work out (e.g. lifting a box).

The lever is the simplest machine used by man. So simple in fact that it is used by other primates as well; you might have seen pictures of monkeys using sticks to lift up boulders so they can get at the tasty ants. We are going to talk about levers a bit in the following section as it builds on our understanding of moments and work and because it provides more insight on the way the musculoskeletal system works. You could say our skeletal system was a simple system of levers, but that would be to diminish the human body.

A lever consists of four components: a rigid beam, a pivot (or fulcrum), effort and load (Fig. 4.16).

The main purpose behind the design of a lever is that it provides something called **mechanical advantage** over the object you are trying to move, be it a child on a seesaw or the door of a safe.

Mechanical advantage is simply the ratio of load to effort. Consider a burglar trying to prise open a safe; the lock on the safe is held by a steel bolt which is capable of resisting forces of 2000 N. A person is unlikely to generate this size of force; however, by using the principle of moments and a lever (in this case a crowbar) inserted into the lock, they can (see Fig. 4.17). If the lock can resist 200 N and is 0.1 m from the fulcrum of the crow bar, then 200 Nm (2000 N × 0.1 m) must be applied to open it. If a robber applies a force of 133 N at a point 1.5 m along the crowbar (from the pivot point), he can generate the necessary 200 Nm required to bust the lock and steal the jewels:

Applied force (133 N) × Perpendicular distance
from fulcrum (1.5 m) = 200 Nm.

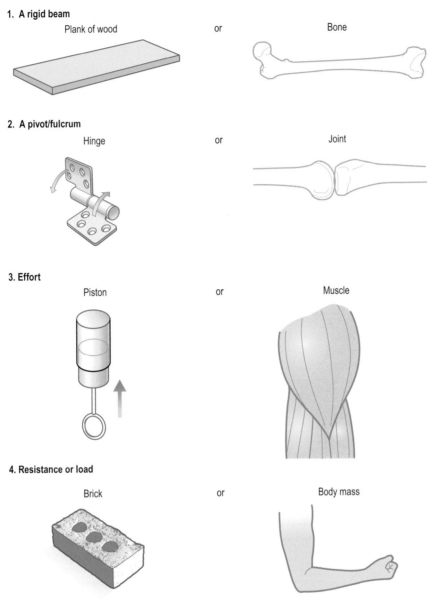

1. A rigid beam

Plank of wood   or   Bone

2. A pivot/fulcrum

Hinge   or   Joint

3. Effort

Piston   or   Muscle

4. Resistance or load

Brick   or   Body mass

Fig. 4.16 Components of a Lever and Some Examples.

So, the load that had to be overcome was 2000 N and effort (push) was 133 N which means the advantage was 15 times (the same as the ratio of the perpendicular distance). The mechanical advantage comes from the ability to locate the effort force further away from the pivot than the load. The use of the lever made the job 15 times easier. However, you have to push it 15 times further.

A wheelbarrow is another example of a machine that helps you perform work. Let's say a 20 kg load of wood is sitting in a wheelbarrow and has to be moved. The mass of the wood creates a moment about the wheel axis (which acts as the fulcrum) of 98 Nm (20 kg × 9.81 [gravity] × 0.5 m [distance from fulcrum]); see Fig. 4.18. To lift the load therefore requires a force to match or exceed this. The

FURTHER INFORMATION 4.4 External Mechanical Work Versus Physiological Work Measurements

When we performed these calculations we just looked at the displacement of the CoM. This approach does not take account all of the other work which goes on in the body. For example, we have to overcome intrinsic joint stiffness and hold body parts steady (e.g. the head and trunk) while other parts move; we even perform work just maintaining balance.

Calculating the movement of the CoM also does not consider input from existing potential and kinetic energy from previous step. These calculations, based solely on displacement of CoM, then represent 'external' work. A different approach to calculating work is not to look at output (movement of CoM) but rather input, the energy consumed in performing the action. This can be measured directly by recording physiological markers, specifically the volume of oxygen consumed during the activity.

There have been numerous papers written on this subject which have compared these two measurements: the direct cost of all the body activity according to the amount of oxygen consumed and the actual mechanical work performed by the body. This comparison provides an estimate of efficiency.

For example, research investigations have reported that the efficiency of walking (mechanical output divided by physiological cost) is around 0.25 (i.e. 25% efficiency). This means that for every 100 units of energy used by the body to walk only 25 units have been transferred to mechanical work on moving the body. The remaining 75% has been used for other functions and converted to other forms of energy, heat for example.

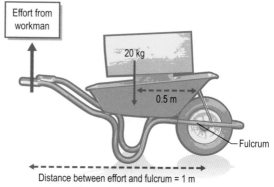

Fig. 4.18 A Wheelbarrow.

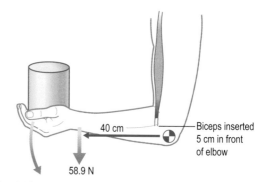

Fig. 4.19 How Much Force Do the Elbow Flexors Have to Produce to Hold the Tin of Tomatoes?

force the workman applies is located 1 m from the fulcrum (i.e. double the distance that the load is from the axis) which means to create the 98 Nm (moment of the wood) only requires a force of 98 N (half the weight of the wood). Therefore the mechanical advantage is 196.2/98 = 2.

Try the next question yourself.

A man is holding a 2 kg tin of chopped tomatoes in his hand. The combined mass of the tomatoes and his forearm is 6 kg which produces a force of 6 × 9.81 = 58.9 N. This force is located approximately 40 cm from the elbow with the forearm horizontal. The combination of force and distance from joint creates an extension moment (trying to straighten the elbow) of 58.9 N × 0.4 = 23.5 Nm. The elbow flexors (muscles that bend the elbow) apply an opposing flexor moment; however, the muscle is attached much closer to the joint, 5 cm. This means to hold the tomatoes, the elbow flexors have to produce a force of ____? (Answer at end of chapter.) (See also Fig. 4.19.)

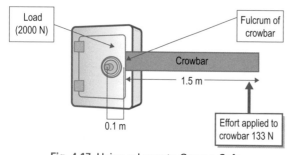

Fig. 4.17 Using a Lever to Open a Safe.

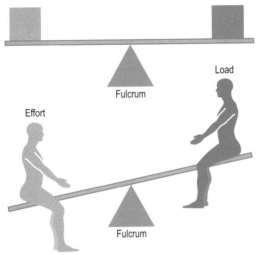

Fig. 4.20 Type 1 (One) Lever.

CATEGORIES OF LEVERS

Right, so now we know that levers are simple machines and that they help you perform work. The more distance from the pivot you can place your effort (compared to the load) the greater the mechanical advantage. You may have noticed from the questions that levers are arranged in different ways that alter their mechanical advantage; in fact there are three arrangements of lever.

The first type, type 1, is the classic seesaw (or teeter-totter if you live in the United States; Fig. 4.20) arrangement where the effort and load are located on either side of the pivot. Mechanical advantage is then dependent on how far away each is from the pivot.

There are not many examples of this type of lever in the human body; perhaps the most obvious is when you nod your head (Fig. 4.21). The neck is the pivot for this movement, the pull of the neck extensors is the effort and the load is the mass of the head (it has more mass toward the front).

The second type of lever is where both the effort and load/resistance are located on the same side (Fig. 4.22). An everyday example of this is the wheel barrow (see Fig. 4.18). Can you think of any other examples?

Because of the way a type two lever is arranged, the effort force will always be further away from the pivot than the load, so it will always be at a mechanical advantage. Again there are few examples of this lever arrangement in the human body; textbooks typically refer to the movement of going up onto the balls of your feet.

The tables are turned for the third-class lever. The effort and load are still located on the same side but this time the load is furthest away from the fulcrum (Fig. 4.23).

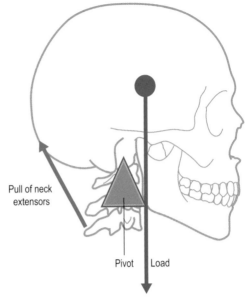

Fig. 4.21 Nodding as an Example of a Type 1 Lever.

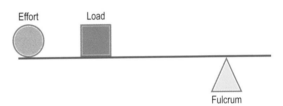

Fig. 4.22 Type 2 (Two) Lever.

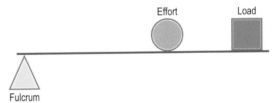

Fig. 4.23 Type 3 (Three) Lever.

This is a little like a baseball player striking a ball. Can you work out where the load, effort and pivot are when a batter hits a baseball? Think about the ball as the load and hands as the effort. Although this may vary, you can think of the pivot as the shoulder. Now you can put them in order and work out that the category of lever is third class.

This lever arrangement is very common in the human body (Fig. 4.24 and try Activity Box 4.6).

ACTIVITY BOX 4.6

Roll your sleeve up and look at your arm. Find the centre of the elbow from the side (the fulcrum). Now find the effort; this could be the biceps at the front or triceps (elbow extensors) at the back of the elbow. Now identify where the load is; this is the mass of the forearm which is around 2–4 kg and is located at the CoM '(about a third of the way along a line between the elbow and the tip of the fingers).' When you extend your arm, for example reaching out for a pencil, what type of lever arrangement are the triceps working in? (Answer at end of chapter.)

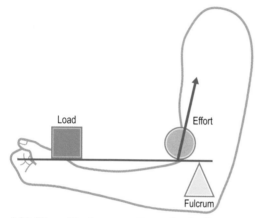

Fig. 4.24 Elbow Flexion as an Example of a Type 3 Lever.

Consider the following items and state which type of lever they are (clue: just identify the fulcrum, effort and load; then it should be obvious):

1. Crane
2. Scissors
3. Bottle opener
4. Drawbridge of a castle (Activity Box 4.7)

Movement Ratio

Given what we have just said about mechanical advantage for the third-order levers and how common this arrangement is within the human body, an obvious question might be why have we evolved what appears to be an inefficient system, where our effort must be larger than the load?

The reason is something called movement ratio. This is the ratio of the **distance moved by the effort** (at the point of application) and the **distance moved by the load.**

Let's take the example of opening a door. We have used mechanical advantage in putting the point of application of our pull furthest away from the pivot, so as to use the least force; however, this also means that we have to pull

ACTIVITY BOX 4.7

Place the levers below (Fig. 4.25) in order of their mechanical advantage (easiest for the effort) (clue: you may need a ruler).

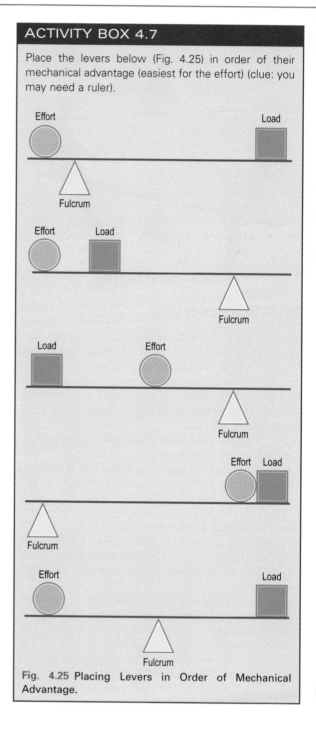

Fig. 4.25 Placing Levers in Order of Mechanical Advantage.

the door handle a greater angular distance than if we pulled next to the hinge. If we did apply our pull close to the hinge, it would certainly be harder in terms of force, but we wouldn't need to pull as far. Muscles are inserted close to joint centres for this reason; they don't have to shorten as much to create the same change in angle as if they were placed far away, but they have to pull harder.

To illustrate this let's get back to the lifting a weight example. By shortening the biceps muscle by a few centimetres the elbow can move through 30 degrees. If the muscle was inserted further along the bone toward the load, its mechanical advantage would be increased but it would have to move through a larger distance (Fig. 4.26). We need to be able to execute movements relatively quickly; therefore muscles are inserted at a mechanical disadvantage to achieve greater range and speed.

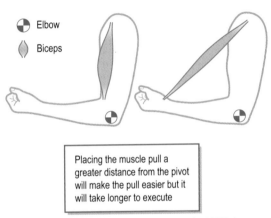

- Elbow
- Biceps

Placing the muscle pull a greater distance from the pivot will make the pull easier but it will take longer to execute

Fig. 4.26 Movement Versus Mechanical Efficiency.

More Advanced Machines

Levers are an example of a machine that can help you perform work. During the Industrial Revolution, simple lever machines were replaced with more sophisticated machines capable of doing heavier and faster work, particularly in trades that required the movement of large loads, for example mining, shipping and farming. Many of these machines were first invented by the ancient Greeks. Some of these machines are used in sport and rehabilitation, although sometimes their objective is not to the make the task easier but harder!

PULLEYS

The pulley is a machine that consists of a wheel with a free (minimal friction) moving axle about which the wheel spins. The wheel has a groove around its circumference and a rope which fits into the groove. It works because the rope grips the wheel and causes it to turn. It has a long nautical history where it is called a block and tackle. The basic pulley (type one) is a simple arrangement of a wheel fixed to a stable surface (e.g. floor or wall; Fig. 4.27). A rope is passed through the groove; at one end of the rope is the load/weight and at the other end is the effort.

The purpose of a simple pulley is that it changes the direction of the force. This is particularly useful if you want to lift an object up rather than pushing it up (see Fig. 4.27B). There is no mechanical advantage; the force you pull with is translated directly to the force that pulls the load up. Well, this is theoretically the case; however, some of the force you apply is opposed by friction (see previous discussion on friction) in the movement of the pulley wheel. The sliding friction of the rope through the groove will also produce

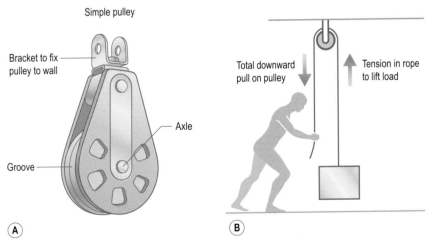

Simple pulley

Bracket to fix pulley to wall

Axle

Groove

Total downward pull on pulley

Tension in rope to lift load

(A)

(B)

Fig. 4.27 (A and B) Type 1 (simple) pulley.

heat which is not terribly useful and something that has to be controlled or it could lead to disastrous results.

Historically, this simple setup served a range of different jobs; however, things became more interesting when pulleys became moveable, not solidly fixed to a stone or tree but able to move via the rope. These are sometimes referred to as type two pulleys and are generally credited to Archimedes (Further Information 4.5). The reason for the excitement is that this arrangement requires much less effort; the trade-off is that more rope has to be pulled to gain the same elevation (a bit like when we moved the biceps along the arm, less effort force but more muscle length has to be used; see Fig. 4.26).

The type two pulley is designed so that the pulley itself can move (not rigidly attached to the wall like a type one;

see Fig. 4.27) when the person pulls the rope the pulley moves up. Now in this situation the force to lift the object is halved; however, the distance you have to pull the rope doubles. So the work (force × distance) remains the same but each pull is easier (useful for heavy loads). Now you might find this arrangement a little awkward, but you can always add another pulley to change the direction.

Now if there are two (moveable) pulleys we can reduce the force required even further, but at the same time the distance the load moves for each pull will reduce. So more pulls but each one is easier (Fig. 4.28).

The simple type one pulley is widely used in rehabilitation. This can be used to assist a movement, for example, shoulder flexion by the pull of a stronger limb (e.g. opposite shoulder extension). It can also provide a means of resisting a movement with the opposite limb creating a greater load (through active resistance) for the exercising arm.

FURTHER INFORMATION 4.5 **History of Levers and Pulley**

Pulleys have probably been around since before records began. Twisting a rope round a rock or tree to help pull or lift something up are likely to have been important methods of moving large objects. There is evidence of this type of pulley being around in the fourth century BC, although surprisingly there is no evidence (although this is still debated) of the ancient Egyptians using them. Makes you wonder how they managed to lift so many huge slabs of rock.

Like so many advances in engineering, Archimedes is credited with the first description of a pulley system. According to the story, in order to win a wager Archimedes designed a series of type 2 pulleys so that he could single-handedly pull a ship onto a beach.

Pulleys in the Human Body

The principle behind the simple pulley has not gone unnoticed by nature. While there are no true replicas of pulleys in the body there are plenty of examples of a change in the direction of a muscle pull being helped by grooves in bones. Consider the action of the quadriceps muscle as it (via the patella) glides over the femoral groove (just like the groove in the wheel of a pulley) so that it can pull on the tibial condyle. This arrangement also increases the perpendicular distance between the knee joint centre and muscle pull, creating a larger moment for the quadriceps (Fig. 4.29).

A similar example can be seen in the long flexors of the fingers. The pull of the muscle tendon is redirected by the tendinous straps attached to the bones so that angular motion across several joints is created by the pull of just one tendon.

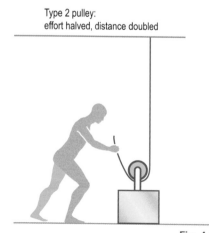

Type 2 pulley:
effort halved, distance doubled

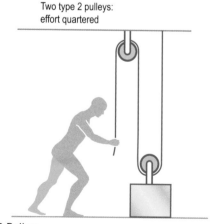

Two type 2 pulleys:
effort quartered

Fig. 4.28 Type 2 Pulley.

This anatomical feature is often described a pulley although it is not a true pulley (Fig. 4.30A). Given our complicated shape it is not really surprising that we have so many changes in muscle direction. Perhaps the closest thing to a pulley in the human body is the action of the peroneus longus which is a muscle positioned on the outside of the lower leg that rotates the foot outwards. The pull of this muscle is redirected by one of the bones in the foot (cuboid) to transfer its pull from the lateral to medial side of the foot (see Fig. 4.30B). The pull causes the foot to rotate (like the spinning pulley) about an axis centred on the sub-talar joint (the joint just under the ankle joint).

THE POWER OF WORK

When we talk about how muscles work, power is an important factor. Although often used synonymously with strength, **power** is actually the rate (or how quickly) the work (force × distance) is being created, so you need to consider time. Power is calculated as the work done divided by the time taken; the units are joules per second or more simply watts (W) after the Scottish inventor of the steam engine, James Watt, who also coined the term *horsepower*.

Let's say you want to lift a box and you have sensibly set up a pulley to do this (type 1). The box weighs 20 kg so you must pull with a force exceeding 200 N (mass of 20 kg × acceleration of gravity which as you recall has a value of 9.81). So you pull down with a force 250 N and the box moves vertically by 35 cm (0.35 m) (Fig. 4.31); this means the work you perform is 250 N × 0.35 m = 87.5 J. If it takes you 5 seconds to perform this elevation, the power you have expended, on average, is 17.5 (87.5 divided by 5) J/s or simply 17.5 W.

So what about muscle power? Just like machines the power of a muscle is its ability to generate work rapidly. You should make the distinction between muscle strength which is simply the ability of the muscle to generate force

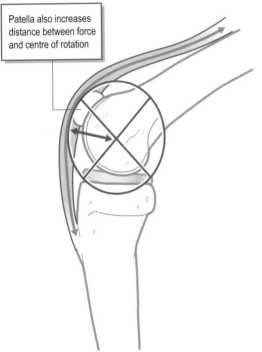

Patella also increases distance between force and centre of rotation

Fig. 4.29 Example of Pulley in Body; Knee.

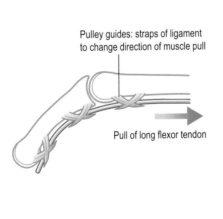

Pulley guides: straps of ligament to change direction of muscle pull

Pull of long flexor tendon

(A)

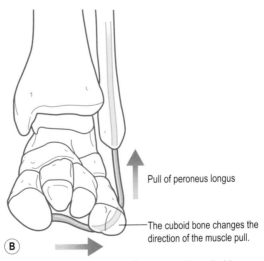

Pull of peroneus longus

The cuboid bone changes the direction of the muscle pull.

(B)

Fig. 4.30 Example of Pulleys in the Body (A) Finger flexion and (B) peroneus longus on the cuboid

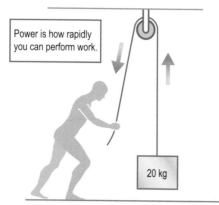

Power is how rapidly you can perform work.

20 kg

Fig. 4.31 Power During a Lift.

(this is also called tension because muscles always pull, you could also think of it as strength) and muscle power which is how rapidly it can perform work.

Let's get back to the standing up from a chair movement. If you recall (see Fig. 4.14) we calculated that during the sit-to-stand movement, the quadriceps muscle group created a moment of 200 Nm which moved the thigh (and therefore the rest of the body) through an arc of circumference 30 cm (an angle of 0.75 radians [0.3 m/0.4 m] or 43 degrees). This meant that 150 J of work (200 Nm × 0.75 radians) was performed by the quadriceps group of muscles. So what about power?

The average time (based on literature) to perform the extension phase of the sit-to-stand movement (thighs horizontal to thighs vertical) is 0.5 seconds. Power, as you now know, is work divided by time; therefore at this speed the quadriceps group would perform:

$$\frac{150}{0.5\,\text{s}} = 300\ \text{W of power.}$$

Interestingly, muscle power has been reported to decrease proportionally more than strength with ageing. Amongst other things, this has manifested in a slower standing-up time from sitting; values of 2 to 3 seconds have been reported. Let's say an older person takes 2.5 seconds to straighten up; this would mean (if we assume the same values of mass and distance) a power value of:

$$\frac{150}{2.5} = 60\ \text{W}$$

which is a reduction of 80%!

It has been suggested that, for a frail older person, standing up from a chair is as difficult as a maximum vertical jump (jumping as high as you can from a standing position) is for a young person. Let's look at the power required to perform a vertical jump.

Let's say an average person (mass 75 kg) performs a maximal standing jump. They squat down and apply a pushing force to the ground that exceeds their body weight and therefore the body accelerates vertically, lifting off the ground. If we estimate the value of this force is around 2.5 × body weight (to take into account the additional force required to accelerate the body up off the ground), 75 × gravity (9.81) × 2.5 = 1840 N. If this lifts the body by 40 cm then the work done is 1840 × 0.4 = 736 J; this work is carried rapidly (let's say 0.4 s), which means the power is 736 divided by 0.4 = 1840 W.

This is quite a difference from the 60 W expended (theoretically) by an older slow person getting out of a chair. The reason it is suggested to be similar to a vertical jump is that this 60 W represents a similar proportion of the available muscle power in an old person as 1840 does in a younger fit person performing a vertical jump; that is, both are near their maximum!

EFFICIENCY

We have already discussed **efficiency** a little, but it is worth spending a little more time on it because it is a popular theme in human movement studies. By understanding how much energy is lost in the performance of a task, a greater insight into the way the body moves can be gained. Later in the chapter we will discuss the ways in which the human body acts to maximise efficiency; suffice to say we are naturally parsimonious when it comes to movement.

In mechanical terms, efficiency is calculated as the ratio between the work put in (input) and the work done (output). You will come across the term in many areas of life. When buying a car you may be interested in how many miles it does to the gallon; how much energy (in this case the chemical energy created by the combustion of petrol) do you have to input to get the output (displacement of the car—miles). It's quite a challenge to calculate all the ways in which energy can be lost; however, it is fairly straightforward to measure efficiency. It is simply the output divided by the input. This is then expressed as a percentage. Let's get back to our comfort zone when we talk about machines, the seesaw (Fig. 4.32).

We can work out the work required to lift the child. The child weighs 25 kg (so force of the child is 25 × 9.81 = 245 N) and (provided the seesaw is rigid) moves vertically by 0.5 m; therefore the work output is 122.5 J. Let's say the amount of work put in was 125 J (250 N × 0.5 m); therefore 5 N more was required so the ratio would be:

$$\frac{122.5\ \text{(Work output)}}{125\ \text{(Work input)}} = 0.98\ \text{or}\ 98\%.$$

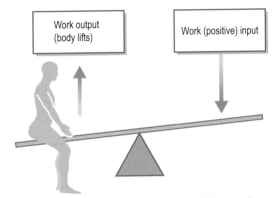

Fig. 4.32 Example of Efficiency, Lifting a Child on a Seesaw.

FURTHER INFORMATION 4.6 The Efficiency of the Bicycle

Simple pulleys and gears lie at the heart of the most popular invention of the human race—the bicycle.[a]

The reason for its popularity is that it satisfies all the basic requirements of a machine: easy to use (well perhaps not for your average 3-year-old), inexpensive, easy to repair and most importantly reduces the amount of work required. In fact the bicycle has been demonstrated to be the most efficient mode of road transport in terms of the ratio between work in and work out.

[a]According to a recent poll carried out in the UK by the British Broadcasting Corporation (BBC), 59% voted for the common bicycle, compared to 4% for the Internet and 5% for the radio.

A value of almost 100% means that practically all the effort put in was converted to work lifting the child. This would be a very efficient machine. But what about the 2%? The process of performing work inevitably means some energy will be converted to another form of energy. For example, overcoming friction, as well as some air resistance, will have resulted in some of the input energy being transferred from accomplishing the movement task.

No system is truly perfect in terms of efficiency. In real life, as a general rule, the simpler the machine the more efficient it is. The type of engine in a traditional motor car, along with the vast number of moving parts, lowers its efficiency to around 40%, so more than half the energy created from the petrol is lost to heat; this is, however, an advance in the old fashioned steam engines which only produced 15% of the consumed energy in useful work. In a simple pedal bicycle the efficiency (Further Information 4.6) is almost ideal with values around 95% to 99%! Although the addition of gears to the modern bike has reduced this

efficiency a little, it represents a very efficient means of transport.

The efficiency of humans has been studied from movement and dietary perspectives. After all, if we know how much energy an activity costs, we can estimate how much energy we need (in terms of food) and perhaps, more importantly, how much we don't need!

The problem lies in calculating a human's energy expenditure. The accepted best way is to use a physiological technique based on the amount of oxygen you use up (consume) while carrying out the activity. The gases you breathe out are analysed (this means wearing a mask) and the percentage of CO_2 calculated and compared with normal percentage in air; this tells us how much O_2 was used and therefore the amount of energy (once you have subtracted the amount used when resting). See Chapter 14 for a more detailed discussion on this.

We will return to the issue of energy and efficiency later when we talk about functional movements and the clever anatomical designs that make us more efficient (Further Information 4.7).

What You Need to Remember From That Bit

Mechanical **work** is the application of force to move a body in the direction of the force. Levers are simple tools consisting of a rigid beam (bone), fulcrum (joint), effort (muscle) and load (body weight/external load) to help us do work. There are three types of lever. The first type places the effort and load on either side of a fulcrum (like a seesaw); the second type sees the effort and load on same side of the fulcrum with the effort furthest away (effort has the advantage); the third class also has the effort and load on the same side, but this time the load is furthest away (load has mechanical advantage).

Power is the rate of doing work (work divided by time) and measured in watts. The power of muscle activity is different from strength and appears to reduce more with age than strength alone.

To finish this section, have a look at the following problems and activities; answers are provided at the end.

Practical Problems on Force and Human Movement

Fold a single sock up into a smallish square and place it inside one of your shoes/trainers so that it will be under your heel when you put the shoe on. What you have done is not too dissimilar (in a Heath Robinson kind of way) to a method used by podiatrists and physiotherapists to reduce load on an injured Achilles tendon (heel chord).

Now stand up and feel the difference between your feet. You should feel a change in how your pressure is distributed at your feet. The CoP (where the ground reaction force is,

FURTHER INFORMATION 4.7   Perpetual Motion Machines

For many years the holy grail in the design of machines was the perpetual motion machine. The idea that captured the imagination of many inventors was the possibility of a machine that could run without an energy source: once started it would continue to move (perform work) forever. Can you imagine how famous you would be in today's energy-stricken world if you came up with a machine like that!

As we have said, a machine performs work, for example lifting a heavy load. To do this, a machine needs energy which is used in two ways: (1) to move the object (kinetic energy being used) and (2) frictional generation of other energy forms (typically heat; thermal energy). If you add the heat energy and kinetic energy together, the total amount expended will equal the energy put in. In other words all the energy can, theoretically, be accounted for, even if only a portion is used for the actual work.

The fact that these machines are actually impossible because they contravene the basic laws of physics, energy input must equal energy output, and there must be some, even miniscule loss of energy from the system, has not deterred some intrepid inventors.

Of course, the so-called perpetual motion machines that do exist only give the appearance of work being done without any obvious input of energy. However, these machines do rely on energy sources. The bobbing of the drinking bird toy (Fig. 4.33) is caused by a process of pressure changes instigated by evaporation and condensation, which are caused by the temperature of the room; it is the heat energy that keeps this amusing toy moving—it wouldn't work in a cold room.

Why not conduct an Internet search for perpetual motion machines and see if you can work out where the energy comes from?

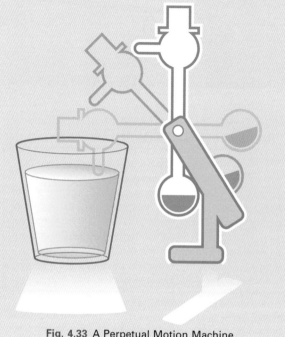

Fig. 4.33 A Perpetual Motion Machine.

on average, located) should have shifted forward a little on the sock side, perhaps under the ball of your foot, but of course this will depend on the thickness of the sock you used!

Can you feel any difference at your ankle, knee, hip, back?

Have a think about how the relationship between your joints and the ground reaction force has changed now that it is being applied further forward on your foot.

Compare both sides; are the same muscles working to the same extent?

For further information on this problem, why not look up the experimental study by Reinschmidt et al. (1994)?

Now that you are standing up, let's move onto a walking problem. Take the sock out of your shoe and stand somewhere that you will be able to walk for a few minutes, for example the corridor and pavement, and make sure the area is clear. Now walk forward for a couple of minutes and

remind yourself and what kind of moments are being created in the lower limb and where they are being created.

Now stop and walk backwards. Have a think about how the forces have changed. The magnitude of the force is likely to be the same, assuming you have not lost mass in the last 5 minutes and you are walking at the same speed as you did in forward walking.

The first point of contact is now the forefoot; how does this change the moments about your ankle and how does this affect muscle activity?

The foot is then gently lowered backward, but which muscle group controls this movement; remember when walking forward that the dorsiflexors (eccentrically) controlled the plantarflexion.

Sometimes to understand a movement problem, it is worth adopting the posture, feeling where the pressure is and how the muscles are working, so for the next problem let's try that. Stand up and bend your trunk forward a little.

Now make a note (in your head is fine) of any changes in the CoP at your feet. How are your muscles working compared to when you were standing straight? Think about how your CoM has moved and how this has altered the moments about your lower limb joints. This time try to focus on your knee; how have the forces and moments changed at this joint when you are bent forward?

Why do you think some people put themselves into this posture when they stand and walk; what possible advantage does it give them in terms of muscle work or altered pressure? Why do you think cyclists adopt this bent posture when they are struggling up hills, crouched over their handlebars?

Ok, let's try another movement problem:

You sit down on a sofa in your friend's house and their very friendly dog comes along and lies under your knees so that your feet are pushed forwards from the sofa. When you come to stand up you find it pretty difficult to do and not because you have consumed too many beers. Can you explain why this has happened? Think about where your mass is and where you are applying the force.

Finally here is another walking problem:

Walking along you come upon a sign that reads 'careful, floor is slippery, danger of falling'.

Being a careful person, you take heed of this warning. Explain why a slippery floor presents a greater risk of falling and then describe how you would adjust your walking pattern to minimise your risk of falling.

Clue: First try it out (but don't actually use a slippery floor, just pretend) and then think about the direction of the forces. Remember that you are applying forces to the ground through your lower limb so the angle it makes with the ground will be important.

The general answers to these problems are at the end of the chapter.

ENERGY DURING MOVEMENT

In the final part of this chapter we will look at energy during movement.

Evolution has fine-tuned us over the generations to be the most physically versatile creatures on Earth. In many ways movement defines us individually and provides the necessary foundation for intellectual development. The way we walk, the hand gestures we use when we talk and the way we hold a cup are expressions of our style and personality.

Even though we have many individual movement mannerisms that help express our individual character we

all, more or less, move in the same way. The predictability of many movements has allowed movement scientists to study and characterise the key elements of movements such as walking, standing up from a chair and reaching for a cup. This has ultimately led to a better understanding, and therefore management, of movement disorders such as cerebral palsy and Parkinson's disease. Sports professionals also use greater understanding of movement to improve sports performance as well as reducing risks of injury.

There are three good reasons for movement patterns being similar:

1. **Anatomy:** We all (more or less) have the same basic body shape and parts.
2. **Environment:** We all have to function in a common gravitational environment, with similar objects, so things like chair height, cup size, height of a tennis net, etc., are the same for everyone. To some degree clothes can also be considered an environmental factor that shapes our movement.
3. **Energy economics:** We are all driven by the same desire to minimise the energy cost of movement. Our natural inclination is to conserve energy.

To a lesser extent, culture, and even mood, shape our movement patterns; this may be the swaggering gait of a cabaret singer or the slow careful steps of a philosopher deep in thought.

In Chapters 6, 7 and 16 we will deal with the first two reasons. The third reason, 'energy conservation', will be explored in this chapter. But first we need to clarify what we mean by energy. Although we have already covered this, it is worth defining clearly again, because it is a critical concept and one that will give you greater depth to understanding human movement.

In mechanical terms, energy is the ability of a body to perform work; mechanical energy exists in two main forms, potential and kinetic energy.

1. **Potential energy** depends on the body's position. So a ball sitting on a table has potential energy due to its height; it has the potential to do some work. If you took the table away, it would travel toward the ground; if you attached a pulley and some string to it, it could pull an object along the table (Fig. 4.34). Because the driving force is gravity, sometimes this is also referred to as gravitational potential energy.

The potential energy (E_p) an object has due to gravity can be calculated simply as:

$$E_p = \text{Mass (of body)} \times \text{Gravity (9.81 m/s/s)} \times \text{Height (metres)}$$

and is measured in joules (see Further Information 4.3).

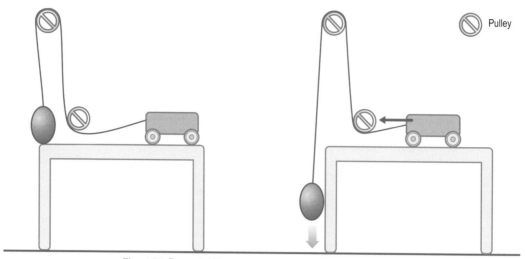

Fig. 4.34 Potential Energy Due to Height Above Ground.

So a man with 70 kg standing on a diving board 10 m above the water has:

$$E_p = 70 \times 9.81 \times 10$$
$$= 6867 \text{ J}$$

Mechanical potential energy doesn't have to depend on gravity; anything which in its current position has the potential to perform work, has potential energy. So a stone placed on a catapult and pulled back has potential energy. A ball filled with air which is placed at the bottom of a swimming pool has the potential to perform work. If you release the ball it would rise to the top and probably lift into the air; if you released the catapult the stone will fly rapidly towards its target.

2. **Kinetic energy** is the capacity a body has to do work due to its motion. Any moving object has kinetic energy. Imagine a golf club swinging toward a ball, without consideration to technique. The faster the club is moving, the greater capacity it has to do work on the ball (move it forwards and up). Mass is again an important consideration; a heavier club travelling faster has greater capacity to move the ball than a light one. The actual calculation for kinetic energy (E_k) is:

$$E_k = \tfrac{1}{2}\text{Mass} \times (\text{Velocity}^2)$$

(See Further Information 4.8.)

A body can change between potential and kinetic energy states. While moving, a body may gain potential energy as it loses kinetic energy and vice versa. Imagine a cyclist on top of a hill. She has potential energy due to her height above the ground (just like the ball on top of the table); as she speeds down the hill she loses height and therefore potential energy but gains velocity, that is, kinetic energy,

as well as heat if the brakes are applied (heat will also occur due to friction between the road and tyre). As the next hill approaches, this kinetic energy is converted back to potential; she gains height but the bike slows down. At the top of the hill potential energy is restored, ready for another speedy descent.

One of the fundamental laws of nature is that energy cannot be destroyed or created. But as we have seen, it can flow from one form to another. During human movement there is a continual exchange between potential and kinetic energy (Fig. 4.35).

The analogy of the cyclists exchanging potential and kinetic energy can also be used during gait. At mid stance (one foot swinging past the other) the CoM is at its highest (like the cyclists on top of the hill); this is converted to kinetic energy as we 'fall' forward and down.

Have you ever seen a child drawing a line along a wall with chalk or a stick while they are walking? If you have, you may have noticed that they leave a wavy line behind; this is not artistic creativity on the child's part but rather a consequence of the body rising and falling during walking. It's this very motion that allows pedometers to count your steps; each lift up counts as one step.

Let's go through the gait cycle together and you will hopefully see what we mean. First of all stand up; at this point your CoM is at its highest (55% of your height, Chapter 3). Now take a step forward; as you do your CoM will fall (both legs are at an angle) by around 5 cm. This 'fall' is just the same as the cyclist speeding down the hill, potential energy converted to kinetic. Of course your body continues to move (kinetic energy) and this energy is used to help the body lift up again to the height you were while standing at the start (highest point); once at the top again your body

FURTHER INFORMATION 4.8 Kinetic Energy and Momentum

You may recall that momentum was the product of mass and velocity which makes it seem quite similar to kinetic energy (½ mass × [velocity²]). But because velocity is squared when calculating kinetic energy, an increase in velocity will increase the body's kinetic energy more than its momentum. Although they are both measures of the physical nature of a body in motion, there are some differences besides their calculations and SI units. Kinetic energy (in fact all energy) is a scalar quantity, it has no direction; momentum on the other hand is a vector so has a direction. An illustration of this distinction is in the collision between two bodies. Let's imagine two pizza chefs standing at either end of a restaurant throwing balls of dough against each other so that the balls collide, stick together and come to a stop in the middle of the restaurant. Before the collision, each dough ball had momentum (mass × velocity); however, because they were in opposite directions, this momentum cancels out so that the combined dough ball has a momentum of zero before and therefore after.

For example, dough ball A has a mass of 1 kg and a velocity of 5 m/s directed from front door to back door (momentum of 5 kg.m/s) and dough ball B has a mass of 2 kg and a velocity of 2.5 m/s directed from back door to

front door (momentum of –5 kg.m/s; I have decided that this direction is negative). So total before collision would be zero (+5 kg.m/s and –5 kg.m/s = 0); therefore total momentum after collision would be zero. If the momentum before was not zero then after the collision the ball would have some momentum. But what about kinetic energy? Before the collision each ball has kinetic energy of 12.5 J each. Energy is a scalar so no negatives; therefore the total energy before collision was 25 J (12.5 J + 12.5 J = 25 J; 25 + 25). The collision caused the dough balls to stop moving (they stuck together), so kinetic energy, unlike momentum, is not conserved, which means no movement. Kinetic energy is instead converted to other energy forms, for example the dough balls will have a higher temperature (thermal energy which is really another form of kinetic energy but let's not get too microscopic here).

So momentum and kinetic energy are clearly related but not equivalent. Momentum is always conserved when bodies come in contact with each other (the net momentum is always the same), whereas kinetic energy can increase and decrease through conversion into other forms of energy; importantly the total amount of energy (in all its states) is always conserved.

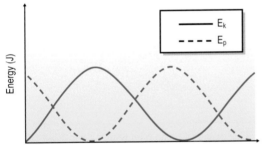

Fig. 4.35 Flow of Energy Between Kinetic and Potential States During Walking.

has regained the potential energy ready for another fall (Fig. 4.36). This swinging pendulum model of walking has been suggested to be very efficient, as it uses existing energy in the body to keep the body moving, so efficient that scientists have tried to recreate this in models called passive walkers (Further Information 4.9).

Elastically Stored Potential Energy

As we mentioned, potential energy can be stored in a piece of stretched elastic material. The energy used to stretch open a spring or rubber band will be returned immediately when

it returns, on release, to its original shape. We will explore this a little more in the next chapter but it follows on naturally from our discussion on energy so far. Nature has incorporated this method of storing energy by developing the elastic properties of connective tissue and tendons in particular; See Further Information 4.10 for a really interesting example. There are also more details on the elastic properties of tissue in Chapters 5 and 7.

Shortening a muscle is quite an inefficient, energy-expensive action, so the body tries to minimise this whenever possible. Fortunately we have connective tissue in our muscle (tendons and muscle harness; see Chapters 6 and 7) which can act as passive springs (no active work) to store kinetic energy during movement; this is a very efficient strategy. This is what the body tries to utilise when walking, a strategy so efficient that the elastic recoil of the Achilles tendon has been estimated to contribute up to 60% of the energy required for normal walking (reference), but how does it do this? Let's have a look at how this happens by looking at the stance phase of gait. In Fig. 4.38 just consider the darkened side, which is the leg that stays on the ground otherwise known as the stance leg.

At the start of the sequence (gait cycle) the forward rotation of the tibia over a foot that is planted firmly on the ground basically winds up the Achilles tendon (and

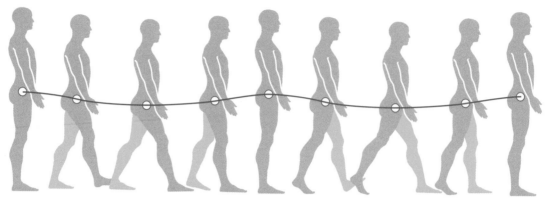

First step: Both feet on ground: Next step lifts   The cycle repeats
CoM lowers   CoM at lowest   CoM again

Fig. 4.36 Vertical Displacement of the Centre of Mass *(CoM)* During Gait.

FURTHER INFORMATION 4.9

Scientists have tried for a long time to perfect models of
walking that use minimal energy. This invariably means
using some kind of pendulum swing to keep the model
moving forward. So the walking commences with someone
lifting the pendulum up, the release of the pendulum
providing the initial power to the walker to take a series
of steps through a series of friction-free hinges (Fig. 4.37).
This is just like an obliging parent pulling back the swing
with their child in it; releasing the swing commences the
cycling pendulum motion of the swing.

Inevitably, without any further pushing, the child's swing
slows down and, despite a lot of tinkering, this also happens
to the passive walking models. This has meant that these
models still need some kind of energy input (like the parent
giving the swing a little push now and again); usually this
is provided by getting the model to walk down a slope,
so the energy comes from gravity.

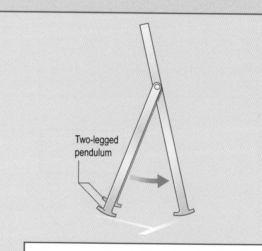

Two-legged
pendulum

There are two pendulums in this passive walker. One of the
pendulums has two points of contact with the ground (two
legs) and the other has only one; this is to improve its
stability. At the point shown, the walker is very stable (all feet
on the ground); however, the two-legged pendulum is about to
advance over the single-legged pendulum (which will act like
an inverted pendulum) driven by the force of gravity.

Fig. 4.37 Example of Passive Walking Model.

other elastic components of the calf) like a spring. As the
body continues to rotate forward the spring is released which
helps to push the body up and forward.

Elastic storage is not just a strategy used during gait;
it contributes to other movements. Let's consider the sit-
to-stand movement (see Fig. 4.39). The initial part of the

sit-to-stand movement involves the individual flexing their
head, arms and trunk forward. What does this do to the
hamstring muscles? Best way to find out is to try it yourself.
While sitting, place both your hands under your thighs and
lean forward reasonably quickly, as if you were about to
stand up.

FURTHER INFORMATION 4.10

The Achilles tendon appears to have developed as a consequence of bipedal upright walking and running. Rather than a weak spot as the unfortunate story of the hero of Greek mythology 'Achilles' tells us, the development of the Achilles tendon is a key evolutionary step. The absence of similarly well-developed Achilles tendons in other primates is a reflection of its importance to human upright gait.

Researchers at Manchester University created a simulation from the fossilised remains of the earliest walking hominid—Lucy—and found the evolution of the Achilles tendon was an important step (excuse the pun) in the development of efficient walking and running. They estimated the tendon probably developed between two and three and a half million years ago.

ACTIVITY BOX 4.8

Can you observe the stretch shortening cycle in other movements or in other muscle groups? Look at the way someone performs a vertical jump or the muscle activity during the triple jump. What about a javelin throw? Are there other muscle groups using SSC during gait apart from the calf muscles?

What you felt (hopefully) was an eccentric contraction (see chapter 6), the muscle is active (tensing under your hand) while lengthening (the hamstrings attach to the pelvis which is moving forward, lengthening the muscle). This eccentric contraction controls the forward movement of the trunk but it also helps the muscle to store elastic energy (see Fig. 4.39). The added tension within the muscle due to the contraction makes the 'muscle spring' even stiffer. So if you stretch a muscle while it is under tension, it will release with even greater force; if this recoil is timed with a concentric contraction the muscle will be able to create very large forces indeed.

This behaviour of muscle is known in the sports world as the stretch shortening cycle or SSC for short. It has been well studied in animals, turkeys in particular, which, due to their proportionally large amounts of tendon, are now known to be pretty efficient runners (Roberts et al., 1997; Activity Box 4.8).

Sports coaches and physiotherapists design exercise programmes to train this property of skeletal muscle. Plyometric exercises start with a stretching phase consisting of a eccentric contraction immediately followed by a rapid concentric contraction; the classic example of this is jumping down from a step. On landing from the jump, the extensor muscles of the lower limb (muscles that straighten the hip, knee and ankle) are stretched and eccentrically

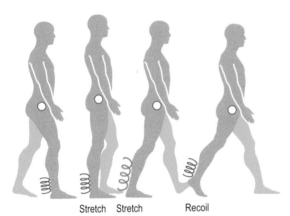

Stretch   Stretch   Recoil

Fig. 4.38 Storing Elastic Energy in the Calf Muscles to Assist Forward Movement of the Leg When Walking.

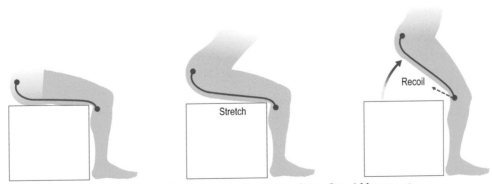

Stretch

Recoil

Fig. 4.39 Using Elastic Storage During the Sit-to-Stand Movement.

ACTIVITY BOX 4.9

Hold the thumb of your right hand with the thumb and index finger of your left. Now stretch it down towards your forearm (Fig. 4.40). You probably won't be able to make it touch your forearm but just bring it down enough so that you can feel a stretch on the back of your wrist. Let go.

The spring-back of your thumb comes from elastic energy stored in your connective tissue. Now do the same thing but this time push a little against your thumb being stretched down (basically try to resist the stretch a little). This time when you let go you should have found your thumb/wrist bounced back further and faster, an illustration of the added effect an eccentric contraction can have on elastic recoil.

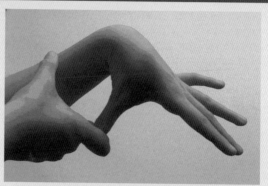

Fig. 4.40 Stretching thumb to forearm.

contract; this action is immediately followed by a powerful extension of the same muscles to accelerate the body up. Repetitions of this activity are said to train the elastic recoil ability of these muscles, useful in sports that include explosive movements such as volleyball and the high jump (Activity Box 4.9).

ENERGY CONSERVATION

The word conservation implies there is something to lose but we know that energy cannot be created or destroyed. So what we mean by conservation is really retention of energy that is useful to the task. The heat given off by a car engine doesn't really help the car move forward (just provides a nice warm surface for cats, once parked). Some of the mechanical energy needed to move the car has been lost to heat, not retained for its task.

Mechanical engineers and scientists have long strived for a machine or system of machines that conserve their energy in a single useful form. The perpetual motion machine was an engineer's holy grail for many centuries, leading to pretty amazing machines (see Further Information 4.7). However, in practice these machines could not exist since there is always some energy exchange to heat or light through friction or air resistance.

This idea of the *human machine* attempting to minimise the loss to other energy forms was behind the explanation of human gait proposed by Inman and Eberhart more than 60 years ago (Inman and Eberhart, 1953). The basic premise of this theory of walking efficiency was that the body minimised movements not directly involved in the forward translation of the body, that is, to minimise the movement

of the body's CoM. They considered up-and-down and side-to-side movements to be inefficient, since they were not in the direction of travel. So they thought, what does the body do to reduce these movements?

They explored this idea through thought experiments (as opposed to experimental testing). They thought: what if there were no joints in the lower limb apart from the hip and that this worked like a simple hinge? They described this as a calliper gait, like opening and closing a pair of scissors.

This model of gait appeared highly inefficient, with the body moving a lot to the side as well as up and down. Why not try it yourself; obviously you can't get rid of your pelvis, knees and ankles, but you could try to keep your knee straight and your ankle in neutral (the way it is when you stand normally). It is quite difficult to walk this way, but if you managed you might have noticed a lot more swaying, up and down and side to side, mainly because it is difficult to swing your straight leg through.

This provided Inman and Eberhard with a basis to explain the movements of the lower limb in what became called the **Determinants of Gait**. They proposed six movements of the lower limb that made walking more efficient, of which we will describe two; please go to the original work to discover the other four.

THE DETERMINANTS OF GAIT

Stance Phase Knee Flexion

During the stance phase there is a slight flexion of the knee. This keeps the body low as it travels over the standing foot, minimising the up-and-down movement.

Pelvic List

As the foot impacts with the ground the pelvis lists (drops) downward on the opposite side. This, it was proposed, minimises the vertical movement of the body. The best way to think about this one is to consider what would happen if your pelvis didn't drop.

Try it; walk about with your hands on your pelvis (slide your hands down the side of your trunk until you get to the bones—iliac crests). You should feel the pelvis lift and drop in time with the feet striking and then pushing off from the ground. Now just focus on initial contact, and try to keep your pelvis up (don't let it drop down); the effect, as you hopefully found, was that your body remains higher and shifts more out to the side.

The advent of sophisticated motion analysis systems has allowed these determinants to be tested under laboratory conditions. It appears that most of them have little impact on the vertical and lateral movement of the body's CoM; in fact the one thing that prevents excessive vertical displacement of the CoM is lifting your heel off the ground at the end of stance phase, a movement which limits the amount of drop your body goes through at the end of stance (Kerrigan et al., 2000). Again, the best way to demonstrate how this works is by trying it out; as you take a step forward your heel will lift off the ground on the opposite side. Now try to keep your heel on the ground; what happens to your body?

This greater drop of your body is not a good idea because now you have to lift it up again at the next step.

Ok, so if, as we already stated, our movements are shaped by the need to conserve energy, the determinants of gait have not provided a full explanation of how this energy conservation occurs during gait; so what mechanism do we use to limit the energy cost of walking? Well you already have the answers; firstly we use the energy efficient pendular motion of the swinging leg and inverted pendulum during stance phase (body pivoting over the fixed foot) just like the passive walkers (see Fig. 4.36). These motions are assisted by 'tendon springs', the Achilles tendon being a good example of this, which release elastic energy created during the motion and stored with the connective tissue (tendon mainly). See Kuo (2007) for a review of these mechanisms.

Despite these efficient body tissues and movement strategies we still need active tension to be generated in the muscles; you can find out exactly how muscles generate this tension in Chapter 6.

What You Need to Remember About Energy?

The last section covered human movement from the perspective of energy. We looked at what energy was, considering its two basic forms, potential and kinetic energy. We examined how the body fluctuates between potential and kinetic energy and how it makes use of elegant strategies (usually involving pendulums) and elasticity of 'muscle springs' to be as energy efficient as possible during movements, with gait and sit to stand being offered as examples.

ANSWERS TO QUESTIONS POSED IN TEXT

Transfer of momentum from horizontal to vertical during the sit-to-stand movement.

The momentum of the trunk, which is mainly horizontal, is transferred to the lower limbs through the action of the hip extensors (gluteus maximus and hamstrings). As the trunk flexes forwards these muscles are more and more wound up, like springs. They do what any spring would do when it is pulled at one end, they pull on the other end, which means extending (straightening) the thigh, which helps to lift your body up. Clearly this transfer is not sufficient to accomplish the vertical movement, so you also need input from the knee extensors (quadriceps) as well as active shortening of gluteus maximus and the hamstrings. Nonetheless this is a highly efficient use of the body's momentum.

By bending the leg as it swings, the moment of inertia of the leg is reduced (therefore easier to swing) but it also helps in clearing the ground, an important factor in avoiding a trip fall.

Answer to Question 2

$$\text{Magnitude of force} = \text{Mass (105 kg)} \times \text{Acceleration (9.81)} = 1030\,\text{N.}$$

The work done is 1030 N multiplied by 1.7 (displacement) = 10,104.3 J.

Answer to Question 3

$$\text{Displacement} = 3 \times \text{Circumference} = 1.2\,\text{m}$$

$$\text{Rotational force} = 90 \times 0.064 = 5.76\,\text{Nm}$$

$$\text{Work done} = 18.75\,\text{radians (526 degrees)} \times 5.76$$
$$= 108\,\text{J of work}$$

Answer to Question 4

To hold the tomatoes steady, the elbow flexors have to produce a force of at least 23.5 Nm, otherwise the arm will fall down.

$$23.5\,\text{Nm} = 0.05 \times ?$$

Therefore 23.5/0.05 = 470 N!

Answer to Question 5

The batter hitting the baseball is an example of a third-class lever:

Fulcrum (shoulder) – effort – Load.

This arrangement will always place the load at a mechanical advantage; that is to say it has the advantage of a longer lever compared to the effort which you could say is at a mechanical disadvantage, being closest.

Categories of Levers

There are many types of cranes in existence but in essence they are all work on the same principle of levers providing mechanical advantage so it easier to lift an object. Modern cranes are generally type three levers. Scissors are an example of a first-class lever; the effort (you pressing) is on one side of the pivot and the load (paper etc.) is on the other; scissors can also be described as a double lever since there are two of them working together. A bottle opener is an example of a second-class lever; your effort is at one end, the pivot point is at the other and the load/resistance is between the two. Finally the drawbridge of a castle is a type two lever; the load (mass of the bridge) is placed between the pivot and the effort (where the chain is attached).

Answer to Activity Box 4.6

The triceps are actually working as a type 1 lever; effort (attachment of triceps) is behind the joint and the load (mass of arm) is in front.

Answers to Practical Problems on Force and Human Movement

Inserting a sock under your heel shifted the CoP forwards; the CoP can be considered to be the point of application of the ground reaction force (GRF). By moving this forwards, it will alter the moments acting about the lower limb joints. When standing normally (i.e. no sock under your heel) the GRF lies slightly (4 or 5 cm) in front of the ankle (see Fig. 2.25), causing a small dorsiflexing moment (i.e. your ankle feels like it wants to bend) which is counterbalanced (otherwise you would fall forward!) by a plantarflexing moment (see Fig. 3.24) provided by the muscles behind your ankle (also known as the plantarflexors). Moving the CoP forwards increases the size of this dorsiflexing moment, which, unless you don't want to fall forwards, means much more activity in the plantarflexors, which you may feel after a while.

Walking backwards means the forefoot strikes the ground first (as opposed to the heel); normally the heel strike creates a plantarflexing moment because it is located behind the ankle (so there is corresponding activity of the dorsiflexors). Hitting the ground with your forefoot, however, means this will be reversed, so you will get a dorsiflexing moment and consequently (like the last question) more activity in the plantarflexors. Because the foot is being lowered when you hit the ground, the muscles perform negative work; they are still active to control the moment but are allowing the joint to move (in a controlled manner) in the opposite direction.

Bending forwards (stooping) when you are standing alters many things which you can easily feel. In very basic terms you have moved your CoM forwards; if you think about your stability, this may make you unstable, but really you would have to bend forward a lot to make you topple forwards because a lot of your base of support (feet) is in front of you. Why not try it for yourself; stand up and see how far forward you need to bend before you begin to feel like you are falling forward. The problem with stability and this posture comes when you start to walk.

During gait, at the point of impact with the ground, the body decelerates (change in momentum); this deceleration starts at the foot and moves up the body (like a wave of deceleration) so that the upper body continues to move forward a little after the foot has stopped. This doesn't last long and the body quickly reverts to the efficient upside down pendular motion with the body rotating forwards over a fixed foot. The problem comes when you have already moved the CoM forwards (when you are in a stooped posture), this continued motion of the body after initial contact risks a forwards instability (you might fall forwards) with the CoM now much closer to the front limit of the base of support. Again why not try this; bend forwards again, at your hip, and walk; you may experience a sensation of toppling forwards when your foot lands; this might reveal itself in an increased urgency to take the next step.

Now some individuals are forced into this flexed/stooped posture because of a spinal condition; however puzzlingly, it seems that some people deliberately adopt this posture. This is a strategy not borne from vanity or efficiency but rather a specific impairment of the lower limbs. If you lose enough strength in your quadriceps muscle (through injury or disease) it means the body is unable to resist the large flexing moment created by the GRF vector projecting behind the knee joint. By moving the CoM forwards, the GRF is less angled so it comes closer to the knee joint, creating a smaller moment so less is required from the knee extensors (quadriceps). Why not try it out and see what you think; a similar change in knee moments could be achieved by hitting the ground with your forefoot first but I will leave you to work out how that works; remember trying things out helps a lot.

Trying to stand up with your legs further forward than normal (because of a friendly dog) will feel like much harder work than normal simply because you are moving your body a greater distance forward (work is force × distance). To make this bigger jump you need to generate larger moments about your lower limb joints as well as more contribution from your upper body (throwing arms forward etc.). Because of the more forward location of the ground reaction force, the moment at your knee may be extensor (GRF orientated in front of your knee), whereas normally it would be flexor.

We have all come across the slippery floor situation so we all know that to avoid slipping we do two things, usually.

We slow down and we take smaller steps; these two not necessarily related strategies reduce the risk of falling by altering the size and direction of force applied by your body to the ground. By slowing down, the required change in momentum at initial contact is much reduced so the force magnitude is reduced. By taking smaller steps the angle of the GRF is more vertical (like you are stamping your legs straight down); therefore the horizontal component (which will cause your slip) will be reduced. Reduced magnitude and reduced angle of the GRF means less chance of slipping.

SELF-ASSESSMENT QUESTIONS

1. In your own words describe what we mean by inertia.
2. Momentum is
   a. Mass × velocity.
   b. Mass × acceleration.
   c. Mass × velocity squared.
   d. Mass × acceleration squared?
3. Is the following statement true or false? Momentum is a vector.
4. In a balanced (not accelerating) rotating body
   a. The centripetal force is greater than the centrifugal force.
   b. The centripetal force is equal to the centrifugal force.
   c. The centripetal force is less than the centrifugal force.
5. Impulse is
   a. Force × time.
   b. Less than a second.
   c. Force × displacement.
   d. Force × acceleration.
6. Newton's third law of motion is
   a. For every action there is an equal and opposite reaction.
   b. Force = mass × acceleration.
   c. Impulse = change in momentum.
7. Sliding friction can be calculated as
   a. F = μ (coefficient of friction) × N (weight of object).
   b. F = μ (gravity) × N (air resistance).
   c. F = μ (coefficient of friction) × N (mass of object).
   d. F = μ (air resistance) × N (weight of object).
8. Work is
   a. Force × distance squared.
   b. Force × acceleration.
   c. Force × mass.
   d. Force × displacement.
9. A lever consists of
   a. A rigid beam, an effort and a load.
   b. A rigid beam, a pivot and an effort.
   c. Mass, a pivot and an effort.
   d. A rigid beam, a pivot, an effort and a load.
10. A type 2 lever has
    a. The effort and load on either side of the fulcrum.
    b. The effort and load on the same side as the fulcrum with the load furthest away.
    c. The effort and load on the same side as the fulcrum with the effort furthest away.
11. What type of lever arrangement is the most common in the body?
    a. 1
    b. 2
    c. 3
12. Power is
    a. The same as work.
    b. Work divided by time.
    c. Work multiplied by time.
    d. Work multiplied by time squared.
13. Mechanical potential energy due to gravity can be calculated as
    a. Mass (of body) × gravity × height squared.
    b. Mass (of body) × gravity divided by height.
    c. Mass (of body) × gravity × height.
    d. Mass (of body) divided by (gravity × height).
14. Is the following true or false? Energy can sometimes be lost.
15. Can you name one of the six determinants of gait?
16. Which of the six determinants has empirical evidence?

REFERENCES

Inman, V.T., Eberhart, H.D., 1953. The major determinants in normal and pathological gait. Am. J. Bone Joint Surg. 35 (3), 543–558.

Kerrigan, D.C., Della Croce, U., Marciello, M., Riley, P.O., 2000. A refined view of the determinants of gait: significance of heel rise. Arch. Phys. Med. Rehabil. 81 (8), 1077–1080.

Kuo, A.D., 2007. The six determinants of gait and the inverted pendulum analogy: a dynamic walking perspective. Hum. Move. Sci. 26 (4), 617–656.

Newton, I., Halley, E., 1744. Philosophiae naturalis principia mathematica, vol. 62. Jussu Societatis Regiae ac typis Josephi Streater, prostant venales apud Sam. Smith.

Reinschmidt, C., Nigg, B.M., Hamilton, G.R., 1994. Influence of activity on plantar force distribution. Clin. Biomech. (Bristol, Avon) 9 (2), 130–132.

Roberts, T.J., Marsh, R.L., Weyand, P.G., Taylor, C.R., 1997. Muscular force in running turkeys: the economy of minimizing work. Science 275 (5303), 1113–1115.

Flow

Andy Kerr and Philip Rowe

OUTLINE

LEARNING OUTCOMES

After reading this chapter, you will be able to:
1. Define stress and strain.
2. Describe the relationship between stress and strain.
3. Explain viscoelasticity.
4. Describe the different kinds of connective tissue and their mechanical properties.
5. Explain the effect of ageing, immobility and injury on the properties of connective tissue.
6. Provide a scientific explanation for stretching techniques.
7. Define density and pressure.
8. Describe how gases and fluids flow.
9. Describe how the properties of fluids and gases can be used therapeutically.

INTRODUCTION

Up to this point, when we talked about the action of force on a body, we considered that body to be rigid, it didn't stretch or get squashed when the force was applied. Of course, this is not the case with the human body; we have many soft bits that squash and stretch when they are pushed and pulled. The forces that squash and squeeze tissues, such as our skin, bone or tendon, might be a sudden single impact from a fall or repeated applications during a cyclical activity like running or using a keyboard. Understanding how our body copes with these different types of force application is fundamental to understanding injury and repair. In this chapter you will be introduced to the principles of material science before applying this knowledge to the tissues of the human body. We have called this chapter *flow* because it describes the way tissues in the body tend to behave when loaded. Similar principles also apply to the way gases and fluids move around the body, which will be the focus of the last section of the chapter.

The body is a wonderful piece of engineering. Aeons of natural selection have resulted in the human body being constructed from a range of materials that are designed for specific functions; for example, bone provides a rigid beam for muscles to create moments, whereas skin provides a stretchable, protective, waterproof barrier. Imagine if these characteristics were swapped? Abdominal expansion after a large dinner would feel pretty uncomfortable with rigid skin while stretchy bones would pose quite a few problems for those of us hoping to actually get out of bed in the morning.

Understanding how materials, in general, behave when forces are applied to them is a good starting place for this chapter. This will allow us introduce some of the key principles before we move on to understanding how these principles apply to human tissues.

BASICS OF MATERIAL SCIENCE

Engineers have long been interested in how materials cope with force. If you are building a bridge you need to know that the materials you use can endure the repetitive compressing (squashing down) loads from cars and lorries as well as high winds, which will push and pull the bridge at different speeds and in multiple directions. The same could be said for clothes designers; they need to know just how far the elastic in your pants can stretch and how often, before it fails.

It should be no surprise to know that the mechanical properties of most materials have been scientifically tested. Material science has its own principles, and of course terminology, which can be applied just as appropriately to the human body as to concrete pillars in bridges or the elastic

in your pants. After all, just like engineers, we need to know why and how they fail and perhaps more importantly how to repair them. Let's start this understanding with a couple of important terms.

Stress

When speaking about materials, **stress** is the force applied to a material per unit area; that is, force divided by area, which means the units are Nm^{-2}. The observant amongst you will have noticed this is the same as pressure. Although the terms stress and pressure could be considered synonymous, in this context for clarity we will just use the term stress.

Stress can be applied to a material in many different directions:

Compressive Stress

Compressive stress is a pushing stress. It is pushing vertically down onto the surface of the body so that it is at right angles to it; that is, perpendicular (Fig. 5.1). For example, if you put a balloon between your hands and squeeze it or when you sit on top of an overfull suitcase to try and close it.

Many structures in the body experience compressive stress. Think of the bones in your leg being squashed by the weight of your body while you are standing, or if you are sitting, consider the weight of your head arms and trunk squashing the skin of your buttocks. Gravity certainly causes a lot of compression. Perhaps the most easily illustrated example of compressive stress is in the spine where the vertebral bodies and intervertebral discs have to endure a long day of being squashed from the mass of your head arms and trunk, in sitting and standing (Fig. 5.2).

Tensile Stress

Tensile stress is a pulling stress. Like compressive stress it is also applied perpendicularly to the surface of the body

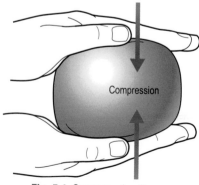

Fig. 5.1 Compressive Force.

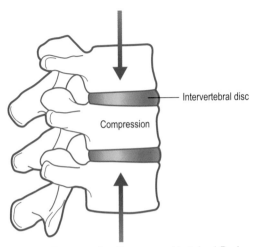

Fig. 5.2 Compression Force on a Vertebral Body.

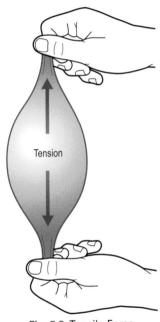

Fig. 5.3 Tensile Force.

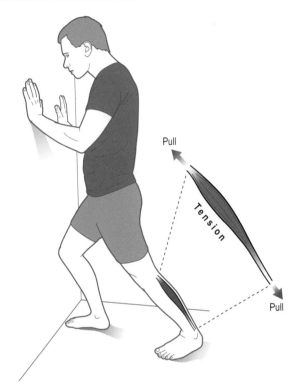

Fig. 5.4 Tensile Force on a Muscle.

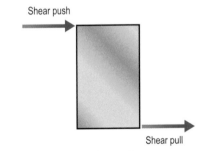

Fig. 5.5 Shear Stress.

but this time it is directed away from the body, for example, if you pulled a spring open or stretched a balloon or elastic band (Fig. 5.3).

When you think about it, lots of the bits in your body are subjected to pulling stress, tendons endure tensile stress with every muscle contraction. This even occurs when the body part is moved passively (Fig. 5.4). Next time you are walking home from the supermarket holding bags of shopping in both hands at least you will now know that the uncomfortable feeling in your shoulders is due to the tensile stress produced by the downward pull of the bags.

Shear Stress

Shear stress is a little more difficult to explain. It can be either a push or a pull, but it is applied **parallel** to a specified plane of a body. So, it acts parallel to a given surface rather than perpendicular to it as in the case of tensile and compressive (Fig. 5.5). Try Activity Box 5.1; it might help you to understand.

ACTIVITY BOX 5.1

Applying shear stress causes individual layers of a material within the body to slide over each other (even if this is microscopically). Get a large book like one of the Harry Potter tomes. A deck of cards would also work (although not as well) if gambling, not reading, is your preference.

Lie the book on a roughish surface (so it won't slide) and press along the top of the front cover as indicated in Fig. 5.6. If you do it correctly you should see the pages of the book slide on top of each other, stopped eventually by the binding. Be careful not to push too far back because you will damage the binding.

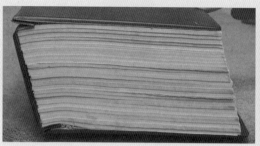

Fig. 5.6 Shear stress, Activity Box 5.1.

Shear stress is experienced by lots of different body structures depending on what you are doing. For example, think about yourself right now sitting on a chair. If you slide down the chair, a little of the skin on your back (if you were resting on a backrest) and buttocks will experience shear stress, the top surface being stretched, and the layers underneath sliding on each other, just like the pages of the book (see Fig. 5.6). If friction is minimal and the layers are allowed to slide, then fine; however, if there is friction between the layers there is the possibility they can become crumpled, causing damage and loss of function.

Basically, if one body slides across the surface of another then shear stress will result. The parts of the body that experience this most often, and with high forces, are the joint surfaces. The articular cartilage that lines the joint surfaces is designed specifically to cope with shear stress. 'It attempts' to cope with shear stress by reducing the friction between the layers as they slide over each other; this reduces any crumpling effect (more on this later).

Most joints don't function as a simple hinge joint (Fig. 5.7), there are additional rotations (spin) as well as translation (sliding) forward/backward and side to side (Fig. 5.8). This is covered in more detail in Chapter 7. These movements are important to the mobility (and health) of the joint, but create **shear forces** on the joint surface.

Bending stress is a mixture of compressive and tensile stress. Imagine sitting on a beam of wood balanced between two chairs (not sure when you would do this but try to imagine). You would expect the beam to bend a little in the

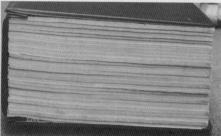

Fig. 5.7 Hinge.

middle (depending on its flexibility and your mass) (Fig. 5.9). What's happening in the beam is that the top layers of wood are being pushed together: compression, while the bottom layers are pulled apart: tension. This difference means that the layers of the material must slide on each other, that is, shear stress must also occur during bending.

Bending forces are a frequent occurrence for bones in the body. Consider the head of the femur when loaded (Fig. 5.10).

Torsional stress or rotational stress. You could think of torsional stress like the twisting force you might use to break off a bit of soft candy or a chunk of French bread. This twisting motion actually results in shear stresses at different points on the body and in different directions (Fig. 5.11).

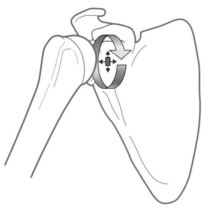

Fig. 5.8 Translation and Spin of the Humerus in the Shoulder.

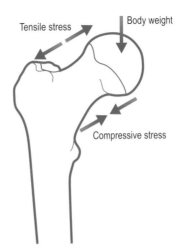

Fig. 5.10 Stresses on Head of Femur.

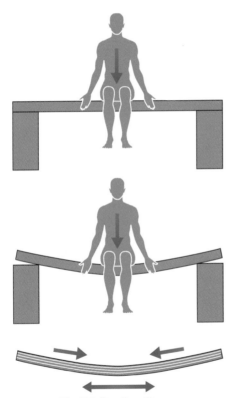

Fig. 5.9 Bending Stress.

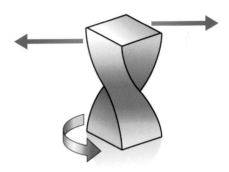

Fig. 5.11 Torsional Stress.

Let's see if you can remember all that with a quick test. Identify the type of stress in the following situations.

A. The foot when running

When your foot strikes the ground while you are running it is typically the metatarsal heads (ball of feet) that touch the ground first (although this does depend on how fast you run).

So what kind of stress do you think the tissue (skin, bursa, tendons and fatty pads) under the metatarsal heads experiences at foot strike?

As the foot strikes the ground there will be large forces generated as the momentum of the body is rapidly reduced. This braking force will be felt in different directions (vertical, side to side, and forwards and back) because the momentum of the body existed in these directions. The vertical and anteroposterior directions are shown in Fig. 5.12.

- What kind of stress does the anteroposterior (parallel) component cause at the metatarsal heads?
  - Bending
  - Torsional
  - Shear
  - Compressive
- What kind of stress does the vertical component cause at the metatarsal heads?
  - Bending
  - Torsional

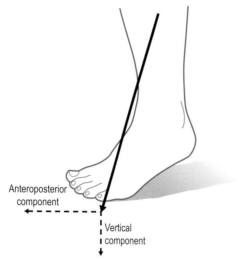

Fig. 5.12 Forces at the Metatarsal Heads When Jogging.

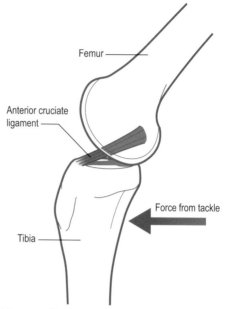

Fig. 5.13 The Anterior Cruciate Under Stress.

- Shear
- Compressive
- What could happen with repetitive application of these stresses?

B. A blow to back of knee

Imagine you are attending a game of soccer. You see a particularly bad tackle with one player kicking the back of the knee of another player causing his tibia to slide forward on the femur.

- What type of stress is experienced by the articular surface from the movement of the tibia?
- What type of stress does the anterior cruciate experience? The anterior cruciate is a strong ligament that is orientated to prevent the tibia sliding forward, as indicated in Fig. 5.13.
- What do you think could happen to the anterior cruciate with this kind of stress? Answers are at end of the chapter.

Now look at Activity Box 5.2.

Ok, we have talked about different kinds of stress, now let's consider the effects of stress.

Strain

Strain is another word that is used by many professionals; for example, a medical doctor might say 'you have strained your ankle ligament' as well as everyday language: 'the last couple of weeks have been a real strain'. In material science, it specifically relates to the change in shape of a body, this could be lengthening, which is positive strain; or compression, which is negative strain. It is calculated by dividing the change in dimension, for example, length, by the original dimension.

So basically, strain is the relative change in shape of a body under stress.

For example, let's say you have an elastic band which is 12 cm long when unstretched (lying on the table in front of you). You pick it up and stretch it between your hands (tensile stress) and of course it increases in length let's say to 17 cm, which means it changes by 5 cm (17 to 12 cm). The strain then would be 5 (change in length)/12 (original length) = 0.42, which we convert to a percentage, so the strain would be 42%.

This strain, caused by tension, is called tensile strain, as there was an increase in length. An important part of this process is the change in the energy state of the elastic band; now that you have stretched it, it has potential energy due to its elasticity. If you let it go it would ping back. Every child knows this as they draw their catapult back ready to launch another attack. We call this elastic potential energy. See previous chapter for a review on the way we store elastic potential energy to help us walk more efficiently.

Compressive strain occurs due to compressive stress. The stress acts on the body to reduce its size. Calculating this is a little trickier than tensile. Imagine you find a bit of children's play putty and you try to get it back into its container, except it is already full, so first you need to make some space in the container by pushing down (compressing) (Fig. 5.15).

Let's say the height of the putty in the container before was 10 cm. You press down and it reduces to 8 cm. There

ACTIVITY BOX 5.2

When you have your next meal make it a big burger, or any big sandwich, and when you bite down onto it think about the stress you are applying (Fig. 5.14). Compression at the front where you bite and tension at the back where it probably opens up. This will probably result in the ketchup or other content falling onto the table or, more annoyingly, onto your lap. This has occurred due to the difference in pressure between the front and back of the burger; we will look more at movement within the body due to pressure differences later in the chapter.

Does this hamburger analogy bring to mind any part of the body?

The intervertebral discs experience much the same pattern of stress application, but in this instance, it won't be the ketchup that moves, it will be the centre of the vertebral disc: the nucleus pulposus. This can result in low back pain.

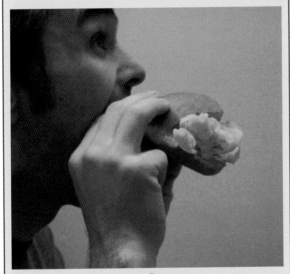

Fig. 5.14 Stress of Eating a Burger.

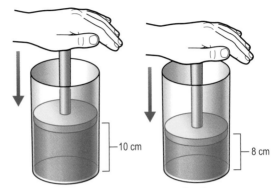

Fig. 5.15 Compressive Strain.

ACTIVITY BOX 5.3 **Energy From Compression**

There is also energy stored due to compression. Get a bicycle pump (a syringe would also work; Fig. 5.16). Put your finger over the end of the pump and press the piston in. What you are doing is compressing the air; the movement of the chamber is the compressive strain. When you can go no further, take your hand of the piston.

What you should have found was that the piston bounced back. This is due to the stored potential energy within the compressed air. The same effect works for a bouncing ball; as it collides with the ground, the force compresses the ball (Fig. 5.17). This energy is then released to push it into the air. Some similar mechanisms are used in human movement (see Chapter 4).

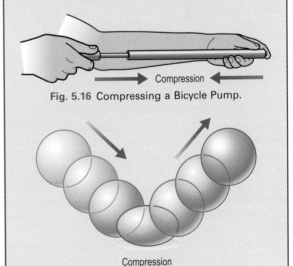

Compression

Fig. 5.16 Compressing a Bicycle Pump.

Compression

Fig. 5.17 Compression of a Bouncing Ball.

was a reduction in height. Compressive strain is therefore 2/10 cm giving 20%; however, this is a negative value because it reduced in size. (Try Activity Box 5.3.)

Shear strain is more difficult to describe. It is measured by the amount of slide that occurs between the layers in the layers. This would be an extraordinarily difficult thing to measure at each layer so the body is regarded as one. The strain is more or less regarded as the overall change in the angle of the body due to the displacement (slide) of all the layers (Fig. 5.18).

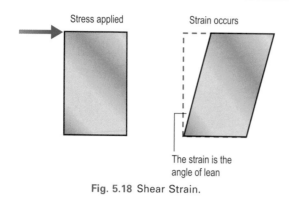

Fig. 5.18 Shear Strain.

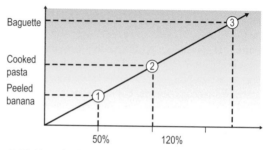

Fig. 5.19 Stress–Strain Relationship With an Elastic Band.

Now we understand stress, which is like force, and strain, which is the change in shape of the body, compressed, lengthened or distorted in some way. The way that a material strains when stressed will depend on many things: how much material there is, what the material consists of, at a microscopic level, and how it is organised. Clearly it is important to understand this relationship between stress and strain. It can tell us why and how the material will break down and how we can best restore its function.

Stress–Strain Relationship and Stiffness

Ok, let's get that elastic band back (unless you broke it with too much stress). We are going to be a bit more empirical (measure things) here and plot a graph. You probably don't have any special instruments to measure the amount of stress we will apply, but you can measure strain with a simple ruler. Put your finger through one end of the elastic band and hook it onto the ruler so that this end of the rubber band is fixed. Hold the other end with your other hand. Record the length when you are just holding it there, pulling slightly perhaps to straighten out any folds. We are now going to explore the stress–strain relationship by stretching the elastic band (Fig. 5.19).

TABLE 5.1 **Recording the stress strain relationship**	
Stress	**Strain (increase in length)**
1	1 cm
2	
3	
4	

Fig. 5.20 Hypothetical Stress–Strain Relationship of an Elastic Band.

But first, in the absence of proper instruments, we have to come up with a way of quantifying (putting a number to it) how much pull (tensile stress) we apply. How about using food analogies? So, apply the following stresses to the elastic and record the length of the elastic band at each stress application in a table that looks like Table 5.1.

Stress 1. Pull on the elastic band with the amount you would need to pull apart a soft peeled banana.

Stress 2. Pull on the elastic band with the amount you would need to pull apart a piece of cooked pasta.

Stress 3. Pull on the elastic band with the amount you would need to pull apart a French baguette.

If you then plot these values you might get something that looks like Fig. 5.20

In Fig. 5.20 stress has been plotted up the Y axis and strain along the X axis. Remember that strain has been converted into a percentage: the change in length divided by the original length and multiplied by 100. If you join up the points you will have constructed a stress strain curve. These curves are the cornerstone of material science and the subject of a lot of research. They provide a lot of information about a material. They tell you the **stiffness** of a material. **Stiffness** is a word used generally to mean inflexibility. It's more or less used in the same way in material science but has a more precise definition. It is the ratio between stress and strain; that is:

Stiffness = Stress/Strain.

This is also known as Young's modulus and is often represented by the letter E.

For those among you who prefer pictures to equations, this ratio is the same as the gradient (angle) of the slope. In Fig. 5.21 there are three stress strain curves including our rubber band. The higher the slope the stiffer the material. This is because there is less movement along the X axis (strain) for the same or greater stress (movement up the Y axis). So material A is stiffer than B, and B is stiffer than C (which could, e.g. be our rubber band).

Let's look again at a typical stress strain. The graph below (Fig. 5.22) is the stress strain graph of a copper wire. As you can see the graph has two different slopes divided around the point Y. This is the yield point when the material starts to give; it is essentially tearing. Before this point the material is undamaged, and if you stopped stressing it before the yield point it will return to its original shape and properties; this is the **elastic** phase. The change in length during this period is down to separation at atomic level, the bonds weaken a little or may separate allowing some movement but not a great deal. So, the slope is higher at this stage, that is, 'it is' stiffer.

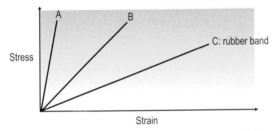

Fig. 5.21 Stress–Strain Plots of Materials With Different Stiffness Values.

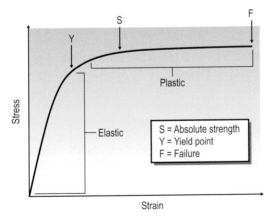

Fig. 5.22 Stress–Strain Curve of a Copper Wire.

After the yield point, the material behaves differently; this is the **plastic** phase. The material behaves a little like plasticine in this phase; it has lost a lot of its stiffness allowing quite a lot of lengthening and, like plasticine, it won't return to its original shape or properties when you remove the stress. If you stress material beyond the yield point into the plastic phase, you have basically damaged it. It now has irreparably broken atomic bonds, and it won't be the same again.

The way that stress is applied will influence the stress–strain relationship. In particular how fast it is applied alters the stiffness of the material. To understand this let's conduct a short experiment.

Get a cheap plastic shopping bag (or just a piece of very thin cheap plastic) and hold it in both hands. Now pull as quickly as you can (i.e. apply a rapid tensile stress). If you are strong enough and the bag is cheap enough you should have torn the bag. Now get another bag and perform the same movement, only this time do it slowly; build up the strength of your pull slowly. This time you should have found that the bag lengthens (or strains) more.

So, why did the bag strain more when the stress was applied slowly? The answer lies in something called **viscosity**. This relates to the ability of all materials to **flow**; the **more** viscous it is the **less** ability it has to flow. Water is not very viscous, steel is highly viscous (but it can still flow!). Without getting too involved in the chemistry, it's to do with how strongly the molecules in the material are bonded together as well as how closely they are packed together.

When materials (gases and fluids included) flow they do so by one layer gliding on the one below (Fig. 5.23). This is called laminar flow (think of a steady stream from a tap) as opposed to turbulent flow where the layers all mix up (like a tap turned on full or the white water of a river). We are going to talk a lot more about gases and fluids later in the chapter.

The ability to flow is an important feature of materials and one you can exploit when trying to stretch out bubble gum or a muscle (we will start talking about human tissues soon—all this food talk can be distracting). The plastic bag demonstrated its viscosity when you applied the stress slowly; the material literally flowed. Of course, you don't want too much flowing going on in your plastic bag, otherwise you would be dragging your shopping bags along the ground

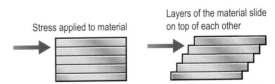

Fig. 5.23 Layers of a Material Glide (Flow) on Each Other.

by the time you got home. Clearly it would be advisable to use paper bags, which are more viscous (i.e. they won't flow so well) and more environmentally friendly!

Other Properties of Materials

Another important characteristic of materials and one which is critical to engineering is **fatigue.** You may have heard of metal fatigue in relation to a building or the wings of an aircraft which are constantly checked for signs of fatigue. Fatigue is structural damage (which could be minor, e.g. microscopic splits) resulting from repetitive application of stress. This is analogous to stress fractures in a very physically active person.

Material strength: this is the amount of stress a material can endure before breaking. It is also known as the absolute strength (see Fig. 5.22) and is essentially the highest point in a stress strain graph.

Thixotropy: this is a really interesting property of materials and one that many sports and rehabilitation practitioners can exploit (even unwittingly), so pay attention.

You have probably struggled to get to that last bit of tomato sauce stuck at the bottom of the bottle. You might try to use gravity by tipping it up but nothing is moving, so you give it a good shake and tip it up again. This time it begins to flow. The sauce has become **less resistant** to flow (i.e. less viscous) out of the bottle, because you agitated it. This property of the sauce is called thixotropy and is not just a special property of sticky sauces. In fact, most materials behave in this way, at least to some degree.

What is happening is that the energy you have transferred to the material, by shaking, has unbonded molecules and possibly uncurled coils of long-chain molecules, making them more able to slide against one another, so the layers move on top of each other more easily. Put another way, there is less friction between the layers. There are lots of materials that behave in this manner; clay, for example, is thixotropic, which poses problems for houses made of clay especially during an earthquake. The walls of a shaking house will soon start to slide down.

The word thixotropy, comes from the Greek language, the word 'thixis', which means to touch/manipulate and 'tropy', which means to change, so thixotropic means a substance that changes due to being handled.

Of course, another way to make a material flow more easily is to heat it up. This is still thixotropy. If you get a bit of sticky tack (e.g. blue tack) in your hand and start to roll it around in your hand it will soon become more malleable 'as it warms.' This property of a material may not always be desirable; the steel cables in a bridge would be useless if they started to strain more easily in summer. Tarmac that starts to flow in the warm weather plays havoc with traffic. So, you have to know 'how much' the material you are

interested in changes viscosity when heated. But there are also obvious advantages: just think of the difference in your flexibility after a warm bath compared to when you wake up after a night camping in the Scottish Highlands, more on this later.

Summary of Material Science Basics

Materials are not rigid, they change shape (strain) when force (or rather stress) is applied. Stress can be applied in different directions: compressive, which squashes; tensile, which stretches; shear, which crumples; and torsional, which twists the material. These stresses can exist at the same time; for example, if a beam bends there is a combination of compressive, tensile and shear stresses. Strain is the amount that the material changes shape as a result of the stress.

The amount of stress needed to cause a certain amount of strain tells you how **stiff** a material is. Stiffness is the ratio between stress and strain, or 'simply' stress divided by strain. This is also known as modulus of elasticity or Young's modulus.

If a material returns to the same shape after a stress was applied then the stress was within the material's elastic phase; if more stress is applied and the material has changed its shape on release then the stress was in the plastic range. So, there is a limit for applying stress, after which the material will undergo permanent change. This limit is also called the yield point.

When stress is applied to materials over time then the material is allowed to flow. This depends on it is viscosity (resistance to flow), which can change with temperature and agitation; a property known as thixotropy. Some materials flow more easily than others.

CONNECTIVE TISSUE

We have talked about materials generally, but what about the materials that make up our bodies? What they are made from and how they behave when loaded is exactly what we are going to cover next.

Composition and Mechanical Properties of Connective Tissue

The human body is built from a range of different tissues. Some are highly specialised, like the brain and eye; and others are more basic (if you can call them that), like ligaments and skin. The way in which these biological materials behave is not so dissimilar to the materials we have talked about so far, with some obvious differences, such as the ability to repair itself. So, let's get on with talking about the materials that make up the human body.

The structure and strength of the body comes from connective tissue. This includes a range of materials such as bone, tendon, ligament, capsule and skin. Connective tissue also provides the strength and structure for our organs, such as the pericardium of the heart or the walls of blood vessels and the lungs. As we are more interested in posture 'and' movement we will focus on the dense connective tissues of the musculoskeletal system, what it consists of and how it behaves when stressed.

Connective tissue contains of three basic ingredients that vary in amount according to the function of the structure.

Ground Substance

Ground substance is a shapeless gelatinous goo that surrounds the connective tissue fibres and cells. It is a loose combination of carbohydrates, proteins and water (lots of water). The purpose of this goo is both to nourish and to lubricate the connective tissue so that the fibres can easily slide over each other. It is the ground substance that gives the connective tissues its viscous (and thixotropic) properties.

Fibres

There are two main fibres in connective tissue: collagen and elastin, with collagen being the most prevalent.

Collagen Fibres

The word collagen derives from the Greek word for glue (Kolla) and source (gen). Quite literally it is the substance that gives us glue (after it is has been boiled up!). In addition to producing glue, boiling up collagen also gives us gelatine, the basic ingredient of those delicious gummy sweeties. It's the conversion of collagen to gelatine when you roast some meat that makes the meat tender. Collagen is also now widely used for a variety of beauty treatments, for example, plumping up lips and smoothing wrinkles. Useful stuff indeed.

There are many types of collagen (approximately 28) although most are classified into four types (Table 5.2 for details). They are constructed slightly differently from each other according to the type of function they perform. The basic unit of collagen is the tropocollagen molecule; this is formed from three intertwined polypeptide chains (Fig. 5.24), which are a series of joined-up proteins. The best way to describe how the collagen fibres are constructed from this basic unit is to liken it to how rope is constructed. The basic units of rope (threads of either cotton, hemp or jute) are bunched together into yarns. The yarns (usually there are three, although bigger ropes may use more yarns) are then twisted together to make the rope (Fig. 5.25). So, the strength of rope comes from the way it is woven together; individual threads may break but the rope will still be intact.

Collagen is more or less made the same way as rope: tropocollagen fibres bunched into microfibrils, which are then organised into subfibrils, and ultimately the *rope* of collagen. A notable difference between rope and collagen is that at the subfibril level of organisation the gooey substance (ground substance) separates the subfibrils. This confers different mechanical qualities on collagen compared to rope, giving it a greater ability to flow when placed under stress. We will talk more about this later.

The organised structure of collagen gives connective tissue its shape and a lot of its strength. The volume of fibres varies according to how strong the tissue 'needs' to be. So, tissue requiring a lot of strength, such as a tendon, will have a lot of collagen tightly packed together, whereas other tissues that do not have to accommodate these large stresses will have less collagen, and 'will, perhaps, be more loosely organised.'

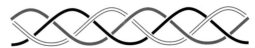

Fig. 5.24 Intertwining Tropocollagen Molecule.

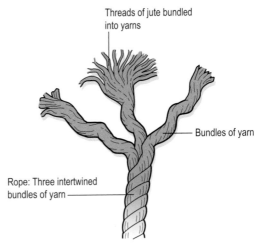

Fig. 5.25 Rope Is Made From Intertwined Bundles of Thread.

TABLE 5.2	Main types of collagen	
Type	Location	Function
1	Tendon, skin, artery walls, scar tissue, bones	Tensile strength and shape
2	Articular cartilage, fibrocartilage	Strength, including shear and compression
3	Granulation tissue	Early scaffold during tissue repair
4	Lens of eye and basal membrane	Structure and strength

Elastic Fibres

Connective tissue must also be elastic; to stretch a little when stressed and be able to return to normal when the stress is removed. Although collagen has some elastic qualities, most of the elastic properties of connective tissue comes from elastic fibres. These fibres are present in many connective tissues to varying degrees, depending on how much elasticity is required. Think about all the bits of your body that are repeatedly stretched and then immediately return to their original size, for example, skin, lungs and blood vessels.

Can you think of any other part of the body that regularly undergoes a change in shape before snapping back?

Elastic fibres are primarily made of bundles of elastin, which is a kind of coil of various amino acids; this coiled shape mean the fibres will return to their original shape after being stretched. You could think of them as small, but fairly weak springs. They can be arranged either in a haphazard manner or more regularly, according to the direction that they are regularly stretched in, which will depend on the function of the tissue. For example, skin requires elasticity in multiple directions, whereas a tendon has a single direction of stretch, that is, along the direction of the muscle pull.

Cells

Finally, there are three main cells in connective tissue that perform a range of functions critical to the health and continued development of the tissue. These cells are:
1. Fibroblasts, which produce the fibres '(collagen and elastin)' and ground substance.
2. Macrophages, which are phagocytes; basically, they are little cannibals eating up any dead cells and other debris resulting from an infection or tissue damage.
3. Neutrophils (white blood cells) are the cells that arrive first at a site of infection, attacking and neutralising microbes. Some types of white blood cells will also produce the necessary antibodies to fight infection.

These basic constituents of connective tissue appear in different amounts and arrangements in our connective tissues, in the same way that different amounts and types of wood might be used in the construction of a building. The steel used to make the spring in a child's toy has been worked into a specific shape, but it is still the same steel used in the construction of an aeroplane. The same material in different volumes and shapes serves many different functions.

With this in mind, let's look at some of the main bits of connective tissue in a bit more detail starting with the largest part of our musculoskeletal system, the skin.

Skin

It might be worth starting this section with a quick demonstration. Straighten your arm out with palm up. Now pinch about 1 cm of the skin on your forearm and pull it so that your skin lifts a little from your arm, but not enough that it hurts you. Now let go. You applied a tensile force to the skin and on release it immediately returned to its shape without any harm. This is elasticity. Try to do the same thing at different locations on your forearm and try different directions of pull. Neither should matter; your skin will always snap back when you remove the stress no matter in which direction you pulled it. This means the mechanical property of skin is isotropic: it's the same regardless of direction. Anisotropic, on the other hand, is where the strength and elasticity are better in one direction than another.

Understanding the ability of the skin to recoil after being stretched has obvious implications for professionals working in burns and plastics, as well as cosmetic surgery. However, it is also relevant to those of you interested in increasing joint flexibility. The skin around a joint has to be flexible enough for the joint to move.

To demonstrate this, grab a handful (well, as much you can) of the skin on the front of your elbow while it is bent. Now try to straighten it. Inextensible scar tissue will cause a similar restriction in joint movement. You may also be interested in understanding how skin is damaged during sports participation; the skin on the sole of the feet, for example, experiences large compressive and shear forces during many sports. Of course, the same could be said for the hands during racket sports, rowing, rock climbing etc. There are lots of good reasons to better understand skin, so let's get on with looking at what skin is made of and what its function is.

Skin has three layers: the epidermis, dermis and hypodermis. The topmost layer, the epidermis is mainly concerned with providing a protective (and weatherproof) barrier for the body, rather like a biological Gore-Tex.

Beneath the epidermis lies the dermis. This is the layer where the real mechanical characteristics of skin are contained. As well as glands and hair follicles, the dermis contains an irregular pattern of dense connective tissue. Its irregularity is important as skin needs strength and elasticity in different directions; remember, we called this isotropy. So no matter which way it is pulled and pushed it will have the same strength. The final layer, the hypodermis, is a transient layer that connects the skin to the underlying fat tissue.

The fat underneath the skin not only helps to keep you warm in winter, but also it has some mechanical properties, particularly in coping with compressive stress at contact points. This is best illustrated by the calcaneal fat pads, which are positioned under the heel to perform like springs when the heel strikes the ground, allowing some cushioning to parts of the body that experience large compressive stresses, a bit like the springs in a mattress (Fig. 5.26). Chapter 17

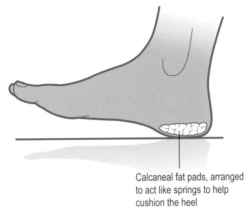

Calcaneal fat pads, arranged
to act like springs to help
cushion the heel

Fig. 5.26 Calcaneal Fat Pads at Heel Strike.

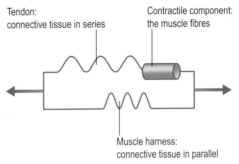

Tendon:
connective tissue in series

Contractile component:
the muscle fibres

Muscle harness:
connective tissue in parallel

Fig. 5.27 Hill's Model of Muscle.

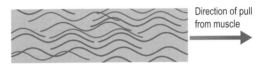

Direction of pull
from muscle

Fig. 5.28 Collagen Arrangement in Tendon.

includes a case study looking at other mechanisms the body uses to reduce these forces.

Muscle

Experiments have demonstrated that the structure most likely to cause a loss of flexibility at joints is the muscle; shortened muscles are frequently found in clinical conditions, such as arthritis and stroke, as well as affecting performance in sport and increasing the risk of further injury. Therefore, it is worth spending a little time on the structure of muscle, particularly the connective tissue components.

Muscle can be separated into two different functional parts: (1) the contractile part and (2) the connective tissue part, which gives the muscle its passive mechanical properties. The contractile component is the part that creates tension within the muscle through the bonding and unbonding of the myosin protein to the actin protein. The resulting tension is translated to the bone via the tendon. In chapter 6, we will look more closely at how muscles actively contract, but for now let's stick to the passive connective tissue.

The connective tissue in muscle is in two places: (1) at the end of the muscle, that is, the tendon, which is also called **series connective tissue** because it lies at either end, and (2) the muscle harness, which is made of sheaths of connective tissue that wrap around the contractile component, and is sometimes called the **parallel connective tissue** because it lies parallel to the muscle fibres. This name also differentiates it from the tendon (series connective tissue). This structure of muscle is shown diagrammatically in Fig. 5.27. Because it was first described by the English physiologist Archibald Vivian Hill, in 1938, it is known as Hill's model of muscle. We will look at muscle structure and function in more detail in the next chapter.

Tendon

The primary function of a tendon is to transfer the pulling force of a muscle to the attached bone. This may be to create a moment big enough to move a joint through an arc of movement or enough tension to maintain a bone's position whilst another part of the body performs an action.

In accordance with the principle that the shape and structure of a tissue is dictated by its function (form follows function) the collagen fibres of a muscle tendon are both densely packed (to provide strength) and arranged in straight lines according to the direction of the tensile stresses placed on the tendon (Fig. 5.28) from the muscle pull.

You may have noticed in Fig. 5.28 that although the collagen fibres are lined up parallel to each other, they are wavy and not straight at all. This wavy pattern is widely observed in connective tissue (particularly tendon) and is referred to as the 'crimp'. It creates a specific feature of the stress–strain curve called the toe region, which we will talk about shortly. As we have said, a tendon needs to be strong and stiff enough to transfer the tensile forces, created by the muscle, to the bone. However, it also needs to strain (or give) to some extent when pulled and then be able to return to its original shape (and mechanical properties) when the pull ends, that is, it has to have elasticity. This is an important characteristic of a tendon as it allows the body to absorb some of the forces created during movement, thereby reducing the potential risk of damage from large forces. As it returns to its original shape the released elastic potential energy can be used to assist the muscle in generating tension.

The way the body uses the elastic energy stored in tendons is now understood to be an important property of the

ACTIVITY BOX 5.4

As we have said, being at the end of the muscle, the tendon will experience large amounts of tensile stress. Take the tendon of the gluteus medius (hip abductor) for example (Fig. 5.29). Stand up and abduct your leg (lift your leg out to the side). The muscle shortens, thanks to the contractile component. This pulls on the tendon, which is fixed to the greater trochanter of the femur. This force overcomes the leg's inertia and it lifts up. As the leg lifts off the ground, the muscle then has to create forces to contend with the adducting moment caused by the mass of the leg (centred approximately at the knee) moving out to the side away from the hip joint.

Now keep your leg out to the side. Just like the plastic bags containing your shopping, you don't want your tendon to start lengthening despite the tensile stress from the muscle pulling it up and the leg pulling it down. The tendon must be stiff enough to resist this persistent tensile stress. How much more stress can the tendon take? Would it make any difference if you performed the movement 20 times? And what would happen if you held it there for 15 minutes (aside from the muscle fatigue)?

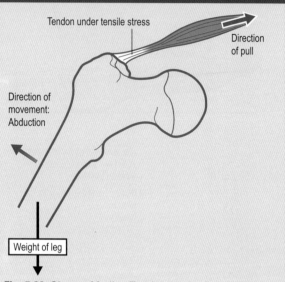

Fig. 5.29 Gluteus Medius Tendon Under Tensile Stress.

musculoskeletal system. Although difficult to measure in live humans, the elastic energy stored in the Achilles tendon, and the ligaments and tendons of the arch of the foot, has been estimated to contribute around half of the mechanical work of walking (Alexander and Bennet-Clark, 1977, Ker et al. 1987), this was also discussed in Chapter 4.

When you apply a passive stretch to a muscle, most of the change in overall length occurs outwith the contractile part of the muscle, that is, in the tendon and muscle harness (Herbert et al. 2002), which is something to bear in mind when you are next stretching someone's muscle.

The only way to answer the questions in Activity Box 5.4 is to look at the stress–strain relationship of the human tendon through experiments like our previous stress–strain experiment with the rubber band. Experiments on human tissue are typically done on dead tissue (for obvious reasons); nevertheless, they offer valuable information for those of you engaged in improving flexibility as well as restoring muscle function.

Fig. 5.30 shows a typical stress strain relationship for human tendon. In many ways it resembles the stress–strain relationships of other materials, for example, copper wire (see Fig. 5.22). It has a yield point and elastic and plastic phases, but it's generally more complex with extra phases. Let's look at it in more detail (see Fig. 5.30), starting at the bottom of the slope, which is called the toe region.

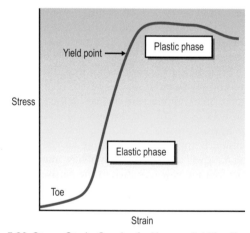

Fig. 5.30 Stress Strain Graph of a Human Achilles Tendon.

The toe region is a consistent finding in studies of the tendon and the ligament in particular, but is not really found in nonbiological tissues. In the toe region there is a less stiff (more compliant) response to stress, that is, the tissue elongates more easily. It appears that during this phase the tissue loses its crimp (see Fig. 5.28). It is a bit like pulling the ends of a sheet to stretch it over a bed; in doing this, any creases or folds in the sheet smooth out, just like the crimp in connective tissue. Some studies suggest that the force required to uncrimp a tendon is similar to the amount experienced during normal activities (Maganaris and Paul, 1999, Buckley et al. 2013). You can imagine the tissue moving in and out of its wavy pattern as you move around.

The elastic phase is similar to that described for other materials; that is, as more stress is applied, gradually more and more fibres become involved. You could imagine a tug of war team. The competitors take up the slack in the rope (uncrimping of the tendon), and then as the two teams begin to pull, more and more team members become engaged in the battle; this is the elastic phase. It is important to remember that during these first two phases (toe and elastic) the tissue has not been damaged, and that when the stress is taken off the tissue will return to its previous shape AND its previous properties, that is, you haven't changed its shape or weakened it. You can use the slope of the stress–strain curve during the elastic phase to calculate the stiffness of the tendon, dividing stress by strain.

The curve begins to change at the yield point. We have reached the point where damage to fibres is now taking place and the tissue begins to lose its ability to resist the stress, like an Indiana Jones film with the hero halfway across the bridge and the rope begins to fray and unwind. He knows there is only a little time left before the bridge breaks and he plummets to the ground. The tendon is no different; continue to apply the stress and the tendon will break. After the yield point, if you take the stress away the tissue will be permanently damaged (well as least until it repairs itself). It is weaker, less stiff and possibly longer. Of course, making the tissue longer may be your intention, and we'll talk a bit more about this later.

The Muscle Harness

This may not be an expression you are familiar with but it is a useful way of describing the connective tissue that surrounds the contractile units in parallel, as opposed to a tendon, which is at the end of a muscle (i.e. in series). In yet another well-organised structure, muscle fibres are parcelled together by connective tissue into fascicles; groups of fascicles are then held together by more connective tissue (the endomysium), which are further bunched into bigger groups by yet more connective tissue (the perimysium); and finally, a sheath of connective tissue surrounds the whole muscle; this is the epimysium. Together all this connective tissue makes up the muscle harness. The word harness is useful here because it holds the muscle together and helps channel the force created by the muscle, just like a horse's harness. In many ways it behaves like the tendon. Although strength is its main attribute, the muscle harness also behaves viscoelastically; that is, it can flow when stressed over time and returns to its original shape when the stress is removed.

Bone

Let's move on to bone. This is a really interesting biological material, providing rigidity to our body, protecting our vital organs, and providing rigid beams for our muscles, to create and control movement. These are just bone's mechanical functions. Within the cavities of bone there is storage space for calcium, red and white blood cells, and platelets, which are all vital to the health and function of our body. However, as this is a book about movement, let's concentrate on the mechanical properties of bone.

There are many types of bones in your body, and lots of them (>200). We can't look at them all, so we will consider a typical long bone, such as the femur, and uncover some of its makeup so that we can understand its mechanical properties. But first, let's start with the basic composition of bone.

Bone is primarily formed from osseous (another word for bone) tissue. This is made from a combination of collagen and hard minerals (calcium, magnesium and phosphate), which make the bone rigid. Bone tissue is arranged into two broad types:

Spongy or cancellous bone (also called trabecular) is situated on the inside of a bone. It is arranged into a network of struts, a bit like scaffolding (except on the inside). Because of this arrangement it is very light (only around 20% of total bone mass) but crucially it is still strong. This natural design has long been imitated by engineers. You only need to glance at the Forth Road bridge in Edinburgh to see this. Perhaps there are buildings or bridges in your area that imitate the crisscross struts of cancellous bone.

Hard compact bone provides the hard, white outer layer of bone, surrounding the cancellous bone. It is very dense (packed closely together), so it is a very tough structure, good for withstanding impacts as well as the pull of muscles, so this part of the bone serves a protective function. When you think about it, the structure of bone is a bit like a Malteser chocolate sweet: a shell of hard, compact chocolate on the outside and a light honeycomb inside, with lots of little struts, see Fig. 5.31.

So, what are the mechanical properties of bone?

The compact bone (hard outer shell) on the outside makes bone very tough, which is great for resisting direct blows (to protect your brain and internal organs), as well as shear and bending stress from external forces and the pull of tendons and ligaments. The matrix network of the cancellous bone means it is light (essential for efficient movement). However, because it is constructed from minerals as well as collagen, it is rigid, making it very good at resisting compressive forces without deforming. Bone is not so good, however, at resisting tensile forces and because of its high mineral content it is relatively brittle; that is, although it

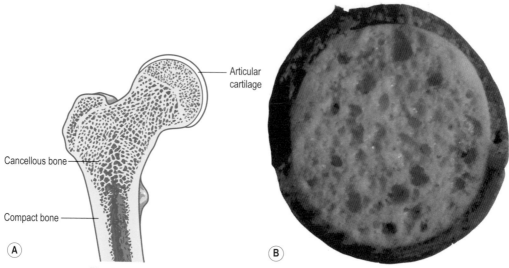

Fig. 5.31 Types of bone (A) and a Malteser (B) of Bone and a Malteser.

has high strength it cannot flow as well as tendon and skin, so it cannot absorb a lot of energy. It is therefore more prone to complete disruption—fracture.

Articular Cartilage

At the ends of bone is the articular cartilage. Articular cartilage is a highly specialised connective tissue constructed from chondrocytes (cartilage cells), collagen and water. It doesn't include either blood vessels or nerves. It has three main functions:

- Withstanding compressive loading
- Distributing load; and
- Decreasing friction

It achieves these functions with its structure, which echoes that of skin. It is arranged into four zones. The top zone (tangential layer) has lots of water and thin collagen fibres laid parallel to the surface in multiple directions (like skin). The chondrocytes in this top layer are flat and packed reasonably close together. The orientation of the collagen is important to cope with the shear forces as the bones glide on top of each other. The high water content in this zone helps to reduce friction in the same way that a layer of water in an ice hockey rink makes it even more slippery.

In the next zone (transition layer), the collagen fibres become less parallel, and are directed more obliquely up and down with the chondrocytes more rounded. This helps the tissue to cope more with compressive forces. The third zone (radial layer) is engineered to absorb a lot of the compressive strain, for example, from weight bearing, with the chondrocytes arranged vertically into columns or stacks, and the collagen fibres lined up alongside them. The final

zone (calcified cartilage) marks the transition between cartilage and bone (Fig. 5.32).

Tissue Remodelling

One of the most fascinating aspects of bone (and indeed all connective tissue) is its ability to remodel. This ability was first described in bone and was called Wolff's law after the 19th-century Austrian physician, Julius Wolff. Basically, this law states that bone adapts to the forces placed on them. Bone tissue is constantly being created and reabsorbed; this is called bone turnover. It's a bit like filling a bath with the plug out. As you pour water in, it drains away down the plug; a point can be reached where the amount of water going in the bath equals the amount going out, so the water level remains the same. You could change this state of equilibrium level by turning the taps or changing the size of the plug. In the same way, bone can adapt to a change in the forces it habitually experiences by increasing (opening the tap and closing the plug) or decreasing (closing the tap and opening the plug) the amount of bone tissue. It is worth stating that this adaptability of connective tissue lasts a lifetime.

If you place more stress regularly on one arm (e.g. if you take up javelin throwing or ten-pin bowling) then the bones of the that side will adapt to these additional forces by laying down more bone tissue (the taps open more and the plug closes a bit). Of course, the opposite can also happen; a decrease in force (e.g. having your arm in a sling) will trigger a reduction in bone density (the plug opens more and the tap closes a little), see Further Information 5.2 for a description on how astronauts cope with this problem. This ability

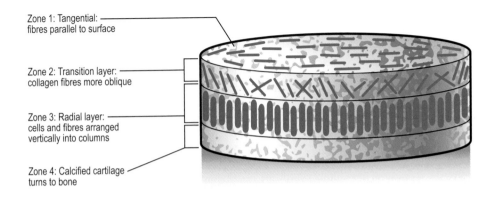

Zone 1: Tangential:
fibres parallel to surface

Zone 2: Transition layer:
collagen fibres more oblique

Zone 3: Radial layer:
cells and fibres arranged
vertically into columns

Zone 4: Calcified cartilage
turns to bone

Fig. 5.32 Zones of Articular Cartilage.

FURTHER INFORMATION 5.1

The field of palaeopathology has profited greatly by this ability of bone. This is a field of archaeology that concerns itself with studying human (and animal) skeletal remains, looking for signs of disease (like arthritis) as well as patterns of bone formation that might give some clues on the individual's occupation; for example, degeneration of the lower back might indicate someone involved in a lot of lifting. These skeletal markers of occupational stress have been used to identify people who used a hoe (like a spade) for farming due to the overdevelopment of the bone where the toe flexors attach, indicating that these muscles were very strong, which might have resulted from a lot of spade work. Similar approaches have been used to identify archers and hunters.

of bone became evident through careful examination of the cadavers of different people, modern and ancient (Further Information 5.1).

This turnover of bone tissue has more than one purpose: it also helps to regulate the level of calcium in the body. Bone turnover is also important in the repair of damaged bone tissue; bone is laid down at the site of damage (like a fracture) until the structure has become stable again before reducing and remodelling the additional bone.

The same thing occurs in other connective tissue, skin, tendon etc. These tissues are smart; they sense if more strength is required to cope with a change in the forces they experience and make the appropriate increase in the amount and organisation of the collagen fibres.

This ability of connective tissue to adapt to the forces they routinely experience is constantly exploited by sports

and rehabilitation professionals. We will talk about this at the end of the chapter, but for now think about what you are doing to connective tissue when you alter someone's posture, increase the volume of an athlete's training or place insoles in a shoe to alter the pattern of pressure in their feet.

There are a number of factors that affect the properties of connective tissue. In this next segment we are going to look at the effects of immobility, maturation, ageing, stretching and temperature.

Inactivity (Immobilisation)

We have already mentioned the role that activity/exercise has on connective tissue. The forces produced by activity provide the stimulus for bone growth, but what happens if you, or part of you (e.g. your arm or leg) are prevented from being active?

When immobilised, muscle quickly adapts to the position it is kept in. It does this by altering the number of muscle fibres (the contractile part) it has in series, the number of links in the chain. Like the captain of a tug of war team putting more or less men (or women) into the team, so it becomes longer or shorter. Basically, if a muscle is immobilised in its shortened position it will decrease in length. The connective tissue also adapts. Without the guiding stimulus of force, any new collagen produced in ligaments and tendons will be arranged haphazardly, and will be less dense and less regular when immobilised, like a squadron of soldiers dismissed at the end of a parade. While on parade they were all lined up, and were strong and organised. On the signal to dismiss they fell apart, and moved off in different directions. Connective tissue therefore becomes weaker. The tissue also becomes less flexible. This may seem a contradiction (weak and stiff) but the stiffness develops from more cross connections between the fibres as well as a loss of water in the ground substance through lack of movement.

Experiments have demonstrated that this weak and stiff connective tissue resulting from immobilisation takes up to 18 months to be fully restored (Martin et al. 2015).

Factors that make immobilisation worse are:

1. Prolonged and complete immobilisation.
2. Immobilisation following an injury, particularly if there is still swelling.
3. If the immobilised person is also old.
   (See Further Information 5.2.)

Maturation

As children mature the stability of the bonds within the tropocollagen molecules in collagen increases. Stronger bonds make the collagen more resistant to tensile stress. There are also increasing amounts of cross-linking between collagen fibres as children grow, which not only further strengthens the connective tissue but also makes it less flexible. Musculoskeletal tissue in children is typically more compliant because of the greater amount of water in the ground substance as well as having immature (less bonded) collagen fibres.

Effect of Ageing

The effect of ageing on connective tissue is actually quite similar to the effects of immobilisation; indeed, some people have argued that it is not ageing in itself but rather reduced levels of activity in older people that causes a lot of the so-called age-related deterioration in the musculoskeletal system.

Generally speaking, as we age there is a decrease in collagen turnover (creation and absorption of collagen). Collagen becomes thinner and is present in reduced amounts. The collagen fibres also become more attached to each other—cross-links—which can be helpful in stiffening up materials but also prevents them straining. This is compounded by a loss of water content in ground substance, which makes the tissue less capable of elongating.

Consequently, tissue becomes weaker and less able to lengthen, that is, it is more brittle and less able to absorb energy. However, just like immobilised tissue, these changes can be reversed, to some degree. For example, one study of older adults demonstrated a 65% improvement in stiffness following 14 weeks of exercise (Reeves et al. 2003).

Try Activity Box 5.5 and see Further Information 5.3 to find out more.

Effect of Recent History

It is traditional, and globally observed, that athletes stretch before a sporting activity, particularly if the activity requires

---

FURTHER INFORMATION 5.2

One of the many problems faced by astronauts/cosmonauts is the effect that lack of gravity has on their bone density. The main force that acts as a stimulant to bone development is our body weight, for which (if you remember from Chapter 3) we need gravity. Consequently, space flight has been shown to cause a decrease in bone density of around 2% per month. Not only is the bone less dense, but also the cancellous bone (the internal scaffolding) will start to lose its regular structure. This weakened bone obviously exposes space explorers to fractures, particularly when they have to contend with Earth's gravity again. (It takes up to and probably more than a year for bone strength to fully recover.) So, to combat this problem, gravity is simulated on board the spacecraft, but not with any fancy spinning things you might have seen on the Sci-Fi channel, but rather with strong rubber bands. Astronauts are instructed to run on treadmills while these bands press them down on to the treadmill to create greater forces, which simulates gravity to stimulate more bone to be laid down and less absorbed.

ACTIVITY BOX 5.5   Ageing as a Dried Banana Skin

Next time you eat a banana, keep the skin and put it on a cloth to dry. At first the skin is compliant, so you can stretch it nicely; it will break but can take quite a bit of stress first. Leave it for a week or so and don't worry about the smell—it will add a wholesome organic aroma. Now try to stretch it: it won't give (as it is stiff by now) and will break easily. I am not saying this is exactly what happens to tissue from ageing and immobilisation, but it has similarities.

FURTHER INFORMATION 5.3

Ehlers Danlos disease is caused by an alteration in the process of constructing collagen fibres. There is less collagen produced and it is of poorer quality. Consequently, connective tissue is weak and easily deformed. This means joints are hyperflexible (hypermobile) and the skin is extremely stretchy. This can result in premature degeneration of the musculoskeletal system (e.g. osteoarthritis) and predispose the individual to joint dislocations and other injuries. In its most severe presentation, Ehlers Danlos can cause premature death due to the damage of major blood vessels weakened by the lack of strength from good-quality collagen.

great flexibility like gymnastics. The reasons given for doing this include:

1. Improving performance.
2. Preventing injury during the game.
3. Preventing longer-term injury.

Although this may seem intuitively correct, there is very little evidence supporting these claims. Indeed, there is some evidence to contradict them. However, stretching before participation in sport does seem sensible; perhaps it was ingrained into us at an early age. So, let's take a scientific look at this problem by looking at the effect stretching has on the stress–strain relationship. Although taken mainly from animal studies, it appears that repetitive, or cyclical, loading of tissue when stretching causes a gradual decrease in its stiffness and strength. It becomes more compliant and weaker, which is not terribly good for preventing injury or enhancing performance, particularly in sports where strength/power are a key part.

Fig. 5.33 demonstrates this effect. Stretches 2 and 3 show a greater amount of strain (i.e. they move further along the X axis) but are less strong (i.e. less stress on the Y axis).

Temperature

Research tells us quite clearly that the temperature of the tissue being stretched is important (Petrofsky et al. 2013). You probably already knew this from your physical education classes when you went through the routine of warming up before a sport.

When connective tissue is cold there is an increase in tissue stiffness, probably due to an increase in the viscosity (stiffness) of the ground substance. This is a bit like when you freeze your home-baked bread. Fresh out the oven it is soft and malleable, but after several hours in the freezer it is hard and brittle (i.e. it will break without bending), try Activity Box 5.6. This happens with cold connective tissue as well; there is an increase in the risk of rupture because the tissue can't give. This quality of connective tissue to alter its viscosity with temperature is called thixotropy, which we mentioned earlier.

On the other hand, if you increase the temperature of connective tissue too much, the bonds in the tropocollagen helix uncouple. So, if you apply stress there will be greater strain and the tissue will reach rupture faster.

Clearly if you increase the temperature of connective tissue too much you will destroy the cells. To achieve this level of destruction you need to exceed temperatures of 40°C so don't worry, an exercise-based warm-up will not do this; you would have to do some serious boiling.

You may have noticed that connective tissue responds the same way to an increase in temperature as it does to repetitive loading. This is not a coincidence. Exactly the same thing is happening to the tissue due to the energy transfer from the heat or from repetitive movement, a change in viscosity of the ground substance (thixotropy) and possibly a change in the bonds of the tropocollagen molecule. This means that a moderate increase in connective tissue temperature either from repetitive movement or direct heat source, such as a bath, will make stretching easier. Let's now have a closer look at how we actually perform a stretch, because we all do it differently.

The Science of a Stretch

It might be a good idea to start this section with a practical exercise, one that demonstrates the difference between two characteristics of stretching: creep and stress relaxation.

Stand up and place your hands on the front of your thighs. Now keep your knees straight and slide your hands down your legs as far as you can. You will you eventually feel the tight, perhaps uncomfortable, feeling in the back of your thigh, which of course indicates that your hamstring muscles have reached their maximum length (in a conscious state anyway). Stop at this point and make a mental note of the sensation. This is the physiological length of the muscle. Ok, now keep the same position and count slowly to 20. By the end of this time you should have felt a marked decrease in the uncomfortable tight feeling. What has happened is

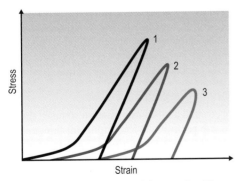

Fig. 5.33 Cyclical Loading of Connective Tissue.

> ### ACTIVITY BOX 5.6
>
> Get a lump of sticky tack, like blue tack, and cool it down (put it in the freezer for an hour or so). Take it out and try to pull it. You should find that it has become more resistant to stress (stiffer) and will snap apart quite easily. Keep pulling it and playing with it until it warms. After a while you will have noticed that it will stretch out more easily, that is, it has become less stiff. Connective tissue has the same property.

that there has been a decrease in tension within the muscle. This is called **stress relaxation**.

Now wait approximately 20 minutes for the effect of the stretch to fade. During this time, you could have a think about what happened during stress relaxation. Why does tension reduce when the muscle was held at its physiological length?

After the rest, repeat the same thing only this time when you feel the tissue decrease in tension stretch down a little further, repeat this stretch a couple of times. You should find you are able to reach further down because of an increase in the length of your tissues. This is called tissue **creep**.

In both stress relaxation and creep, the same process has occurred; when you reached your limit the collagen fibres were allowed to slide past each other a certain amount. Without further stress this would result in a decrease in tension within the muscle (there is also a nerve reflex—Golgi tendon reflex—which relaxes a tense muscle), which is stress relaxation. However, if you decided to maintain the stress by stretching further, this movement of the collagen fibres will manifest in an increase in tissue length, which is tissue creep. The differences between stress relaxation and creep are demonstrated in Figs 5.34 and 5.35, respectively.

Do you think there are any negative implications for tissue creep? (See end of chapter for discussion of this point.)

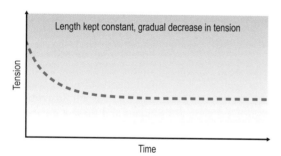

Fig. 5.34 Stress Relaxation.

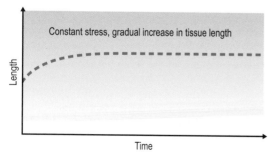

Fig. 5.35 Tissue Creep.

Changes in the length of tissue due to creep are short lived, because the collagen begins to revert back to its original shape. Elongation in tissue from creep will last anything between 30 and 90 minutes, depending on what you are doing during that time. If you are moving around it tends to last longer; if you have complete rest it will not last as long.

If you are interested in improving someone's flexibility by increasing the length of the connective tissue, tissue creep is only a short-term solution, although this may be useful to improve performance. To gain a lasting change we need to alter the habitual daily stresses that the tissue goes through. This means, for example, the forces a tendon experiences, the range of motion a joint goes through and the length that a muscle is held in. We can call this the tissue's mechanical background (what it regularly experiences) and you can alter it by a simple change in someone's sitting posture, tennis serving technique, step length of their gait etc. Some health and sports professionals impose a change in the tissues' daily stress by using splints or braces that maintain the posture of a joint and therefore the length of surrounding tissue. More on this later.

One thing we haven't talked about is how fast you apply the stretch. Remember tearing the strip of plastic (or plastic shopping bag, see earlier in chapter). It's the same for connective tissue: if you apply the stress too rapidly it doesn't get a chance to comply with the stress by straining. It will therefore reach its yield point rapidly and permanent damage will occur. Applied slowly and the tissue is allowed to strain. This is the viscoelastic property of connective tissue: its ability to flow over time. A greater increase in length is possible with a slow application of stress before any damage occurs. This is particularly the case with stiffer tissues, for example, older tissues. See Fig. 5.36.

Now, of course, permanently lengthening a tissue may be your aim, in which case a rapidly applied stress (e.g. a physiotherapist or chiropractor manipulating a joint; applying high velocity thrusting movement to a joint) might be appropriate. However, you need to consider the fact that damaged tissue will trigger an inflammatory response resulting in new (potentially stiffer) collagen being laid down as scar tissue. If you do not follow up the manipulation with a daily range of movement exercises (changing the mechanical background) to maintain the new length, you will quickly be back at the starting point.

Summary of Connective Tissue

We have covered a lot of information so far in this chapter, so it is worth recapping a few important things about connective tissue. Connective tissue consists of three basic ingredients: ground substance, fibres (collagen and elastin) and cells that create new fibres (fibroblasts); and it helps repair damaged tissue (macrophages and neutrophils). The

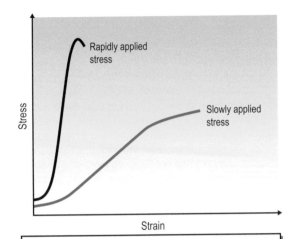

In the rapidly applied stress, although more stress can be applied (higher up the Y axis), it reaches the breaking point much sooner. When the stress is applied more slowly the tissue adapts, more strain can be achieved before the yield point is reached.

Fig. 5.36 Response of Connective Tissue to Slow and Fast Stress Application.

mechanical properties of connective tissue vary according to the amount and pattern of collagen, which gives the tissue strength; elastin, which improves tissue elasticity; and the viscosity of the enveloping ground substance, which allows the tissue to flow (viscoelastic) by lubricating the fibres. These mechanical properties alter with age, physical activity, temperature and recent history.

We know that a warm-up helps tissue lengthen by reducing the viscosity of the ground substance. This is achieved through a rise in temperature, either from repetitive movement or direct heat. Even though creep is different from stress relaxation, with new length gained through creep and reduced tension being achieved with stress relaxation, the mechanism is the same. Increased length from creep lasts only a short period (about the duration of a game of football); to maintain a change in length the everyday mechanical background of the tissue has to change. Finally, we know that connective tissue responds stiffly to a rapidly applied stress, reaching breaking point quickly, whereas a slowly applied force can gain greater change in length, by flowing, before reaching the point where damage occurs.

FLUIDS AND GASES

In the final part of this chapter we will continue with the theme of understanding how things flow, but instead of the body's connective tissues we will consider fluids, such as our blood, and gases, such as the air we breathe. Outside of the body, understanding how fluids and gases behave when forces are applied is helpful to therapists designing a water-based exercise programme (hydrotherapy) and to better understand the postures and equipment involved in high-speed sports, such as cycling.

Fluids and gases are forms of matter that continuously change shape when stresses are applied to them. The behaviour of gases and liquids are surprisingly similar. Objects can float (or sink) in both liquids and gas, and they can both create drag, so it is useful to consider them together.

Relative Density

Let's begin with floating. To understand why and how some objects float we need to introduce a few principles and definitions. Namely **density** and **relative density (RD).** All bodies have **density** which is the amount of mass confined within its volume. We talked about this in Chapter 3 when we discussed the centre of mass. Density then is simply the mass divided by the volume; that is:

$$\text{Density (P)} = \text{Mass (kg)}/\text{Volume (m}^3).$$

Density tells you how spread out the mass is within the body shape. Liquids have a low density (the molecules are more spread out) compared to solids; for example, the density of pure water is 1 g/cm³, whereas mercury is denser (the molecules are packed more closely together) with 13.6 g/cm³. Other notable densities are copper at 8.89 g/cm³, wood at around 0.5 g/cm³ (depending on the type) and ice at 0.92 g/cm³, which, you may note, is lower than pure water. Gases are even less dense: air, for example, has a density of 0.0012/cm³. See Fig. 5.37 for an illustration of the differences.

RD is the ratio between the density of a particular substance and the density of a reference substance. For liquids, the reference liquid is pure water (density = 1 g/cm³) and for gases it is dry air at sea level at a temperature of 20°C (density = 0.0012 g/cm³). So, for example, the RD of copper is 8.89; that is, it is 8.89 times more dense than water and 7408 times more dense than air.

Anything with an RD >1 (heavier than pure water) will not float in pure water, so copper (8.89) will not float, whereas wood (0.5) will float, although there is a broad variation in the RD of wood according to type. This value also tells you (as a percentage) how much of the body will be under the water. With an RD of 0.5 a lump of wood will have 50% of its mass under the water. As you may recall, ice had a density lower (0.92) than water, which is why you only see the tip of the iceberg: 92% is under water and 8% is above. The human body has an RD a little higher than ice but still less than 1; with a value around 0.96, 4% of the body will float, but which 4%?

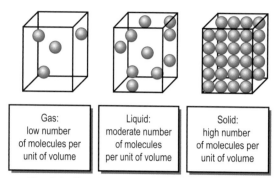

| Gas:
low number
of molecules per
unit of volume | Liquid:
moderate number
of molecules
per unit of volume | Solid:
high number
of molecules per
unit of volume |

Fig. 5.37 Density of Gases, Fluids and Solids.

ACTIVITY BOX 5.7   Are You a Floater or a Sinker?

The next time you visit a swimming pool try this experiment. Find a quiet corner where the water is relatively calm. Hold onto the side and slowly lie down on your back while still keeping hold of the side. Take a deep breath and slowly let go of the side. Did you sink straight away? Which part of you went down first? Some people's legs slowly sink a little under the water before coming to a stop, they are floaters. Now do the same thing but this time before you let go of the side push all the air out your lungs. You should find you sink a lot faster; without air your RD has increased. This is one of the techniques used to estimate body fat, with as much air out of your lungs. Whether you float or sink comes down to how much body fat you have. The actual technique (hydrostatic weighing) is a little more complex, but essentially amounts to the same thing.

If you try to float in a swimming pool (not exactly pure water but it is difficult and expensive to get enough pure water to float in) you may not find that 4% of you stays above the water; you might, instead, completely sink. The value, 0.96, is an average value; people vary considerably. You might even say we can be categorised as sinkers or floaters (see Activity Box 5.6), depending on whether our densities are above or below that of pure water. The other problem is that this is an overall value for the human body; different parts of our body have different densities.

Basically, your musculoskeletal system (bones, muscles, tendons etc.) are denser than water (RD >1), and fat is less dense with an RD around 0.9. In addition, you retain just over a litre of air in your lungs at all times, which of course means your lungs will be less dense than water. Therefore, if you lie on your back in a swimming pool you will probably find that your legs will sink (a lot of bone, tendon and muscle). However, your chest (lots of cavities, fat and air) will float. In fact, because the back of your chest contains the most lung tissue, this is the part that is most likely to float, which is why you see 'dead' people floating on their front in those grisly scenes at the start of crime films. When you learned to swim, you may have started with the mushroom position (face down in water, wrapping your arms around your bent knee), which is the most stable position (easiest to maintain) because the 4% that wants to be out of the water (upper back) is out the water; however, it is not a particularly sustainable position (Activity Box 5.7).

Exactly the same principle applies for gases: if you are lighter than the air around you, you will float; heavier and you will sink (or rather you won't float). But don't worry, with a density almost 800 times greater than air, there isn't much chance of you spontaneously floating away. Hot, moist air is even lighter than normal dry air, so it will rise, which is something the Montgolfier brothers exploited in their early attempt at flight. However, density alone can't explain why planes (which are definitely heavier than air) can stay up in the sky; we also need to understand the patterns of pressure within fluids and gases and how differences in pressure can cause pulling and lifting forces.

We have already talked a bit about pressure in Chapter 4 when we considered solid bodies in contact with each other, for example, your feet on the ground. The pressure at your feet was measured as the force divided by the contact area. Pressure within a fluid is not, unfortunately, as easy to measure because there are so many contact points—the stuff just keeps moving about.

Hydrostatic Pressure

The molecules in a fluid or gas are not as tightly constrained as they are in solids; they are freer to move around, colliding with each other as they do (Fig. 5.38). These collisions work in just the same way as a large impact; force is exerted over a surface area resulting in pressure. But because these pressure points are so small they aren't, individually, very important; however, taken together all these pressure points create a generalised pressure, which is felt on the surface of the material containing the fluid or gas. It's a bit like the corn popping in your microwave or pot; all those bits of corn crashing into one another create pressure, which usually results in the lid coming off the pan or the bag (if you use microwave popcorn) expanding.

Now, if we consider a fluid at rest (e.g. a glass of water) the pressure within the water is the same no matter which direction you consider. If you take a single point in the water there will be pressure acting on it from every direction,

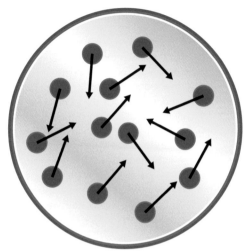

Fig. 5.38 Movement of Molecules in Gases and Fluids.

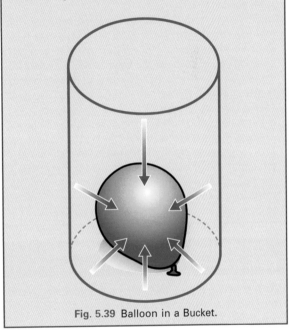

Fig. 5.39 Balloon in a Bucket.

but one direction will not be greater than the other, otherwise the point would be moving. This means that pressure within static water has no direction, which means it is not a vector quantity. This is called hydrostatic pressure: the pressure of a fluid when at rest.

As you will have noticed, in Activity Box 5.8, the deeper a body (e.g. the balloon in activity box 5.8) is pulled under the water the more crushed it becomes, but we said previously that the pressure was the same throughout. Well, it has the same direction throughout but not the same magnitude; pressure in a fluid increases with depth. The weight of the column of water above an immersed point (like our balloon) presses down on the water below, this downward force is simply the mass of the water multiplied by gravity. Unlike solids, the gases and fluids can be compressed (remember when you compressed air in Activity Box 5.3), which results in an increase in density (more molecules packed together) and therefore more pressure (less space = more collisions = more pressure). A bit like when yet another person tries to get into an already packed elevator, there is less space and more contact among the people. It's the same for the balloon, the increased pressure squeezes the balloon more, which it's thin rubbery material can't resist and it collapses (see Further Information 5.4 on how early deep sea divers conquered this problem).

This relationship between pressure, density and water depth can be expressed by the equation:

$$Hydrostatic\ pressure = d \times g \times h$$

where d is the fluid density, g is gravity and h is the height of the column of water (or depth if you like).

The next couple of activities allows you to explore some properties of fluids, pressure, temperature and volume (Activity Boxes 5.9–5.11).

Density and Pressure Summary

Density is how closely packed together stuff is. If something is denser than water, it sinks; less and it floats. The human body, on average, just about floats. Water pressure increases the deeper you go. If you stand up to your neck in water, there will be more pressure at your feet than at your neck (see Activity Box 5.9). Temperature can also affect pressure:

ACTIVITY BOX 5.9

When you are next at your local swimming pool, stand in the shallow end up to your shoulders. Stay there for 5 minutes, trying not to look suspicious. During this time the higher pressure at your feet compared to your top pushes more blood than normal up into your chest and abdomen. This is exactly the same way that the air was pushed upwards when you immersed the balloon in the bucket (see Activity Box 5.7). This increased volume of blood centrally can constrict your breathing. You will probably not feel this because it is only a small change but if you had an existing problem with your breathing, being immersed in water may cause you to become short of breath. The increased pressure also increases the rate that your bladder fills (so you need to go to the toilet sooner).

Being immersed in water can have benefits too; for example, the higher pressure at your feet may help disperse any swelling around your ankle if you had an ankle injury. Perhaps the most obvious benefit of immersion is reduced loading through your joints due to buoyancy (which we will talk about in the next section). This is particularly helpful if you are trying to gradually reintroduce loading through injured parts of the body, for example, during the rehabilitation of a lower limb fracture. As a rough guideline, if you immerse yourself up to:

the top of your shoulders = loading reduced by 90%

the bottom of your breast bone (sternum) = loading reduced by 66%

to your hip bone = loading reduced by 50%.

ACTIVITY BOX 5.10   Pressure and Temperature

Now pressure is also dependent on temperature. Turn the heat up and the molecules move around more; there are more collisions and therefore more pressure (think of the popcorn). This can be best illustrated with an experiment. Blow up a balloon (if you have any left) and note its size (use a tape measure or draw round it). Now pop it in the freezer for a couple of hours. When you take it out you will notice that it is much smaller. Put it on a table and watch what happens. The change is all to do with temperature since the amount of air within the balloon has remained the same. At room temperature the air particles are smashing into each other and pressing against the side of balloon; at low temperatures the particles lose their energy and move less; and with nothing pressing against the side of the balloon it collapses.

ACTIVITY BOX 5.11   Pressure and Volume

Blow up a balloon but not to the point of bursting—just reasonably well inflated. You have pushed a lot of air molecules into the rubber balloon. The pressure from all these molecules moving about is being felt by the walls of the balloon and this internal pressure causes it to expand. Now put your hands around the balloon and squeeze so that the balloon gets smaller (without bursting). The volume (the space occupied by the air molecules) reduces so there will be more impacts among the molecules, which increases the pressure of the walls of the balloon—a pressure you should be feeling.

FURTHER INFORMATION 5.4

The increase in hydrostatic pressure with depth has always presented a barrier to deep sea diving (as well as the lack of an air supply of course). To prevent the diver being crushed (like the balloon in your bucket) or at the very least finding it very difficult to breathe, suits were designed as early as the 16th century to withstand high pressures. The most important development was making helmets out of hard metal, which protected the brain and eyes, and allowed the diver to breathe out (Fig. 5.40).

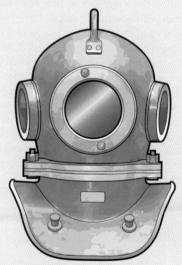

Fig. 5.40 Metal Diving Helmet.

higher temperatures, higher pressure (provided the stuff is contained within the shape).

Archimedes Principle, Buoyancy and Pascal's Law

The difference in pressure of an immersed object between the top (low pressure) and bottom (high pressure) causes something called upthrust, better known as **buoyancy** (Fig. 5.41). If you have a long, thin balloon and squeeze it more at one end than the other the air moves along to the unsqueezed end, bulging that end out more (see Activity Box 5.9). It may even jump out of your hand like a bar of soap. This is essentially **Pascal's law** in action: a change in pressure (like you squeezing the balloon) is passed on to the rest of the gas or fluid and to the surfaces of the container. This also explains buoyancy, which is a force we all know from our times in the swimming pool; this is the force that works against us if we try to touch the bottom of the pool. This is the force that caused Archimedes to leap out of his bath shouting 'Eureka!' (Further Information 5.5). On entering his bath, Archimedes displaced a certain amount of water; the more he displaced the greater the upward thrust (buoyancy). This has since been known as the **Archimedes principle:** that an object immersed in water creates an upward thrust (buoyancy) equal to the weight of the displaced water. You will have experienced this effect in Activity Box 5.7; the more of the balloon that was immersed the greater the force pushing it up. Buoyancy can be very useful in rehabilitation by providing a means of resisting movement as well as supporting painful limbs (see Activity Box 5.8).

Pressure

The way that a contained fluid (or gas) behaves when pressure is applied to it (passing on the change in pressure to the rest of the fluid) provides an effective way of coping with high pressure points. For example, a chair cushion filled with gel will evenly distribute pressure created at the hip and pelvic bones of someone sitting, which is a useful characteristic for anyone at risk of damage due to prolonged periods of pressure high enough to disturb the blood flow to an area, for example, bed-bound patients and wheelchair sportsmen. Pascal's law is also the principle underpinning the use of air pockets in the design of running shoes and the introduction of gel pads to the gloves and saddles of cyclists, to distribute pressure evenly, thus avoiding high points of pressure. This pressure-relieving mechanism is not something that has escaped nature; for example, the fat pads of the heel work in a similar way to distribute pressure when the heel strikes the ground during gait (see Fig. 5.26).

Air Pressure

Now here is an interesting point and one that might help you interpret the weather report or at least the barometer in your grandfather's house: air pressure works in the same way as hydrostatic pressure.

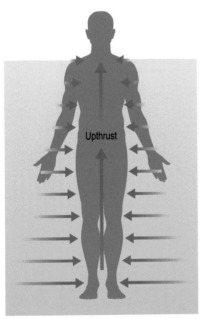

Fig. 5.41 Pressure Difference on an Immersed Body Causing Upthrust.

FURTHER INFORMATION 5.5
Archimedes of Syracuse

Archimedes was a pretty stunning individual in terms of the inventions and discoveries attributed to him. He lived more than 2000 years ago in a port called Syracuse, which still exists, in southeast Sicily. He died aged 75 years during a war with the Romans while, legend has it, trying to protect his scientific instruments. He spent most of his time solving mathematical and engineering problems. Among his inventions were the Archimedes screw, which is a method of transporting water uphill using a pipe with an internal helical winding system that literally scoops up the water. The simplicity and effectiveness of this design has stood the test of time and is still used today by farmers in some parts of the world, as well as draining the polders in the Netherlands.

As we have already mentioned in this chapter Archimedes also discovered the principle of buoyancy—a discovery inspired by a local ruler's need to measure the quantity of gold in his crown!

As you sit there reading this book you are being crushed by the air above you. Just like the water in the bucket, air increases in density the deeper it gets, being most dense when it is next to the earth's surface. This is measured by a barometer. So, if you go too high up, such as in a plane, the density of air might get so low that there aren't enough oxygen molecules around for you. This is why the air inside a plane is pumped through the fuselage to keep the pressure the same as it was (more or less) at ground level.

The difficulty with air is that it is not contained, so air pressure might be greater in one direction compared to another, which causes air to move. So, we get areas of high pressure and therefore low pressure, and the system attempts, but never succeeds for very long, to reach pressure equilibrium, that is, the same pressure throughout (Further Information 5.6).

Mechanics of Flow

We have considered fluids and gases at rest—all the forces in balance. If there is an unbalanced force (e.g. the heart pumping blood, a fan pushing air or you squeezing one end of a balloon) then fluids and gases will move. They flow. This movement occurs in layers, with one layer of the fluid sliding over the one next to it (this is exactly the same as shear strain, see Activity Box 5.1). This movement in layers is called **laminar flow**; the main factor, which affects laminar flow, is the stickiness between the layers, which is the same as viscosity (resistant to flow) that we talked about earlier in the chapter. So, the layers of treacle, for example, will slip over each other more slowly than water. The layers next to the containing surface (artery wall, sides of swimming pool etc.) will move the slowest; they kind of stick to the sides, whereas the layers in the middle will move the fastest. This type of flow is demonstrated in Fig. 5.42A.

FURTHER INFORMATION 5.6

Differences in air pressure are important to sailors; it's one of the factors that creates wind (the others being the spinning motion of the Earth and the temperature differences—the latter of which cause convection currents). There is an area around the equator called the Doldrums, which is essentially an area of stable low air pressure caused by the high temperatures. Without a nearby area of high pressure there will be very little wind. Consequently, sailing ships could be marooned for days or even weeks. This has led to the use of the phrase 'down in the Doldrums' to mean inactivity or even a state of despondency.

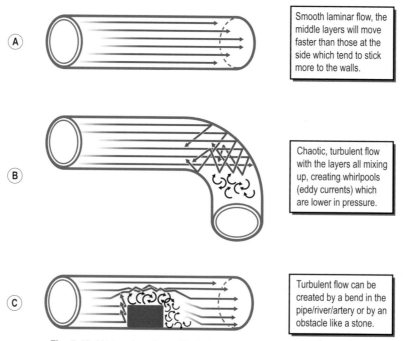

Smooth laminar flow, the middle layers will move faster than those at the side which tend to stick more to the walls.

Chaotic, turbulent flow with the layers all mixing up, creating whirlpools (eddy currents) which are lower in pressure.

Turbulent flow can be created by a bend in the pipe/river/artery or by an obstacle like a stone.

Fig. 5.42 (A) Laminar flow. (B) Turbulent flow. (C) Turbulent flow.

You can imagine this movement in layers like the lanes of a motorway. The lane on the inside moves slowly with greater movement in the overtaking lanes so the fastest cars travel in the lane closest to the central reservation. Just like the motorway, laminar flow continues smoothly until it comes across an obstacle or is forced to make a change in direction. This causes the layers to start mixing (like cars changing lanes), producing what is called **turbulent flow** (see Figs 5.42B and 5.43C).

Drag

The turbulence your moving hand produces in a bucket or bath of water (Activity Box 5.12) creates a force that acts in the opposite direction to the motion; this force is called **drag**. Drag only occurs when a body (brick, bike, bird etc.) travels through a liquid or gas. If you sit, unmoving, in a very quiet swimming pool you won't experience drag. Drag comes from a couple of different factors. Firstly, there is friction between the moving body and the water/air molecules. In this case friction works in exactly the same as it did on land: the rougher the surface, the greater the coefficient of friction

---

ACTIVITY BOX 5.12

Next time it rains heavily take a trip to your nearest river (once the rain has abated) and from a safe vantage point observe the way the river flows. Place a stick into the river close to the bank, and note how fast it moves; this is the slow lane of the river. Now throw another one into the middle, this is the fast lane. If you have ducks inhabiting your river you will notice that they don't swim up the middle of a river; intelligently they use the slow lane to move upstream.

If you haven't got a river close by, or it is still raining, then try this alternative.

Fill your bucket or bath again with lukewarm water, around about 30 cm of depth should do it. Now, unlike the river, this is a contained liquid, but we can still observe laminar and turbulent flow by moving objects through it, in this case your hand. So, place your flat hand in the water and move it sideways keeping your fingers pointing down as if you were imitating a shark's dorsal fin. The water moves smoothly around your hand, laminar flow. Now turn your hand so that you are pushing the water with the palm of your hand. This time you should see some frothy water and little whirlpools (also known as eddy current) behind your hand; this is the result of turbulent flow—the layers of water mixing with each other. Adjust the speed of your hand; you should find that the faster it gets the more turbulence is created.

(see Chapter 4). So, if you want to reduce drag, make the surface of your body smooth; you don't have to look far to find evidence to support this. Consider the skinsuits worn by competitive swimmers and cyclists, which are designed with reducing friction in mind. Can you think of another example of something made with its outer surface smooth to reduce friction? When you think about it, anything that goes fast is designed in this way, that is, with smooth surfaces.

The other main cause of drag is the shape of the body moving through the water/air, this is called **form drag.** Remember in Activity Box 5.12, there was more turbulence created when you turned your hand round so you were 'pushing' the water with the palm of your hand. Your hand, or any other moving object, is literally pushing the layers apart so that it can occupy the space where the air/water molecules used to be; the more water the more difficult it is to prise the layers apart. It's a bit like when you take a walk in the woods at the peak of summer, you have to push apart the overgrown plants that are obstructing the path you are walking down; the more plants there are, the more difficult this task is. If you are squeezing along an overgrown path you shape your body so that it is narrower at the front (e.g. you may turn sideways). This means you are pushing against less vegetation, and it doesn't have to move as far (so less effort). Moving through water or air is exactly the same, after all they both still contain mass, which has to be pushed aside.

As an object hits the water/air a large front end will mean more water/air is pushed aide (like a very wide person trying to move down your overgrown path). It will also mean the layers of air/water will mix up (see Figs 5.42B, 5.42C nd 5.43) causing turbulence. So, the trick is to gradually separate the layers of water so they continue to flow in layers over the object. By presenting a narrow front surface that gradually slopes back, the layers can flow over the object with minimal disruption. Again, this principle is behind the design of many fast-travelling bodies/objects, for example, the nose cone of a rocket. This principle is also followed in sport; for example, divers enter the swimming pool with their arms stretched out and their head tucked to minimise disruption of the water, they are trying to slip between the layers of water, in fact they are scored on exactly this ability.

Although bodies and machines have been designed to be more aerodynamic, or hydrodynamic if going through water, they can't completely avoid drag and the worst bit is that the faster they move the greater the drag. No wonder so much design time is spent reducing friction and improving the shape.

Bernoulli's Principle

Speed affects the amount of drag by something known as **Bernoulli's principle**, which states that pressure will reduce the faster the water or air moves. As you probably noticed when moving your hand through the bucket (Activity Box 5.12) the turbulence created is located behind the moving object; move it fast enough and you will probably see eddy currents (see Figs 5.42B and C). Because the water is moving much faster now that it is turbulent the pressure decreases; this drop in pressure pulls (perhaps sucks is a better word) the body backwards.

Again, this is something you will be aware of in everyday life and especially with things that move fast. Imagine yourself walking along a pavement and a large lorry whisks past you; depending on the speed and size of the lorry you will experience some sensation of being pulled towards the back of it (this is sometimes referred to as the wake or slip stream). The pulling sensation is caused by this area of low pressure immediately behind the lorry caused by the fast-moving turbulent air (Fig. 5.44).

Another example of this can be observed in the spring time at your local river/pond. At this time of year, you might observe the train of ducklings flowing along in the water

behind their mother. They aren't really as fast as their mother, they are just using this sucking effect from the fast flowing, turbulent, water behind their mother to help them keep up. Being pulled along in your parent's wake is probably quite an enjoyable experience, until the day you decide to move off in a new direction.

Drag is usually described as a horizontal force, pulling backwards on an object that is moving through air/water. However, it can also act vertically; the wings of a plane are shaped so that the air flows faster above the wing than below, as you now know this creates a low pressure above the wing that sucks the aircraft up. This is the same as drag, but when it acts perpendicularly (at right angles) to the motion it is called lift. Now you know a little about aerodynamics why not have a go at Activity Box 5.13.

Blood Flow: Haemodynamics

As we are all dealing with the human body, when we talk about flow we need to talk about the main thing that flows around our body: blood. Blood is more viscous than water, so it tends to move that bit slower; well it would if it didn't

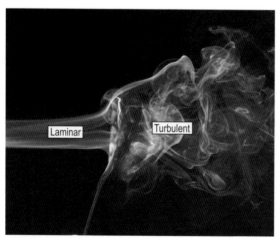

Fig. 5.43 Laminar and Turbulent Flow From a Burning Match.

ACTIVITY BOX 5.13   Aerodynamics and Cycling

Next time the Tour de France (or any other bicycle race) is on the television, make a note to watch it. Professional cyclists put into place all the principles of aerodynamics. See if you can observe any of the following:
1. Smooth, skin-hugging clothes.
2. Bikes smoothed with the joints in the frame rounded.
3. A low riding position with their back flat and crouched over their handle bars.
4. A back wheel that is filled in with a disk.
5. Helmets shaped like a teardrop at the back.
6. Riders cycling very closely behind each other.
7. Shaved legs.

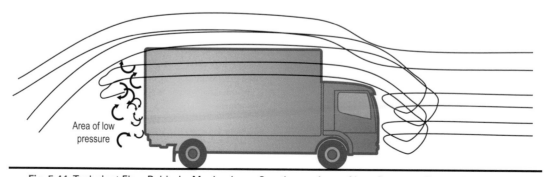

Fig. 5.44 Turbulent Flow Behind a Moving Lorry Creating an Area of Low Pressure; Bernoulli's Principle.

have a pump (your heart), which periodically (once every second or so) increases the pressure. Blood flow through arteries behaves the same way as other liquids: laminar flow until obstacles are met, the artery narrows or there is a change in direction (e.g. moving around bent joints). These situations will create turbulence, which, as we now know, lowers pressure; if there is too much turbulence you need to turn up the pump to keep the same blood pressure. So, if you want to keep turbulence to a minimum you will need to keep all your joints straight!

The shear stresses on arterial walls created by blood flow have been implicated in the development of atherosclerosis (the leading cause of death in the western world), due to gradual damage to the endothelium wall of the artery and consequent inflammation. Higher stresses are observed at locations where there is arterial branching or bifurcation, and therefore resultant turbulent (nonuniform) flow (Cecchi et al. 2011).

See Further Information 5.7 for a bit of ancient history on flow.

Summary Fluid Dynamics

Objects float or sink in gas or liquid depending on their RD. The pressure within a static liquid has the same direction throughout but will increase with depth. Pressure can be altered by volume and temperature. Pressure differences within a liquid cause upthrust (buoyancy), which can be used by therapists. Pressure within a liquid is evened out; this is called Bernoulli's principle and can be used to reduce specific areas of high pressure. Pressure differences within gases and liquids causes movement that tends to be in layers (laminar), but can become turbulent (layers mix) if flow is rapid or an obstruction is met. Turbulent flow causes areas of low pressure; this is one of the factors behind drag (a force opposing forward motion)—the other being friction.

Therapeutic Flow

To finish this chapter on how tissue, fluids and gases flow, we thought it might be useful to look at the way these principles are applied therapeutically. We will look at three examples: serial splinting, hydrotherapy and finally a look at a respiratory technique.

Dynamic Wrist Splints

Splints are external devices that correct or support a part of the body by applying and modifying force. In the final chapter we will look at a case study that uses a splint over the ankle and foot to improve walking, but for now let's consider dynamic wrist splints, which are widely used, particularly by occupational therapists. These are, essentially, moulded plastic sleeves that wrap around the wrist and hand (Fig. 5.45) sometimes with wires that create additional forces (Fig. 5.46). Their purpose, typically, is to apply tensile

FURTHER INFORMATION 5.7

Flow was well understood by the ancient Egyptians. Life depended on controlling the water flow from the Nile through the basic, but effective, irrigation and damming system, which still sustains a huge population. Transport along the Nile during the time of the Pharaohs was also so much easier if you understood air flow so that you effectively positioned the sails on your Felucca (Egyptian sailing boat).

Finally, the Egyptians had an understanding, albeit grisly, of body fluids. The process of mummification involves the draining of the body fluids into jars. The Egyptians understood that this took time and could be helped by gravity, which conjures up a pretty grisly image.

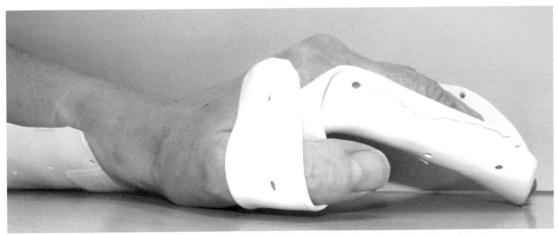

Fig. 5.45 Wrist Splint Moulded to Hand to Help Maintain Functional Position of Wrist.

stress to shortened tissue. Because they are worn for pro-longed periods they work on the viscoelastic properties of connective tissue, that is, stress applied over time to give the tissue an opportunity to flow. Orthodontists use a similar approach when they fix braces to teeth; low load, prolonged duration means the tissue won't be damaged and any changes in the length (or position in the case of teeth) are more likely to be permanent.

The make-up of the dynamic splint is quite interesting from a biomechanical perspective. First the plastic sleeve (see Fig. 5.45) is 'thermodynamic'; this means that when it is heated it becomes very compliant (in exactly the same way that your own tissues are more flexible when warmer, just more so with this type of plastic) and, on cooling will become stiff again. This allows the therapist to mould the sleeve carefully around the wrist/hand so that the joints are fully supported. If you are going to apply force to a body part (even low loads over long periods) it is important to make sure the force is evenly spread, otherwise there is a risk that some parts will experience higher pressure with resulting damage to the skin. A tight-fitting sleeve is also important to avoid the splint moving up and down, which creates shear stress on the skin. Prolonged applications of shear stress are likely to result in skin damage—just like the blisters caused by your feet sliding up and down in shoes that are too big for you.

Second in the make-up of a dynamic splint are the wires (see Fig. 5.46), which apply a force in a specific direction. The wires can be tightened a certain amount every time the patient sees the therapist so that the tensile stress is maintained (we don't want any slacking off). If you recall, this was called tissue creep.

Hydrotherapy

The therapeutic benefits of water have been widely used for thousands of years. In rehabilitation, water provides a versatile medium suitable for a broad range of individuals—from older patients to young athletes. Buoyancy and drag can be used to construct exercise programmes that start with assisting and supporting movement and end with strenuous resistance. Let's consider the biomechanics of one technique.

In the Halliwick approach to hydrotherapy turbulence is used extensively to assist the patient. One example of this is where the therapist stands behind the patient who is lying on their back in the water, perhaps supported by floats (Fig. 5.47). The therapist then begins to walk backwards, while providing some support to the patient's head (always reas-suring the patient as they go). The water between the therapist and patient becomes turbulent with a resulting drop in pressure (Bernoulli's principle), which pulls the patient towards the therapist (try Activity Box 5.14 if you don't believe me).

The purpose of this technique is to develop confidence and balance in the water, so patients move through the water without much help from the therapist. They may then begin to contribute more to the movement by moving their hands and feet. It provides a really good starting point, and hey, if it's good enough for ducklings then it should be good enough for us.

There are many other ways that a therapist can use water to facilitate or resist movement using buoyancy and drag in particular. Have a think about how you might, for example, resist shoulder abduction using buoyancy and drag (there are some suggestions at end of the chapter).

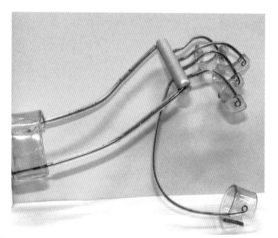

Fig. 5.46 The Use of Wires to Generate Additional Stress Along Specific Directions.

ACTIVITY BOX 5.14

You can try this simple exercise in your bath. Put your rubber duck/toy boat in a bit of calm water (and free of bubbles); put your hand in the water a couple of centi-metres in front of the duck and pull your hand through the water towards you. Do it slowly, and then do it quickly. Did the duck move? If not, then try keeping your hand closer to the duck while you are moving. You are applying Bernoulli's principle to move the duck, creating fast flowing turbulent water that has a lower pressure; this pressure difference causes a pulling force on the duck.

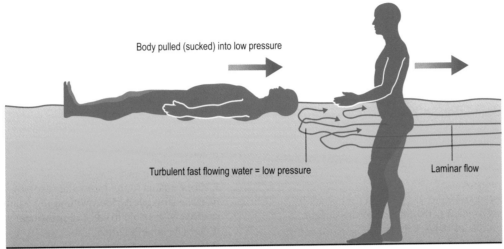

Body pulled (sucked) into low pressure

Turbulent fast flowing water = low pressure

Laminar flow

Fig. 5.47 Using Bernoulli's Principle to Assist Swimming.

Respiratory Technique

Therapists don't just use force on the musculoskeletal system; those working with patients incapacitated with a respiratory condition also use force. The forced expiratory technique (FET), or simply called huffing (for reasons soon to become obvious), is a technique employed by respiratory physiotherapists and nurses to help individuals get rid of excessive or thick mucus lining their airways, which might be affecting their breathing. Basically, the technique consists of one or two 'huffs' (Activity Box 5.15 Fig. 5.48) interspersed between controlled breathing. The purpose is to generate high velocity in the air leaving your lungs, but why would you want to do that if you were trying to get rid of mucus? Two reasons:

1. Higher air speed creates more turbulent air flow and greater shear forces, which could dislodge bits of mucus. It's like a fast-flowing wild river that can take bits of the river bank with it; bits of tree, mud etc.
2. As well as dislodging bits of mucus the shear forces alter the viscosity of the mucus lining the sides of the air tracts acts. This is gained through friction between the air and mucus, which warms it up, like the way you warm your hands up by rubbing them together. The increased temperature reduces the viscosity of the mucus (makes it runnier) making it easier to cough up.

A simple analogy would be cleaning out a blocked drain pipe by pushing fast flowing water through it. When you think about it this is what you do when you cough (fast air flow); the FET is a refined version of this that avoids the trauma of harsh repetitive coughing.

ACTIVITY BOX 5.15 **The Huff**

Get a hand mirror or stand in front of your bathroom mirror. Take a normal-sized breath and when you breathe out do it rapidly with your mouth open as if you were trying to steam up the mirror or warm your hand (Fig. 5.48). The sound you get is a kind of huff, a bit like the way you pant after running, but without the big breaths. Don't be too violent with your breathing out.

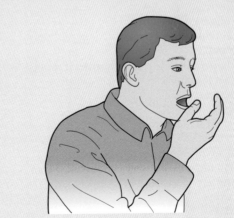

Fig. 5.48 The Forced Expiratory Technique.

SELF-ASSESSMENT QUESTIONS

1. What is the difference between stress and strain?
2. How do you measure tensile strain?
3. Young's modulus is
   a. Strain multiplied by stress.
   b. Stress divided by strain.
   c. Strain divided by stress.
   d. Stress divided by strain squared.
4. Is the following statement true or false?
   A material with high viscosity has a high resistance to flow.
5. Shear stress is
   a. A lot of stress.
   b. Stress applied perpendicular to the surface.
   c. High rate of stress.
   d. Stress applied parallel to the surface.
6. If a material returns to its original size and properties after a stress is removed, the material has remained in its
   a. Plastic range.
   b. Elastic range.
   c. Viscous range.
   d. Viscoelastic range.
7. What type of collagen is contained in tendon, skin, artery walls and bone?
   a. 1
   b. 2
   c. 3
   d. 4
8. What kind of fibre gives tendon its strength?
   a. Elastic
   b. Collagen
   c. Ground substance
   d. Fibroblasts
9. If a material has isotropic properties it means?
10. What is the middle layer of skin called?
    a. Dermis
    b. Epidermis
    c. Fat layer
    d. Hypodermis
11. What are the two types of bone called?
12. Tendon fibres have a wavy pattern called a/an
    a. Crease.
    b. Crimp.
    c. Wave.
    d. Undulation.
13. The collagen in tendons and ligaments are arranged
    a. Haphazardly and densely.
    b. Densely and in same direction.
    c. Loosely packed together and in same direction.
14. Elastic fibres are made of
    a. Collagen coiled up.
    b. Fibroblasts.
    c. Elastin.
    d. Macrophages.
15. What is Wolff's law?
    a. Bone adapts to the forces they experience.
    b. Bone strength declines with age.
    c. Bone is less able to resist tensile force.
    d. Female bone is lighter.
16. Which factor can make immobilisation worse?
    a. Prolonged period of immobilisation
    b. Inflammation
    c. Age
    d. Gender
17. Is this statement true or false?
    Stress relaxation is where there is a gradual decrease in tension within the stretched muscle when it is held at a constant length.
18. Connective tissue consists of three basic ingredients, fibres (collagen and elastin), cells (fibroblasts, macrophages and neutrophils) and
    a. Nerves.
    b. Arteries.
    c. Fat.
    d. ground substance.
19. What is density?
    a. Mass × volume
    b. Volume/mass
    c. Mass/volume
    d. Mass/volume squared
20. If the human body has an RD of 0.96 how much of the body would float in pure water?
    a. 4%
    b. 9.6%
    c. 0.96%
    d. 0.4%
21. Hydrostatic pressure is
    a. Density × gravity.
    b. Density × height (depth).
    c. Density × gravity × height (depth).
    d. Density × gravity/height (depth).

22. Pascal's law states that
    a. D pressure change in a contained fluid or gas is transmitted evenly throughout the gas/fluid.
    b. D pressure change in a contained fluid or gas is transmitted to the bottom of a gas/fluid.
    c. A pressure change in a fluid or gas is transmitted evenly throughout the gas/fluid.
    d. A pressure change in a contained fluid or gas is transmitted mainly to the supporting surface.

23. The movement of a gas or fluid where the layers slide on top of each is called
    a. Layer flow.
    b. Sedimentary flow.
    c. Turbulent flow.
    d. Laminar flow.
24. How does the FET technique assist the removal of mucus from lungs?
25. How can Bernoulli's principle be used to assist swimming?

ANSWERS TO QUESTIONS POSED IN TEXT

A. The Foot While Jogging

What kind of stress does the anteroposterior horizontal component cause at the metatarsal heads?
    Answer: Shear
What kind of stress does the vertical component cause at the metatarsal heads?
    Answer: Compressive
What could happen with repetitive stress application?
    Answer: Repetitive compressions can lead to callus (thickened skin) formation. This is the body's response to this kind of stress. Areas of high compressive stress can lead to corns forming. Repetitive applications of the shear stress can lead to the skin breaking down with inflamed skin and possibly blisters.

B. A Blow to Back of Knee

Imagine you are attending a game of soccer. You see a particularly bad tackle with one player kicking the back of the knee of another player causing the tibia to slide forwards.
What type of stress is experienced by the articular surface from the movement of the tibia?
    Answer: Shear stress
What type of stress does the anterior cruciate experience? The anterior cruciate is a strong ligament that is orientated to prevent the tibia sliding forward.
    Answer: Tensile stress
What do you think might happen to the anterior cruciate with this kind of stress?
    Answer: Tearing of the ligament, usually at its weakest point, which is where it attaches to the bone

Creep

Creep is an effective way of gaining a lot of elongation from a tissue however it makes the tissue less stiff. If this decrease in stiffness occurred at the tendons then this would affect its ability to transfer the force of the muscle to turning the bone, which may have a detrimental effect on performance of a sport or even put the tissue at risk of injury because, for a short period (60 to 90 minutes) it is not as strong as it was. This suggests that a small number of repetitions should be used and that these should not be done before engaging in an activity that involves large forces, such as participation in a sport.

Hydrotherapy Question

Shoulder adduction (bringing your arm to your side) could be resisted firstly with drag. Lying on your back (using appropriate floats) with your arm lying out to the side, move it slowly back to your side. The resistance to your movement came from (1) the mass of the water you are pushing out the way, and (2) drag, mainly from friction. Now do the same movement faster; this will be harder because of an increase in drag (mass of displaced water will be the same) from the turbulent flow created by the faster movement.

There is, of course, a limit to how much you can use drag; after all, you can only go so fast. So, to increase the resistance further you could use buoyancy. From a standing position, with your arm out to the side (so the arm lying on top of the water) pull your arm down to your side; this movement was resisted by buoyancy. To progress the resistance, you can make the arm bigger (so more water is displaced) and make the arm lighter (RD is decreased). This is accomplished nicely with an inflatable arm band; the more air in the arm band, the greater the resistance from buoyancy during the adduction movement.

REFERENCES

Alexander, R.M., Bennet-Clark, H.C., 1977. Storage of elastic strain energy in muscle and other tissues. Nature 265 (5590), 114–117.

Buckley, M.R., Sarver, J.J., Freedman, B.R., Soslowsky, L.J., 2013. The dynamics of collagen uncrimping and lateral contraction in tendon and the effect of ionic concentration. J. Biomech. 46 (13), 2242–2249.

Cecchi, E., Giglioli, C., Valente, S., Lazzeri, C., Gensini, G.F., Abbate, R., et al., 2011. Role of hemodynamic shear stress in cardiovascular disease. Atherosclerosis 214 (2), 249–256.

Herbert, R.D., Moseley, A.M., Butler, J.E., Gandevia, S.C., 2002. Change in length of relaxed muscle fascicles and tendons with knee and ankle movement in humans. J. Physiol. 539 (2), 637–645.

Ker, R.F., Bennett, M.B., Bibby, S.R., Kester, R.C., Alexander, R.M., 1987. The spring in the arch of the human foot. Nature 325 (6100), 147.

Maganaris, C.N., Paul, J.P., 1999. In vivo human tendon mechanical properties. J. Physiol. 521 (1), 307–313.

Martin, R.B., Burr, D.B., Sharkey, N.A., Fyhrie, D.P., 2015. Mechanical properties of ligament and tendon. In: Skeletal Tissue Mechanics. Springer, New York, pp. 175–225.

Petrofsky, J.S., Laymon, M., Lee, H., 2013. Effect of heat and cold on tendon flexibility and force to flex the human knee. Med. Sci. Monit. 19, 661–667.

Reeves, N.D., Maganaris, C.N., Narici, M.V., 2003. Effect of strength training on human patella tendon mechanical properties of older individuals. J. Physiol. 548 (3), 971–981.

Human Movement

6

Skeletal Muscle, Muscle Work, Strength, Power and Endurance

Tim Sharp

OUTLINE

LEARNING OUTCOMES

After reading this chapter, you will be able to:

1. Describe the structure and function of skeletal muscle.
2. Explain the physiological processes that occur during a contraction.
3. List and compare the different types of muscle activity.
4. Summarise the adaptations that occur in muscle with an increase or decrease in activity.
5. Differentiate between muscle force, strength and power.
6. Name the factors that influence muscle force production.
7. Explain muscle endurance.
8. Describe the common methods of measuring muscle strength and endurance.
9. Apply the principles of muscle strengthening and improving muscular endurance in the design of a rehabilitation programme.

INTRODUCTION

To understand movement you need a basic knowledge of the parts involved. The skeleton provides the bony frame of the body. This gives us our shape, protects our organs and, more relevantly for movement, provides the attachment and leverage for muscles. There are many individual bones in the body; how they are joined together may or may not allow movement to occur. The place that they are joined is called a joint, and it is the shape of the bones and the type of joint that ultimately dictates if, and what kind of movement, occurs. Running over the joints, attaching via tendons from one bone to the other, are the muscles. These muscles can be thought of as small motors (actuators) that create tension between the bones, either to pull them together, hold them in a specific position or allow them to move apart in a controlled manner. More detail about joints can be found in Chapter 7. This chapter will deal with how muscles work and how changes in muscle can be brought about. It is important to have a basic understanding of the structure and function of skeletal muscle. Before we proceed, try Activity Box 6.1 to get you thinking.

The primary function of muscle is to generate force. The journey to discover how muscles contract to produce force at high speeds is a fascinating one, especially when you consider how small each contractile component is and therefore the need to coordinate lots of contractile components within a single muscle, and then coordinate this with other muscles to produce a precise and powerful movement such as a badminton smash (see Activity Box 6.1). Just as well we don't have to consciously think about it!

To create the tension needed to hold a specific position (also known as posture, which is discussed in more detail in Chapter 8), or create and control movement, it must have components that are capable of contracting (shortening). As well as having contractile elements, muscles also contain noncontractile elements; these form the structural components, tendons to join the muscles to the bones, and sheaths wrapped around the layers of muscle to harness the force. While these are not actively involved in producing force, they transmit the force to the bone and store elastic potential energy to make the process more efficient. These structures (tendon, epimysium, endomysium and perimysium) mainly consist of collagen, which is pretty stiff (useful for transmitting force), but they also contain elastin (in varying degrees), which allows them to return to their original position after a stretch, like a rubber band (Lieber, 2010) (see Chapter 7 for a more in-depth discussion). As these structures link the muscle to the bone it is important that they are not too stretchy as the force would go into stretching the tendon rather than producing movement. So, basically, muscle shortens and pulls the tendon, which pulls on its attachment and produces, or controls, movement.

Before we go any further into looking at the types of muscle work, it is important to understand how skeletal muscle is able to produce a force. This requires knowledge of its structure from the proteins to the gross anatomy. We shall start at the protein level and build up to the gross muscle anatomy.

PROTEIN FILAMENTS

At a molecular level, skeletal muscle is composed of various proteins arranged in a precise fashion. This gives skeletal muscle a distinctively ordered array. There are four proteins involved in muscle contraction; Myosin, which forms the thick filament strand and the three proteins that make up the thin filament (actin, troponin and tropomyosin) (Fig. 6.1). As can be seen in Fig. 6.1B, myosin (thick filament) resembles a golf club, with a long handle and a head; unlike a golf club, the head is attached to the filament via a flexible neck. The thick filament consists of many myosin molecules packed together in a regimented fashion so that the heads project away from the shaft. They are also arranged in an antiparallel fashion, in which some lie pointing one way and others will point in the opposite direction. The heads end up at the ends of the filament, with the shafts in the centre. This makes it look a bit like a double-headed toilet brush (see Fig. 6.1B).

The three proteins of the thin filament are arranged with the actin as a core to the filament, the tropomyosin twisting around the actin, and the globular protein troponin sitting on the tropomyosin every so often (see Fig. 6.1A).

So far, we have two separate filaments—thick and thin—each of which possess specific characteristics. It is these specific characteristics, along with the regimented organisation of the thick and thin filaments, that give muscle its properties. Before looking at the organisation, we need

---

ACTIVITY BOX 6.1   **Thinking About Muscle Work**

To start you thinking about muscle work, think about the badminton smash, or even better watch someone performing a smash in badminton. Think about what is going on around the shoulder joint, just in terms of muscle work.

- Which muscles accelerate the arm forwards, bringing the arm and racket closer to the shuttle?
- Which muscles slow the arm down (decelerate) at the end of the shot?
- Are there other muscles working to hold the posture?

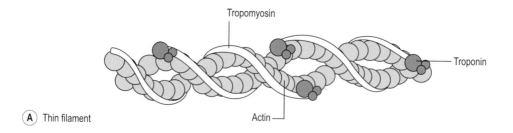

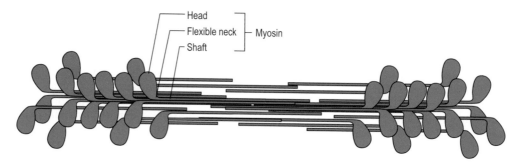

Fig. 6.1 A thin filament (A), showing the double helix of the actin with the tropomyosin and troponin. A thick filament (B), showing the myosin molecules arranged in an antiparallel fashion. The resemblance of the myosin molecules to a golf club can clearly be seen.

to know how these unique characteristics allow the thick and thin filaments to interact.

The actin of the thin filament possesses binding sites for the myosin heads, but these are covered by the spiral strands of tropomyosin. Troponin, which is also attached to the actin and tropomyosin is able to change its shape, and due to its attachments pulls the tropomyosin to expose the myosin binding site. This change in shape occurs in the presence of calcium ions. When calcium ions are released the myosin binding sites are exposed (by the changing troponin shape) and the myosin head is able to attach to the actin. Once attached to the actin, the myosin neck flexes, pulling the thin filament along the thick filament. As can be seen in Fig. 6.2, this flexing has the effect of sliding the thick and thin filaments over each other. Once the myosin neck has flexed, it is released from the actin using energy from ATP (Adenosine Triphosphate) to break the bond; the neck is restored to its original position and is free to bind with the actin again and repeat the process. In effect, the myosin walks along the actin filament. This is a very basic description of the sliding filament theory as first proposed by Hugh Huxley in 1953; further reading is recommended (Triplet, 2015; Astrand et al., 2003). For now, it is enough to appreciate the interaction of the filaments to create a muscle contraction. If you want an analogy to help you remember, think of a rowing action. The

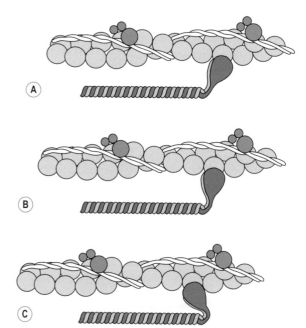

Fig. 6.2 During a muscle contraction, the cross-bridge of the myosin molecule attaches to a binding site on the actin filament (A) and the myosin head rotates (B and C) and pulls the actin filament to the left.

oar (myosin) enters the water (actin) and the rower pulls, moving the oar through the water before repeating these power sweeps over and over again; very simplified, this is the essence of the sliding filament theory of a muscle contraction.

Moving out a little further, the thick filaments of myosin are grouped together in bundles with other structural proteins, such as titin, binding the filaments together at the centre of the filament. These structural proteins, as well as holding the filaments together, space them apart. This space is important, as this is where the thin filaments slide. Typically, the structural proteins where the thick filaments are attached is depicted as a line when viewed from the side. However, a disc is more of a true representation, with the thick filaments running through it and sticking out either side (Fig. 6.3). This disc is known as the M line. The thin filaments are arranged in a similar way; the same type of disc can be found, and this is known as the Z line or Z disc (Lieber, 2010).

So, we have two basic functional structures in skeletal muscle: bundles of thick filaments and bundles of thin filaments. Imagine these two bundles are Lego bricks of different colour; let's say the thick filaments are blue bricks, and the thin filaments are yellow bricks. Imagine taking the blue bricks and placing them in a line with an even gap between each brick. Now place a yellow brick on top of a blue brick so that it bridges the gap between the two blue bricks. If you filled in each gap then you would have alternating columns of blue then yellow bricks. The Lego bricks fit together much like the thick and thin filaments. The difference in a muscle, compared to Lego, is that the filaments have the ability to slide over each other, allowing the columns to come closer to each other. Each thick filament is separated by six thin filaments instead of our Lego model, which had just one (so a stack of six yellow bricks instead of one). This arrangement of alternating bundles of thick then thin

filaments stacked in a long line produces the regimented appearance of muscle tissue and, more importantly, allows the column to change length. If we were to cut our column into sections, splitting each yellow brick in half, so we have a blue brick with two yellow halves on each end, this would represent a sarcomere.

THE SARCOMERE

The sarcomere is the basic functional unit of muscle and is defined by adjacent Z lines. Starting at one Z line travelling along the filaments, we first travel along a light area of thin filaments. This light area of solely thin filaments is known as the I band. Next to this is a darker area where we come across thick filaments as well as thin filaments, and this is the area of overlap. Then there is again a slightly lighter area known as the H zone, where there are just thick filaments, before we reach the M line and then go through the reverse of this to get back to the Z line. The light and dark areas of the sarcomere are clearly visible in Fig. 6.4. As well as I bands, H zones, M lines and Z lines, there is also an A band, which is basically the zone that contains the thick filaments (including the H zone and the overlap area with the thin filaments). These bands change size during contraction, indicating that the filaments are sliding over one another, making the sarcomere shorter (Astrand et al., 2003).

The column that we had described earlier of the alternating bundles of thick and thin filaments is repeated many times, making a long, thin, cylindrical column. This is called the myofibril and, as can be seen in Fig. 6.5, it has a striated (striped) appearance. A muscle fibre is made up of lots of myofibrils lying parallel to each other (see Fig. 6.5). The sarcomeres are all lined up, so the entire muscle fibre has a striated appearance. The myofibrils are attached to the next myofibril with more structural proteins that help to

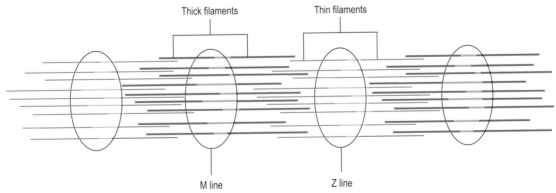

Fig. 6.3 Alternating Bundles of Thin and Thick Filaments in Series. Note how the thick and thin filaments overlap. A sliding of the filaments over one another would bring the M line and the Z line closer together.

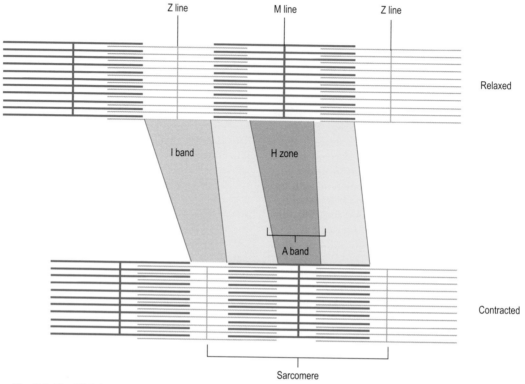

Fig. 6.4 The Divisions Within a Sarcomere and the Effect on the Various Zones During a (Concentric) Contraction.

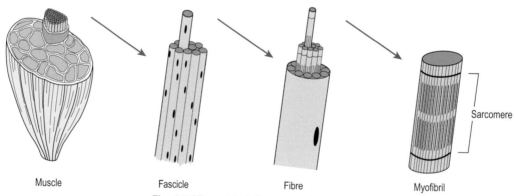

Fig. 6.5 Hierarchical Structure of a Muscle.

transmit the contraction of each sarcomere ensuring that the muscle fibre contracts as one unit. The muscle fibre is, in essence, a single muscle cell and contains all the normal things found in a cell, such as a nucleus, mitochondria and a cell membrane (sarcolemma) (Astrand et al., 2003). The function and abundance of these structures is very important in the production of a contraction but we do not have the

scope to discuss them in detail and don't want to distract you from key learning. There are many good physiological textbooks covering muscle which are worth exploring.

Muscle fibres are surrounded by the sarcolemma and a connective tissue sheath called the endomysium. Anatomically, the muscle fibres are grouped into fascicles, which again have a connective tissue sheath (called a perimysium);

the fascicles are all bundled together to form the muscle, which again is surrounded by a sheath (called the epimysium). The connective tissue sheaths that surround the various divisions of the muscle are all linked together and are important in the transmission of passive forces through a muscle, such as when a muscle is stretched. Fig. 6.5 gives an appreciation of this structure. The sheaths found between the different levels of muscle have different names according to their location, but in functional terms they are a continuous unit. This allows us to appreciate that as the muscle fibres are connected to the various layers a contraction of one part of the muscle will pull all the other parts of the muscle along with it, so the muscle shortens as a whole unit but not all muscle fibres are involved in the contraction. This concept is extremely important in preventing the intramuscular stress leading to damage (Petrof, 1998).

Before we move on to muscle work, there are two important concepts about the arrangement of the sarcomeres in a muscle that are worth mentioning at this point. First, remembering back to the blue and yellow Lego brick construction of a myofibril, the sarcomeres are said to be in series (end to end). As each sarcomere has an ability to change length by a certain degree, the more sarcomeres you have in series the greater the degree and speed a myofibril can shorten (Fig. 6.6). Under certain circumstances, the number of sarcomeres in series can change (Lieber, 2010). This would change the range of movement that the muscle can work through and the speed of contraction. As we will see later, there are other aspects that can influence the speed of contraction.

Second, thinking back even further to the myosin–actin cross-bridged interaction, you may remember that ultimately this is the motor that drives the shortening of a muscle. Each sarcomere has the ability to generate a specific amount of tension. To increase force, you need more sarcomeres pulling side by side and not in a line. The easiest way to imagine this is to think of pulling a car or heavy object. If you see someone pulling a car and you want to help, you can grab hold of the rope and pull on the same rope. More people can join in a tug-of-war type set-up; however, there comes a point when the rope will not be able to take the force of all the people pulling on it. In this situation the only way to increase the amount of force being applied on the car is by adding more people through second or third ropes attached to the car. As sarcomeres are arranged along the line of force generation they can be viewed as the people pulling on the ropes. The greater the number of sarcomeres side by side (parallel) the greater the force generation capacity of the muscle. Fundamentally, the more sarcomeres there are in parallel the bigger the muscle and the bigger the force. This makes sense, as the stronger you get the bigger your muscles become; however, as we will see later, muscle force and strength are two different concepts.

The analogies presented above illustrate how the functional unit (sarcomere) arrangement can influence the muscle's force production capacity. As muscle force production and strength are conceptually different, there are many factors that can affect strength, and this shall be presented in the next section.

We know why muscles have to be developed in terms of strength and endurance when participating in sport at any level. It is self-evident why a shot putter needs strong arms that can deliver a powerful thrust to propel an 8-kg shot 20 m, or a marathon runner needs muscle endurance to run over 26 miles. Although these athletes sometimes appear superhuman, they actually function in the same way as you or I, and the neurophysiological processes they need to build up their muscular systems are essentially the same as those

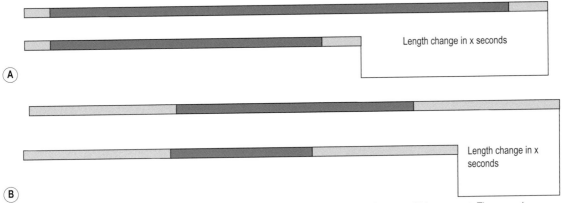

Fig. 6.6 The Effect of the Number of Sarcomeres in Series on Muscle Range of Movement. The muscle with more sarcomeres in series (A) is able to shorten through a greater range and at a greater velocity compared with the muscle in (B).

for someone who has become weak and out of condition through trauma, disease or any other form of disuse, as well as ageing. (Try Activity Box 6.2.)

Did you notice when undertaking Activity Box 6.2 that movement was affected in many, if not all, of the diseases and traumas in your list? This decrease in movement occurs even when the disease or injury does not directly affect the muscles themselves. If a person does not move or moves incorrectly for any length of time, then the muscular and cardiovascular systems will deteriorate. This process is technically known as *deconditioning*. So, just like the top-class athlete, deconditioned patients will need to improve their condition by increasing the strength, power and endurance of the muscles relevant to their functional needs.

In the following section, mechanisms by which muscle work brings about increases in strength and endurance will be discussed. Basic definitions will be given, as well as the physiological process and physical procedures required to produce these changes in condition.

THE DIFFERENCE BETWEEN MUSCLE FORCE AND MUSCLE STRENGTH

Muscle strength and *muscle force* are sometimes used interchangeably. They are, however, two distinct, though related, concepts. As discussed in Chapter 2, a force is an entity that is generated by an action—a push or a pull, for example—or imparted as a kick. The object to which the force is imparted may move or deform. Therefore, a force can be defined as *something that changes the state of rest or motion of a body*.

These forces are a product of the mass of the object producing them multiplied by its acceleration ($F = m \times a$). The unit of measurement is the newton (N).

Forces can be thought of as being either external or internal. External forces are generated outside the body, usually acting on the body, such as gravity, friction or a push from another person. Internal forces are those produced by the muscles. It is the muscle's capacity to produce force that is a measure of the muscle strength. A fuller definition of muscle force would be *the ability of a muscle or group of muscles to produce tension and a resulting force in one maximal*

effort, either dynamically or statically, in relation to the demands placed on it.

The production of the internal force was explained in the previous section. The sliding filament theory explains how the actin and myosin protein fibrils slide over one another and form a series of cross-bridges that pull the sarcomeres together, thus shortening the muscle and producing the force Narici (1999).

MUSCLE WORK

A muscle has to contract to produce a force. The force it produces can be either very small, so that the resultant action is correspondingly fine (e.g. picking up a feather), or quite large, with a result of deforming or moving a large object with a large movement (e.g. throwing a cricket ball across a field). The shortening of the muscles (bringing the proximal and distal attachments closer together) produces the work. If the movement (i.e. the change in length of the muscle) can be measured, this can be multiplied by the force generated to give the work done by the muscle (work = force × distance). The unit of measurement of the work done is the joule (J).

From the definition, it can be seen that the muscle will be doing work only if there is a change in length. If the muscle is getting shorter as it is performing its task, it is said to be performing a *concentric contraction*, and the work done is therefore *concentric work*. If, on the other hand, the muscle is getting longer as it is performing its task, it is said to be doing *eccentric work*, as the contraction is eccentric. The former will be positive work (shortening) and the latter negative (lengthening). Paradoxically, if a muscle is producing an isometric (static) contraction then mechanically no work is being done, as there is no movement. If you hold a weight in an outstretched arm, it will not be long before you can feel the work that you are doing. How can this be so? An isometric contraction using our understanding of the sliding filament theory would not need to make any new cross-bridges to slide over each other as there is no movement, and hence no work done. However, this doesn't explain the increase in tension. It is likely that there are very small changes in length of the muscle fibres both concentrically and eccentrically with the filaments sliding one way then the other; this movement is too small to observe externally. This would also explain the energy requirements for isometric contraction.

The different amounts and types of muscle work, which result from the muscle's ability to alter the forces produced and the direction of its action, are important when we consider the activities that humans have to perform. Time for a short activity—try Activity Box 6.3.

If you analyse the muscle activity in the first example in Activity Box 6.3, it can be seen that biceps brachii appears

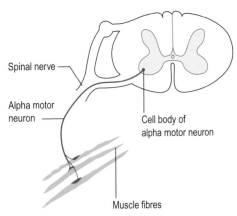

Fig. 6.7 A single motor unit is composed of the motor neuron and the muscle fibres that it innervates. The cell body of the motor neuron is in the anterior horn cell in the spinal cord, and its axon is one of the motor nerves in a mixed peripheral nerve.

to be doing most of the work throughout the movement. As you bring the drink up to your mouth (mainly bending your elbow), the work being done by the muscle is concentric, as the muscle is getting shorter. As you lower the drink, the biceps again performs most of the work, but this time the muscle work is eccentric, as the muscle is getting longer. Energy is also used when the muscle has to contract isometrically to hold the drink to your mouth. As you drink more, the load that you have to move becomes less, so although the type of work that the biceps produces will not change, the required force will decrease. Please note that this isn't a valid excuse to drink more fluid in bars!

In the second example, the muscles of the lower limb are working to produce walking. During gait there is a cyclical change between concentric (e.g. hip flexors during early to terminal swing) and eccentric muscle work (e.g. knee extensors during loading response). If you suddenly have to change the amount of muscle work in order to run for the bus, this is done by producing more force within the muscles, engaging more sarcomeres in series and performing faster contractions.

These two examples show that there is a constant interplay between the type and quantity of muscle work that produces propulsion and control so that humans can perform the manifold functional tasks that are needed throughout the day.

MUSCLE STRENGTH

The two activities in Activity Box 6.3 show the variation in the amount of muscle force needed to carry out the functional activities of everyday life. The same muscles are used concentrically and eccentrically to walk and run, which is just a difference in magnitude and rate, and the biceps are capable of lifting a heavier weight than a pint. The shot putter, on the other hand, needs to use all the force that could be generated in their muscles to give impetus to the shot. Therefore, it can be concluded that a muscle has the ability to change the force generation for different activities. In other words, each muscle has a range of force outputs available to it. How much strength a muscle has to use to perform a task is dependent on many influences.

It can be seen that muscle force is generated by the sliding filament (actin and myosin), whereas strength is the maximal output of the muscle, which includes a contribution from the noncontractile elements. We can vary the amount of force generated according to the task, but our strength is often seen as our maximal force capability. The control of muscle action is tackled in more depth in Chapter 9 (motor control) but an overview here makes sense, and repetition is always good!

RECRUITMENT

As described earlier, muscle is built up from bundles of fibres bound into fascicles (see Fig. 6.5). It can also be grouped into functional units. These units are called motor units. As described and illustrated in more detail in Chapter 9, muscles need a signal in order to contract. This signal is delivered by the alpha motor neurons originating from the spinal cord. A single alpha motor neuron may innervate between 10 and 1000 muscle fibres, depending on the muscle. A single alpha motor neuron and the muscle fibres that it innervates make up a motor unit, which is illustrated in Fig. 6.7. The force produced by a single muscle fibre is very small and quite insignificant. It makes sense to group fibres together so that a single stimulation of a motor neuron will cause a simultaneous contraction of all the muscle fibres in that motor unit (the 'all or nothing' principle), producing a useful amount of force. The motor unit has muscle fibres spread throughout the muscle, so they are not necessarily adjacent to each, which is why it is a functional collective rather than an anatomical one. The amount of force produced by a single motor unit depends on the number of muscle fibres it contains. There is a large variance in the number, because some muscles are associated with delicate and fine movements and some are quite gross. When precise and fine movements are needed, such as in the hand or eye, the motor units contain a small number of muscle fibres; when a relatively high degree of force is required and the movement can be quite gross, such as in the lower limb, there are a high number of fibres in a single motor unit.

MUSCLE FIBRE TYPES

Before considering how muscle force can be precisely controlled, it is necessary to be aware of one more factor that can influence the amount of force that a motor unit can produce. This relates to the different muscle fibre types. It is accepted that in humans there are three types of fibre, and they are classified by either their force characteristics or the isoforms of the contractile proteins (specifically myosin). Luckily, the two classifications are different only in their name. For the purposes of this text, the muscle will be classified according to the protein isoforms: type I, type IIa and type IIb. Table 6.1 lays out the various characteristics of these fibre types. It can be seen that for a given stimulation, type I muscle fibres reach the peak force at a slow speed and produce a low force but are fatigue resistant (FR). Type IIa fibres reach their peak force quicker, produce a greater force per stimulation and are FR. Type IIb fibres produce the highest amount of force in the shortest period of time but have a higher degree of fatigability. Type I fibres are therefore suited to activities that require a low amount of force for a long duration, whereas type IIb fibres are suited to quick, forceful contractions. A single motor unit will contain only one fibre type, and the alpha motor neuron will have functional characteristics that mirror those of the muscle fibre (Lieber, 2010). The motor unit that contains slow fibres will be small in diameter, making conduction velocity relatively low; this type of motor unit is known as a slow (S) motor unit. The motor units that contain type IIa fibres are known as FR motor units, and those that have type IIb fibres have the widest diameter of axons and fastest conduction velocities and are known as fast fatigable (FF) motor units. Each muscle contains a mix of the three types of motor unit in varying proportions according to the functional role of the muscle. Postural muscles (e.g. the soleus) that work to maintain posture will typically have a majority of S motor units, whereas the gastrocnemius has a high proportion of FR and FF motor units. However, the proportions are not drastically different; for example, it has been estimated that the hamstring muscle group has around 45% S motor units compared to 55% FF and FR, and as such is often classified as a 'mobiliser muscle', as opposed to a postural muscle.

GRADATION OF MUSCLE FORCE

As we have seen muscles can vary their force production (remember the reducing pint in the bar?) and past experience is a vital component. Lifting a full glass of liquid is a common activity, so the brain has a good idea of how much strength is needed and therefore how much effort to use to lift the glass. On the other hand, if we lift a closed box expecting it to be heavy, the result may be that the box is thrown up in the air because it is, in fact, empty. The brain had been expecting a heavy load and the muscles had contracted accordingly to match the expected force.

The above scenarios are dependent on the number of motor units used during the muscle contraction. The contraction of the motor unit is termed *recruitment*, and it is this recruitment that enables us to use our muscles to produce fine movements such as writing, larger movements

TABLE 6.1	Examples of Differences Between Muscle Fibre Types.[a]		
Property	**Type I**	**Type IIA**	**Type IIB**
Muscle fibre type	Slow oxidative	Fast oxidative glycolytic	Fast glycolytic
Motor unit type	Slow	Fast fatigue-resistant	Fast fatigable
Motor unit size	Small	Medium	Large
Twitch tension	Low	Moderate	High
Mechanical speed	Slow	Fast	Fast
Fatigability	Low	Low	High
Mitochondrial enzyme activity	High	Medium	Low
Glycogenolytic enzyme activity	Low	Medium	High
Myoglobin content	High	Medium	Low
Capillary density	High	Medium	Low

[a]Note that different terminology exists for types of muscle fibre and motor unit.

such as picking up a glass, or the whole of our strength in putting the shot. So, the task itself, or the load to be overcome, is the main component in determining the force exerted by the muscle. However, as seen earlier, the motor unit has an all or nothing contraction. Therefore there must be a way to grade the muscle force according to the demands. Indeed, the body has two ways that vary the amount of force: motor unit recruitment and the frequency of stimulation.

Motor units within a muscle are recruited in a set order according to the force requirements. For activities requiring a low amount of force, the motor units that produce the lowest force are recruited first (i.e. the S motor units). This has two effects: first, the fibre type is FR and can therefore go on for a long period of time; second, subsequent recruitment of more S motor units results in a smaller step increase in force (Fig. 6.8), allowing for a finer gradation of muscle force production. As the force production increases, the fast FR motor units are recruited next. As the force reaches near maximal, the FF motor units are recruited. However, this cannot be sustained for very long, as they are susceptible to fatigue, and a sustained contraction will be unable to maintain the maximal force output. Note that in Fig. 6.8 the steps associated with the FF units are much larger. This recruitment of motor units follows the Henneman size principle; this is also known as the size principle, as the neurons that are easiest to stimulate are the smaller ones associated with the S motor units and are therefore recruited first. The larger the neuron, the harder it is stimulate, and

therefore more effort is required to produce a contraction of the larger motor neurons of the FR and FF motor units.

The second point is the frequency of stimulation; for any given motor unit, a single stimulation will produce a given force output. We have already seen that if force needs to be increased, recruitment of more motor units will achieve this; however, the motor unit can also produce more force (up to certain point) if the frequency of stimulation increases. A bit like the cox in a rowing boat requesting the rowers to increase their stroke rate. These options give the body more ways of controlling the force output of a muscle. These two methods are both at work during sustained low force contraction; motor units are switched on and off according to demand, and changes in stimulation frequency also occur—both of which can finely tune the force output to closely match the task. This type of activity is typical of everyday activities such as standing or walking.

LENGTH-TENSION RELATIONSHIP

As well as recruitment, other physical properties of the muscle are important in determining strength generation, including the length–tension relationship of the contractile unit. It has been shown that the production of force in the muscle is proportional to the number of cross-bridges that occur between the actin and myosin fibrils (number of oars in the water, to continue the rowing analogy). If few myosin heads are in contact—as when the actin and myosin fibrils are stretched apart, for example—then force production will be decreased. If the fibrils are too contracted, the tapered ends of the myosin filaments push against the Z bands, and again the force that can be generated is decreased (Fig. 6.9). These length–tension characteristics are enhanced by the intracellular titin filaments that run through the length of the myosin protein filament between the Z lines. These titin filaments have an intrinsic elastic property that can alter the propensity of the muscle to contract (Lakomy, 1999). It is tempting to think that during movement when the muscle shortens, the muscle will behave exactly like the graph in Fig. 6.9. In other words, when a muscle is in a lengthened position (outer range) there are very few cross-bridges between the myosin and actin, as the overlap is small, and the muscle is unable to generate much tension. Similarly, if the muscle is in a shortened position, there is too much overlap, and the myosin filaments cannot move any further down the thin filaments as the Z disc is in the way, again limiting the amount of tension. However, the length–tension curve as represented in Fig. 6.9 is valid for isometric contractions only (when no movement occurs); it should be viewed as a series of points rather than a curve.

Clinically the full range of movement through which a muscle works is usually divided into thirds: inner, middle

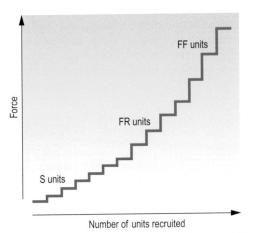

Fig. 6.8 The Regulation of Force by Recruitment of Motor Units. At low forces, only the small, slow (S) units are recruited. As force increases, the larger fatigue-resistant (FR) and then the largest fast, fatigable (FF) units are recruited. The S units have relatively few muscle fibres and the FF units have the most. Therefore the increment in force as a new unit is recreated also varies.

and outer. Inner range is when the muscle is in a shortened position, outer is when it is in a lengthened position, and middle is between the two (Fig. 6.10). So, for an isometric contraction, the outer range is where there is very little overlap between the thick and thin filaments, the middle range is where there is optimal overlap, and the inner range is where the thick filaments run into the Z disc. It has been known for some time that the muscle is weaker in the inner and outer range and strongest in the middle range. Part of the reason is the length–tension relationship; however, the biomechanics in relation to the anatomy plays a large role. The angle of pull of the muscle on the bone changes through the range such that the muscle is usually strongest in the middle range (when the angle of pull is at 90 degrees). For more details on this, see Chapter 4. To be able to appreciate the tension in a muscle during a movement, the distinction between active and passive tension and velocity needs to be discussed.

ACTIVE AND PASSIVE TENSION

In Fig. 6.9, you can see a curved line; this represents the passive tension within a muscle. When a muscle is passively lengthened, the muscle resists the lengthening. This resistance is thought to result from the stiffness in the noncontractile parts of the muscle (tendon, endomysium, perimysium and epimysium) as well as the protein mentioned earlier: titin. When a muscle is taken from midrange to outer range, the passive tension increases slowly initially, and as the end of range approaches the tension increases dramatically (as you have all felt when doing a hamstring stretch). Therefore, as it approaches outer range, the tension of the muscle will increase irrespective of the activity of the muscle. This could be viewed as a mechanism to stop the sarcomere from being overstretched and keep some degree of overlap between the thick and thin filaments, so that a contraction is still possible.

FORCE–VELOCITY RELATIONSHIP

As most muscle contractions are involved in movement, it is important to understand how a muscle behaves during movement. As mentioned earlier, the length–tension relationship is not helpful here, as it is valid only when there is no length change (isometric). If a muscle is allowed to change length during a contraction, it can do so at a variety of speeds. The force–velocity relationship is another aspect that affects muscle strength. Different forces can be generated at different speeds (Fig. 6.11). If the force generated by the

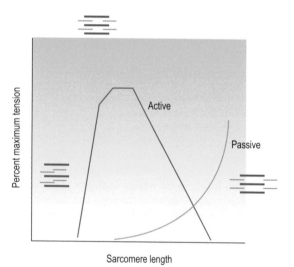

Fig. 6.9 The sarcomere length–tension curve during sequential isometric contractions of a muscle fibre, with diagrammatic representation of the thick and thin filament overlap. The curved line represents the passive tension of the muscle.

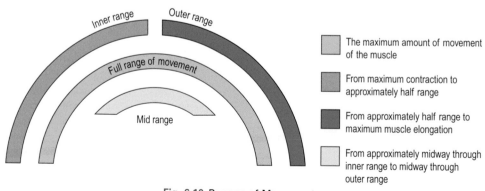

Fig. 6.10 Ranges of Movement.

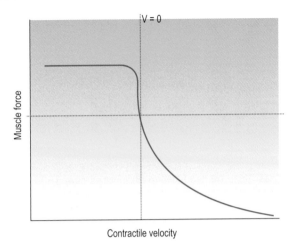

Fig. 6.11 Force–Velocity Relationship Graph. Isometric contraction is represented at V = 0. To the right of this is concentric contraction. As the velocity increases, the force reduces. To the left of V = 0 are eccentric contractions as the velocity of lengthening increases.

muscle is equal to the load, then no movement will occur (velocity = 0, an isometric contraction). If the muscle force is greater than the load, then the muscle will shorten (concentric contraction). The greater the velocity of contraction the smaller the tension in the muscle. It can be seen from the force–velocity graph that concentric contractions do not develop as much tension as isometric contractions. If the load is greater than the muscle force, then the muscle will lengthen (eccentric contraction). This type of muscle contraction generates a greater amount of force than isometric or concentric contractions. Unlike concentric contraction, in eccentric contraction as the velocity of lengthening increases the tension increases, up to a point. This is quite poorly understood, but this relationship is also applicable to the energetics at a molecular level. Therefore this increase in tension is probably because the muscle uses very little ATP to break the bonds holding the cross-bridges.

ANGLE OF PULL

Other anatomical and biomechanical aspects of muscle function will affect the strength generation. The angle of pull of a muscle at the time of its action will affect its strength. The angle of pull of a muscle is defined as *the angle between the segmental axis and the line of pull of the muscle*.

An angle of pull that is nearer to 90 degrees means that more of the resolved muscle force would rotate the segment (vertical component). If the angle of pull was greater or less than 90 degrees, then the distractive or compressive forces

(horizontal component) would increase. This is explained again in Chapter 4.

STABILITY AND SEQUENCING

For the muscle to work efficiently, it should work from a stable base. The strength of the muscle will then be used for the intended movement task and not diverted to ensure that a stable base is maintained. This is very important during early rehabilitation, as the muscles can be very weak. This is quite commonly seen when performing exercises on a gym ball. People often perform weight-lifting exercises on a gym ball for various reasons; however, the weight that they can lift on the gym ball (the unstable surface) is much less than if they adopted the same position on a stable surface. During many functional movements, many muscles have a role to provide this stable base, for example some of the abdominal muscles. These muscles are helped to achieve this stable base and work more efficiently by working in predefined sequences. These sequences are learned as movement is refined during the maturation process or we learn the pattern as a new skill. Chapter 15 explains these processes.

ANATOMY

The gross structure of the muscle is well adapted to provide the appropriate range, direction and force of contraction. The muscles that produce precision movements have fine muscle fibres, whereas the gluteus maximus (big postural muscle), for example, has coarse muscle fibres. How the fibres are structured within the muscle is also important. They are usually parallel, oblique or spiral relative to the direction of pull of the muscle. In muscles, the angle of pennation (the angle at which the fibres join the central spine of connective tissue) of the muscle itself will affect its ability to produce force. The greater the angle of pennation, then the more sarcomeres can be fitted in. This will lead to an increase in strength but a decrease in shortening velocity (Narici, 1999). Examples of the different forms of muscle fibre arrangement can be seen in Fig. 6.12.

The length–tension relationship, the angle of pull, and the sequencing and patterning of muscle action are all most effective in producing greater strength when the muscle is in its middle range. Of course, these biomechanical factors result in efficient strong muscle work only if the neuromuscular and muscular systems are intact. The physiological systems, such as the circulatory system, must also be functioning optimally to initiate, maintain and terminate muscle action. If any of these systems malfunction, as in many pathologies, then muscle strength and subsequent efficient movement are decreased.

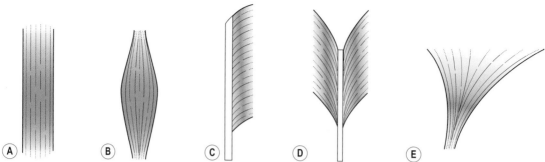

Fig. 6.12 Some of the Common Arrangements of Muscles. Strap (A) and fusiform (B) muscles have a tendon at either end and relatively long muscle fibres that run between the tendons. The muscle fibres are arranged in parallel to, or are very similar to, the angle of pull of the tendon. Unipennate (C) and bipennate (D) muscles have a central tendon into which short muscle fibres are inserted. The fibre direction is different to the angle of pull of the tendon. Triangular muscles (E) display mixed characteristics.

AGE AND SEX

Age and sex also have an effect on absolute muscle strength. It will be seen in Chapter 10 that the changes caused by ageing are complex and are a combination of the physiological process, disease and lifestyle. However, the general consequence is that muscle strength decreases with age, although they remain trainable throughout life. As for sex, a male sarcomere is equal to a female sarcomere. The well-documented differences in muscle strength relates to the difference in the number of muscle fibres, with men, in general, having more.

PSYCHOLOGICAL FACTORS

It is important to remember that as well as the physical and physiological aspects discussed above, there can also be a psychological element to muscle strength. The shot putter will win the gold medal only if they are psychologically prepared, if they have produced enough adrenaline (epinephrine) to produce a maximal effort and the calmness to recreate their optimal technique. Sometimes the apparent limit of physical ability to produce muscle strength is overcome by psychological influences. There is the tale of the mother who lifted a car under which her child was trapped. This superhuman feat was obviously beyond her perceived physical ability.

MUSCLE POWER

In Chapter 4, power is defined as the rate at which work is being done. The unit of work is the watt (W), named after the celebrated Scottish engineer/scientist James Watt. The rate at which a muscle works is termed *muscle power* and

can be calculated by using the following formulae (units in brackets):

$$\text{Power (watts)} = \text{Work done (joules)}/\text{Time taken (seconds)}.$$

(If we remember that work done is force [newtons] × distance [metres].)

Positive power is generated during a concentric contraction, and negative power is generated (or you could say absorbed) during an eccentric contraction. See Padulo et al. (2013) for more details on this. Earlier, it was explained that the velocity of muscle contraction is largely determined by the composition of that muscle (i.e. the fibre type[s] it contains). The type II (phasic fast twitch) fibres that generate large amounts of tension in a short time are geared towards anaerobic metabolic activity and tend to fatigue quickly. The power produced by these muscles will typically be anaerobic (oxygen not required) and will produce high-intensity activity over short periods of time. Type I (tonic slow twitch) fibres generate a low level of muscle tension but can sustain contraction for a long time. These fibres are geared towards aerobic metabolism (need oxygen) and are slow to fatigue. The power they produce is therefore aerobic power. Although there are many ways of classifying power in relation to movement, using aerobic and anaerobic power is useful as it can inform exercise selection for training or rehabilitation.

MUSCLE ENDURANCE

If you think about all the activities you carry out on an average day, there are few occasions, if any, when you use maximum strength, provided you have typical levels of muscle strength, of course. Instead many activities require repetitive muscle action; just think of walking, typing, dancing or playing a musical instrument as examples. The muscle's ability to keep on working over long periods of time is a measure of its endurance and is defined as *the ability of a muscle to sustain repetitive isometric or isotonic contractions.*

In the preceding text, strength was described in biomechanical/physical terms, basically its ability to create force. However, endurance needs to be described from a more physiological perspective. Endurance is dependent on the type of energy pathways used by the working muscle (i.e. the aerobic and anaerobic energy systems). The anaerobic system does not require oxygen to create the ATP necessary for muscle action, but instead manufactures it directly and rapidly from the breakdown of creatine phosphate and glycogen (sugar), which is stored in the muscles themselves; however, this store is rapidly used up (1 to 3 minutes). If muscle work continues, and therefore the need to make ATP continues, this can be achieved aerobically through the metabolism of food stuffs (sugars and fats) transported to the muscles in the blood. The end product of this digestive process creates pyruvate (like concentrated energy), which is broken down further to create the ATP in the Krebs cycle; a critical ingredient for this process is a constant supply of oxygen. Thus oxygen transport from the lungs to the working muscle is a vital part of the aerobic energy system.

During sustained muscle work, waste products such as carbon dioxide, potassium, acetylcholine and lactic acid are being produced. It is just as important for the functioning of this system that this waste is removed from the area. If the waste is not removed, then its build-up will cause the muscle to fatigue, resulting in a reduction in muscle strength and co-ordination. The longer the muscle can resist fatigue, the greater its aerobic capacity (Daniels, 2001).

So, although the body can supply muscles with instant energy, in the absence of oxygen (anaerobic), these stores are limited. Sustained muscle work (i.e. endurance) will depend on the processing of sugars and fats (in the presence of oxygen) to supply the necessary ATP for the filaments to slide over each other and create tension. This aerobic muscle work, although potentially almost limitless, requires time for the reactions to occur, to break down the foodstuffs, especially fats, and to produce the (almost) endless supply of ATP.

FATIGUE

Everyone has felt tired at times when there seems to be a lack of energy at the end of a task or at the end of a long school day. This type of tiredness is really the body's need for sleep and should be distinguished from fatigue, which means an inability of the muscle(s) to perform a task (muscle action) to its optimal ability.

Fatigue can take two forms: *mental fatigue* and *muscle fatigue.* Mental fatigue is a multifactorial state including cognition, sleep deprivation and general health. Muscle fatigue can be caused by several things: depletion of energy source and/or build-up of waste products within the functioning muscle, a decrease in the availability of oxygen, and any disturbances in the contractile mechanisms such as inhibition by the central nervous system and a decrease in conduction at the neuromuscular junction. It is defined as *a diminished response to repeated stimuli characterized by a decrease in amplitude of the motor unit action potential (MUAP) and/ or the inability to sustain a force.* This is a fairly common event and provides the biochemical and neurological stimuli necessary for the development of the aerobic capacity of the muscle. Local muscle fatigue is recognised by the inability to generate force and carry out the full range of movement of the task being undertaken, a decrease in the speed of contraction, shaking or fasciculation (flickering) within the particular muscle, pain and a loss of coordination.

A full explanation of exercise physiology can be gained from many standard texts, but from the brief description above and the preceding text it can be seen that for the muscle to carry out its functions properly there has to be intact neuromuscular, musculoskeletal and cardiorespiratory systems. Failure of any or all of these systems will lead to the muscle being unable to adequately perform its function (Wilmore and Costill, 2004).

MEASURING MUSCLE WORK

To enable us to determine if a muscle is working to its maximum capacity for both strength and endurance, it is important that both these components can be measured. For the activities you looked at in Activity Box 6.4, you should really measure the strength or endurance of the muscle or muscle groups used. This is important for several reasons: first, to determine if there is any deviation from the normal; second, to see if the condition is getting worse, better or remaining the same; third, to give a base measurement to the muscle condition; fourth, to assess whether any treatment you implement is having a positive or negative effect on the muscle; and fifth, to give an insight into the mechanism underpinning any loss of strength. In Chapter 11 we will talk more about the principles of measurement.

Measuring Muscle Strength

Thinking back to the shot putter, it could be seen that the size of the muscle was important in producing strength. People with large muscles are usually stronger than those

---

ACTIVITY BOX 6.4   **Muscle Analysis During Movement**

For two examples of sporting extremes (e.g. a high jump and a marathon) and two examples of everyday activities (e.g. writing and opening a tight jam jar), analyse the differences between each upper and lower limb activity in terms of muscle strength, force, work and power.

 Identify a working muscle in each activity.

 Is it working repetitively (endurance)?

 As a percentage of its maximal strength how hard do you think the muscle is working?

 Is it working concentrically, eccentrically or isometrically?

 If it is a concentric contraction does it happen rapidly (high power generation)?

---

with smaller muscles. Therefore it can be assumed that the larger the muscle, the greater the force that the muscle can generate. This would seem pretty obvious, as the larger the muscle, the more actin and myosin would be present and therefore the greater the propensity for the contractile unit to form cross-bridges.

Physiological Cross-Sectional Area

In gross terms the physiological cross-sectional area (PCSA) of the muscle is proportional to its strength (Jones and Round, 1990). However, this is not a convenient measure as only the anatomical cross-sectional area (ACSA) can be ascertained when measuring the girth of the limb using a tape measure. The true PCSA can be found only through dissection or modern scanning procedures such as ultrasound and MR (magnetic resonance). However, a loose relationship between size and strength does exist (Narici, 1999).

The results of measuring the girth of a limb (taking a tape measure round the circumference) to discover the ACSA must be read with caution, as the whole of the limb may be asymmetrical when compared with the other side due to different growth rates. This would mean that there is difficulty in distinguishing which part of the limb is responsible for any difference, in particular bone or muscle.

Atrophy and Hypertrophy

When the muscle has decreased in size through injury, disease or disuse, it will usually be weaker than normal. This decrease in size is generally due to a loss of muscle mass and is termed *atrophy*. When we build our muscles up in size, we usually find that the muscle is stronger. This increase in size is termed *hypertrophy* and is caused by an increase in the amount of protein in the muscle (French, 2015). Measurement of the PCSA is possible with the use of techniques such as magnetic

resonance imaging, but these are not really practicable in an everyday clinical situation due to expense and time.

Indirect measures of strength by measuring force can be obtained using handheld dynamometers, but these are limited by the strength of the operator. Another valuable tool in measuring force production is the isokinetic dynamometer, although it may be too expensive for many therapy departments. If the muscle is capable of performing its full range of movement, it is convenient to use the Medical Research Council Scale (the Oxford Muscle Grading [OMG] Scale) to measure muscle strength. This is classified on a scale of 0 to 5 (Hollis and Fletcher-Cook, 1999):

- 0, no movement at all
- 1, a flicker of movement
- 2, full range of movement with the effect of gravity eliminated
- 3, full range of movement against gravity
- 4, full range of movement against gravity and resistance
- 5, full range of movement with maximal resistance.

Although useful, the OMG Scale has many limitations, and many variations of this scale have been developed. The main problems with this scale are the ceiling effect (once you get to 5 you can't improve further) and the range of possible strength grades, which can all be categorised as a 4. A potentially more useful measure of strength in a wider context may be the one repetition maximum (1 RM), defined as *the maximum amount of weight a muscle can lift once with proper technique (Fleck and Kraemer, 2014)*. The 10 RM is a derivation of the 1 RM and is *the maximum weight a muscle can lift ten times with a proper lifting technique (Fleck and Kraemer, 2014)*. Both these quantities are found by trial and error, and the technique for finding this is well described in the NSCA's (National Strength and Conditioning Association) strength and conditioning text (Haff and Triplett, 2015). A more subjective measure that is frequently employed is isometric testing. This is carried out by manually resisting the muscle contraction in various positions within its range and not allowing any movement. The resistance used to prevent movement is compared with that of the unaffected side and is subjectively graded on a scale from 0 to 5 on a similar scale to OMG. This method is obviously applicable only if the problem is unilateral and the subject normally symmetrical.

Measuring Endurance

As discussed earlier, there is a greater involvement of physiological processes in muscle endurance. Therefore testing endurance is going to involve physiological testing. Measurements of expired air, heart rate, respiratory rate, blood gases and waste products after maximal and submaximal exercise on treadmills are the procedures usually used (McArdle et al., 2015). These measurements would be fairly difficult in an ordinary department. Pulse rate is a useful measure to give an indication of how hard someone is working generally, but it is not that useful when working out a local muscle's endurance. Although it is difficult to measure muscle endurance directly, measuring the time to fatigue (or number of repetitions to fatigue) and the time to recover will give an adequate estimate of the endurance of the muscle and how it is progressing and regressing. It is also possible to use electromyography, which can show a shift in the frequency of muscle activation when fatigue sets in (Hawkes et al., 2015). The isokinetic dynamometer mentioned earlier also has a facility to measure—indirectly—muscle endurance.

WHEN THINGS GO WRONG

There are times when muscle strength and endurance cannot be maintained. The most common causes of decrease in strength and endurance are injury, disease and disuse. Injury can be to the muscle itself, its nervous or vascular supply, or the skeletal support. Direct trauma that disrupts the contractile unit, such as a muscle or tendon tear, will mechanically affect the ability of the muscle to either produce or transmit force. Disruption of nerve supply will mean that no recruitment is able to take place, and hence no muscle contraction. Disruption of blood supply will mean that energy, in the form of fats and sugars, and oxygen will not be delivered to the muscle, and waste products will not be taken away. This will mean a decrease in the respiratory capability of the muscle and a decrease in its endurance. There are many diseases that affect the muscle or its neurological supply. Muscular dystrophy is an example of a muscle-wasting disease in which the muscle protein is affected. A neuropathy would disrupt muscle stimulation, leading to a decreased contraction.

The examples above would lead to an inability of the muscle to function to its optimal capability. The muscle may also not be used if another body part, proximal or distal to the muscle, has to be kept immobile (as in a joint problem or bone fracture). Pain, muscle spasm, habit and certain psychological factors will lead to weakness caused by disuse. If the muscle is not used, then the actin and myosin protein will be reabsorbed. This will diminish the ability to form cross-bridges; hence the force production and strength will decrease. This decrease in strength is mirrored by a decrease in size, *atrophy*. Therefore the case above will be termed *disuse atrophy*. Concurrent with the reabsorption of actin and myosin, there will also be a reabsorption of the supportive skeletal structures such as bone, tendon and ligament, a collapse and eventual reabsorption of the small blood and lymph vessels. This, together with the decrease and inefficient use of energy stores, will cause a decrease in muscle endurance.

INCREASING STRENGTH AND ENDURANCE

For a muscle to perform any functional activity, it must be able to generate enough force to overcome the resistance of the task. This could be one maximal effort or a series of submaximal efforts over time. For the former, the muscle strength is paramount, while the latter requires both strength and endurance.

Muscle Strength

For a muscle to increase in strength, it simply has to work more. For optimal gains in strength it has to work to fatigue with a load placed on it that exceeds its usual metabolic work rate. This is known as the *overload principle*. This type of training is known as resistance training.

Physiological Processes

If the muscle is stimulated to work hard, then various metabolic and neurological factors stimulate the production of more skeletal muscle proteins (actin and myosin). The myofibrils are increased in length and width. There will be an increase in myocyte (muscle cell) number and size and in the number of sarcomeres, which will increase the strength of the muscle. There will also be a change in the density of the mitochondria (the tiny factories that produce ATP) within the muscle tissue. More muscle glycogen, creatine phosphate and ATP substrate will be stored ready for action. There will also be an increase in the concentration and activity of glycolytic enzymes, myokinase and creatine phosphokinase (the enzymes needed for producing energy) (Maughan and Gleeson, 2004). This adaptation process usually takes 4 to 6 weeks. Although strength can change quite quickly when a programme is commenced, typically these initial changes are due to neurological factors (i.e. the skill/coordination of the movement improves).

Increased Vascularisation

If there is enough stimulation through activity, then increased vascularisation of the area will also occur (up to a 50% increase is possible), and thus the supply and utilisation of oxygen and energy will also change so both strength and endurance will increase (Greenhaff and Hultman, 1999). However, the type of resistance exercise done can increase or decrease the vascularisation of the muscle. This specific response to the imposed demands is known as the SAID principle (Specific Adaptation to Imposed Demands) and is fundamental to getting the right exercise for an individual or situation. More of this later within the specificity section.

Increase in Size

As the muscle increases in strength, it also increases in size, *hypertrophy*. However, it must be noted that initially, increases in strength are not accompanied by a corresponding increase in size. It is thought that recruitment of motor units becomes more efficient, and there is an increase in the number of motor units that are recruited. There also appears to be an inhibition of the antagonist muscle groups, together with a more efficient integration of the synergist muscles (helper muscles, not the prime mover). Some authors believe that hyperplasia, or the splitting of developed fibres, takes place, but this continues to be debated (French, 2015).

Increasing Strength

Muscle weakness is the inability to generate force. If a muscle is weak, then the best method to increase strength is exercise training. Training can be defined as *the facilitation of biological adaptations that improve the performance of specific tasks.*

There are three main categories of exercise that are used to increase muscle strength: assisted exercise, free active exercise and resisted exercise. Assisted exercise could be manual or mechanical and is used when the muscle is so weak that the segment cannot be moved through a sufficient range against the force of gravity. Manual assistance may be given by the therapist (therapist-assisted), by the patient (auto-assisted) or a mechanically (e.g. with a robot or weight support system). The assistance given may be just to eliminate the effect of the force of gravity, so taking the weigh to the limb. Care must be taken that the movement does not become passive.

Mechanical assistance could be assisting the movement by eliminating or decreasing friction; for example, using a sliding board or sling suspension. Pulleys also can be used to facilitate the movement and these days therapy robots also may be available. Such assistance is useful for muscles that have been measured as grade 2 on the OMG Scale. If the muscle has been measured at grade 3 or above, then it can be strengthened by using free active exercise, defined as *exercise without the use of assistance or resistance except gravity* (some people make body weight the exception to this).

Fatigue, and consequently muscle strengthening, can be achieved with active exercise by changing the parameters of the exercise, such as repetition, speed, rhythm and leverage. The exercise can be progressed and regressed by altering the starting position.

Once a muscle is able to move a segment against gravity, the more usual form of exercise used to strengthen muscles is resisted exercise. To be most effective, the resistance must be directed against the movement of the muscle and if possible at 90 degrees to the principle (long) axis of the segment.

The resistance may be given manually or mechanically. Manual resisted exercise can be thought of as *active resistance exercise in which the resistance force is applied by the physiotherapist (therapist-resisted) or the patient themselves*

(autoresisted) to either a dynamic or a static muscular contraction.

The position of resistance is an important consideration, as the further away from the axis of rotation the resistance is given on the segment that is moving, the less effort has to be made by the therapist. This can be explained by considering leverage and the effect the length of the lever arm has on the effort required. As will be seen in Chapter 4, the moment of force is defined as the force multiplied by the distance from the pivot. Therefore, if the distance from the pivot is increased, then to maintain the same moment the force is less. (Try Activity Box 6.5.)

Mechanical resistance is any resistance against which the body can exercise. The main categories are weighted resistance, free weights (barbells, dumb-bells, cuff weights, ankle weights, weighted boots or sandbags), multigyms, isokinetic dynamometer and springs made, for example, from materials such as elastic latex. Exercise cycles, body weight and hydrotherapy may all be used as forms of mechanical resistance.

Resistance Training

When a muscle has to undergo exercise to improve strength, it is usually because there has been a problem, and it is very unusual for this problem to manifest itself as only a decrease in muscle strength. Many other systems may be involved, so we need to approach rehabilitation holistically. Any strength programme will improve both strength and endurance; in other words, physiological adaptations that result in increased strength will increase the endurance capacity. However, as we shall see later there are ways to manipulate the parameters of the exercise programme that emphasises one over the other and it is important to know which factor you are trying to improve. In addition, other factors—such as muscle elasticity, joint range, coordination, balance and cardiovascular fitness—must also be addressed. Although this text does not cover all the elements of programme design within a patient population, it is useful to become familiar with basic training principles and programme design.

ACTIVITY BOX 6.5   Manual Resistance

Work in pairs. One of you sits over a plinth with your thigh supported, acting as the patient. The other one, acting as the therapist, gives resistance to the leg, beginning at the knee and moving down towards the ankle in increments. Think about the force required to resist maximal effort and the effect this has on the patient. What trick movements do you notice when the activity becomes more difficult? How could these be corrected?

Assessment

As always, before you start a rehabilitation programme you need a thorough assessment. Muscle strength, joint range of movement and integrity, pain and functional ability all need to be assessed. This is a good time to work out the 1 RM and 10 RM of the muscle and/or the muscular endurance. Of course, it will depend on your specific situation; the OMG Scale may be more appropriate.

Principles of Strength Training

The fundamental principles of strength training are as follows.

Overload. This is making the muscular system work at a level greater than normal. For strength, this would mean moving a greater resistance and maintaining a contraction for a longer period. The stimulus for muscle growth partly related to the tension generated, therefore it is important to consider this tension varies with speed and at different lengths.

Specificity. It has been shown that training that mimics the activity for which the action is needed is more effective than if they are different (Ackland and Bloomfield, 1995). Conversely, training for one factor (e.g. strength) would not necessarily improve another factor, such as endurance. There is not necessarily an overlap. This is also true for different fibre types speeds of contraction and ranges of activity. Therefore the training needs to be specific for the muscle action, range of movement, type of contraction, energy system and functional need.

Progressive (or principle of diminishing returns). For any given training sessions, a certain degree of adaptation will occur as a result of the training. If the training is simply repeated, then the degree of change will reduce with each session. Therefore the training sessions need to be assessed and progressed regularly to continue strength or endurance improvements (see Progressive Resistance Exercises below). You will probably not have the time to do a complete assessment every week so you should choose a primary outcome (e.g. number of repetitions or 1 RM) for continuous assessment.

Reversibility. Generally it can be said that the adaptations gained through training are lost rapidly once training stops (MacDougall et al., 1980). However, there is a difference between endurance and strength gains. Endurance capacity quickly reduces when activity levels are reduced through either bed rest or cessation of training. However, for strength, other aspects—such as age, genetics and nutritional, hormonal and environmental factors—can all play a role in regulating muscle mass. It has also been suggested that different fibre types respond to decreased use in different ways (Astrand et al., 2003). As a general rule, the maxim 'use it or lose it' applies to the principle of reversibility. If the muscle is not being used to its full capacity, strength gains will be reversed. However, as little as one exercise session per week is sufficient to maintain muscle strength.

Motivation and learning. This is an important aspect of any exercise programme and is discussed in depth in Chapter 15.

Programme Design

As was indicated earlier any muscle work that overloads the muscle will result in changes in the muscle to increase its strength and endurance. However, by choosing the correct parameters for the programme, the emphasis can be changed according to the needs of the individual or to counteract the effects of pathology. When selecting programme parameters, the acronym FITT can be useful (Oberg, 2007). This stands for Frequency, Intensity, Time and Type. The appropriate programme parameters are briefly discussed below, as set out in the American College of Sports Medicine guide to exercise selection for health (Garber et al., 2011).

Frequency. Frequency is how often the programme is undertaken and is generally given as number of times per week. For cardiovascular fitness exercising every day is important, whereas for strength training ensuring a day's rest between sessions is key to allowing for adaptations to be made and for avoiding muscle damage. This means that a frequency of two or three times a week is appropriate.

Intensity. This is an indication of how hard the individual is working. For strength training, the intensity can be easily indicated by the size of weight lifted. The weight itself doesn't indicate how hard someone is working, so to do this we can express this in terms of percentage of their 1 RM. Typically for a strength programme one should work at 80% to 95% 1 RM. This would mean that the individual would only be able to lift the weight a few times. Whereas for a muscular endurance programme, as you need to complete more repetitions, the intensity is generally much lower, closer to 55% to 65% 1 RM.

Time. This is the time duration for an exercise programme, both in terms of activity and rest. For instance, for general fitness and health it is recommended to perform moderate exercise for 30 minutes a day for 5 days a week to total 150 minutes per week (Garber et al., 2011), see Chapter 14 for more on this. For strength training programmes the time for an exercise is indicated by the number of sets and repetitions (reps). The fewer reps the greater the degree of strength involvement. Conversely the greater number of reps the greater the endurance emphasis. As indicated earlier the number of reps is closely associated with the intensity of the work. Equally as important is the rest time between sets. Longer rest periods, 2 to 4 minutes, are used during strength programmes, whereas for muscular endurance 30 to 60 seconds is more usual.

Type. This is the type of activity undertaken. This is closely linked to the exercise goal and is usually the first decision to be taken. If improvements in endurance is the goal then walking, jogging, running, swimming or cycling are options for this goal. For improvements in strength the resistance training is the best option. This may be delivered via free weights or weight machines or body weight exercises. Each of which has its own advantages and disadvantages and is not the place for this text to offer extensive details here.

Exercise programme. So far, we have seen the various choices in parameters and how they may differ for the different components of fitness and health. The table below (Table 6.2) shows examples of the different programmes for muscular strength and muscular endurance.

Progressive Resistance Exercises

These are specific exercise regimens that ensure overload of the muscle is achieved and that generally use weights in a strengthening programme. Progressive resistance exercise is defined as *load or resistance to the muscle as applied by some mechanical means and are quantitatively and progressively increased over time.*

Specific Regimens

Many training regimens were developed during and just after the Second World War to treat the many injured soldiers and to get them back to employment. They were based on the fundamental principles given above, and some are shown in Table 6.3.

Although these programmes are probably not used these days in their original form, derivations are used, and the basic principles underlying them are still valid. Now that you have a bit of information, why not try Activity Box 6.6?

Increasing Endurance

Conditioning is the augmentation of the energy capacity of the muscle through an exercise programme. This is produced by exercise of sufficient *intensity*, *duration* and *frequency*. The methods used to increase endurance differ between the fit athlete and the patient who has become deconditioned,

---

TABLE 6.2   Comparison of Muscular Strength and Endurance Programmes.

Exercise Goal	Sets	Reps	Intensity	Rest	Frequency
Strength	2–3	≤6	80%–95% 1 RM	2–4 min	2–3 × per week
Endurance	2–5	≥12	≤65% 1 RM	30–60 s	2–3 × per week
Hypertrophy	2–4	6–12	70%–85% 1 RM	30–90 s	2–3 × per week

RM, Repetition maximum.

Adapted from Haff, G.G., Triplett, N.T. (Eds.), 2015. Essentials of Strength Training and Conditioning, fourth ed. Human Kinetics, Champaign, IL.

TABLE 6.3   The DeLorme and Watkins Programme (DeLorme and Watkins, 1948), the Oxford Programme (Zinovieff, 1951) and the MacQueen Programme (MacQueen, 1954, 1956).

Name	Regimen	Effect	Conditions
Delorme and Watkins	10 lifts at ½ 10 RM 10 lifts at ¾ 10 RM 10 lifts at full 10 RM	Increase strength	×3 each session, 4 or 5 per week, retest 10 RM weekly
Oxford	10 reps at 10 RM 10 reps at ¾ 10 RM 10 reps at ½ 10 RM or 10 reps at 10 RM then reduced by 5 kg for 10 sets	Increases strength	×5 sessions per week
MacQueen (1)	4 × 10 reps at 10 RM	Hypertrophy	
MacQueen (2)	10 reps at 10 RM 8 reps at 8 RM 6 reps at 6 RM	Power	

RM, Repetition maximum.

ACTIVITY BOX 6.6   Muscle Strengthening

Choose a muscle or group of muscles (e.g. the shoulder abductors) and work out a strengthening regimen if the muscle was assessed as a grade 3 on the OMG Scale. Set aims and objectives for each stage of the recovery and use assisted, free active and resisted exercise. Discuss how you would assess the condition and progress the exercises as necessary.

ACTIVITY BOX 6.7   Muscle Endurance Training

For the lower limb, devise a circuit exercise programme that would improve local muscle endurance for the major groups of muscles. What would you use to continually assess?

---

but the principles of treatment remain the same. The overriding consideration is the overload principle. As for strength training, the muscle must work above its usual metabolic functioning for adaptation to take place.

Intensity for endurance exercises is the rate at which the exercise is carried out. Intensity is easier to quantify if we are trying to improve general cardiovascular endurance. The maximum volume of oxygen uptake (VO_{2max}) is a function of the intensity, and because heart rate and VO_{2max} are linearly related, heart rate can be considered as a function of intensity. So, the intensity of the exercise could be defined through the heart rate. Local muscle endurance is usually measured as the length of time the muscle can function or the number of repetitions of the activity before fatigue occurs. The muscle's ability to recover post exercise is also used as a measure of its endurance. General conditioning is said to occur when the heart rate is between 60% and 90% of maximum, the training zone. For local muscle endurance to increase, the number of repetitions needs to be high but against a low resistance.

The *duration* of an exercise is the length of time for which the exercise is carried out. The greater the intensity, the shorter will be the duration, and vice versa.

Frequency is the number of times that the exercise programme is carried out per week. Although this will vary from patient to patient depending on the assessment, usually a minimum of three times per week is necessary to ensure that physiological adaptations take place (Watham and Roll, 2000).

Endurance Training

When training for endurance, the principles that were used for strengthening still apply. Exercise is still used, but the repetitions have to be greater to ensure that the overload principle is met. Therefore it must be ensured that the aerobic energy system is utilised, so low or even no resistance is used. These exercises can be progressed or regressed with some degree of objectivity by using numbers of repetitions, duration of exercise or a combination of both as markers.

The rest or time interval between sets of exercises also can be used as a method of progression or regression. The rest interval can be shortened as the recovery from fatigue is speeded up.

For the earlier stages of rehabilitation, assisted and free active exercise can be used to increase endurance. As rehabilitation progresses, free active and resisted exercise are used. Now that you have a bit of information about endurance training why not try Activity Box 6.7.

Delivery of Exercise

The programme used to deliver the exercises for increasing strength or endurance could be either individual (patient and therapist) or in a group situation (therapist and class). Each has its advantages and disadvantages. In the one-to-one situation, the therapist could give individual encouragement and ensure that the exercise is being carried out properly. The exercise could be progressed and regressed as soon as applicable, as the therapist would be constantly assessing capability. However, in the group situation, the patient will be motivated by competition with others and the variety of exercise could be greater. Adherence to a group exercise programme is often better than a solo programme, but the evidence is still uncertain and probably varies by individual (McLean et al., 2010).

Circuit training as a group exercise is particularly effective when increasing cardiorespiratory endurance, but it is also very effective for increasing local muscle endurance, as the delivery of oxygen and the ability of the muscle to use it are closely linked (Maughan and Gleeson, 2004). The circuit is made up of a series of well-defined activities with a predescribed rest period between each. The circuit is usually repeated a set number of times with a rest period between each (usually enough time for recovery) (Astrand and Rohdal, 1988).

CONCLUSION

Muscle strength, power and endurance, although described separately, can be seen to be closely integrated and should be thought of as equally important in affecting movement of the musculoskeletal system and ultimately locomotion of the human. We have seen through this chapter that the production of muscular force, movement initiation, and control and continuation of useful integrated and functional movement require an intact neuromusculo-skeletal system. These systems have to be studied through anatomical, physiological, biomechanical and psychological perspectives so that if any are disrupted through trauma or disease we can, after thorough assessment, return them to an optimal condition to perform functional human movement.

SELF-ASSESSMENT QUESTIONS

1. What are the names of the two proteins involved in a muscle contraction?
2. The thick filament consists of
   a. Actin and myosin.
   b. Tropomyosin, actin and tropin.
   c. Actin.
   d. Myosin.
3. What molecule releases myosin from its attachment to actin?
4. What is the basic functional unit of the muscle called?
5. Which is correct?
   a. Bundles of fibres make up a myofibril.
   b. Bundles of fibres make up a fascicle.
   c. Bundles of fascicles make up a myofibril.
   d. Bundles of fascicles make up a fibre.
6. What is the difference between muscle strength and muscle power?
7. What is the difference between and an isometric and an isotonic muscle contraction?
8. What is the difference between eccentric and concentric isotonic contractions?
9. What kind of contraction is about power absorption (negative power)?
10. Is the following statement true or false?
    A type 1 muscle fibre is slow to twitch (contract) and fatigues rapidly.
11. A muscle will produce its maximal force during an isometric contraction in its
    a. Outer range.
    b. Middle range.
    c. Inner range.
12. True or false?
    A force produced by a muscle does not vary according to speed of contraction.
13. Is a female muscle fibre
    a. Stronger than a male muscle fibre?
    b. Weaker than a male muscle fibre?
    c. The same as a male muscle fibre?

14. What is a grade 3 on the Oxford Muscle Grade Scale?
    a. Full range of movement against gravity
    b. Full range of movement against gravity and resistance
    c. No movement at all
    d. Full range of movement with maximal resistance
    e. A flicker of movement
    f. Full range of movement with the effect of gravity eliminated
15. What is a 10 RM?
    a. 10% of maximum
    b. Resistance/weight that can be lifted 10 consecutive times
    c. 10 times the 1 RM
    d. 10 repeated muscle contractions
16. Using your movement analysis and the FITT principles as a guide, design a programme for an individual who wants to improve his strength so that he can climb the stairs. This individual has undergone significant atrophy due to forced inactivity from a prolonged illness. Therefore he has limited muscle strength (Oxford Muscle Grading Scale 3), through his whole lower limb.
    a. Which muscles are key to this functional activity?
    b. What type of contraction is occurring and at what speed?
    c. Is going up the stairs the same as going down?
    d. What physiological adaptations do you want to occur to allow this individual to achieve their goal?
    e. What type of exercise is best to achieve this goal?
    f. What would you choose as the frequency, intensity and time for this programme?

REFERENCES

Ackland, T.R., Bloomfield, J., 1995. Applied anatomy. In: Bloomfield, J., Fricker, J., Fitch, K.D. (Eds.), Science and Medicine in Sport. Blackwell Scientific Publications, Oxford.

Astrand, P., Rohdal, K., 1988. Textbook of Work Physiology. Physiological Basis of Exercise. McGraw-Hill, Singapore.

Astrand, P., Rohdal, K., Dahl, H.A., Stromme, S.B., 2003. Textbook of Work Physiology. Physiological Basis of Exercise, fourth ed. McGraw-Hill, Singapore.

Daniels, J., 2001. Aerobic capacity for endurance. In: Foran, B. (Ed.), High Performance Sports Conditioning. Human Kinetics, Champaign, IL.

DeLorme, T.L., Watkins, A.L., 1948. Techniques of progressive resistance exercises. Arch. Phys. Med. Rehabil. 29 (5), 263–273.

Fleck, S.J., Kraemer, W.J., 2014. Designing Resistance Training Programs, fourth ed. Human Kinetics, Champaign, IL.

French, D., 2015. Adaptations to anaerobic training programmes. In: Haff, G.G., Triplett, N.T. (Eds.), Essentials of Strength Training and Conditioning, fourth ed. Human Kinetics, Champaign, IL.

Garber, C.E., Blissmer, B., Deschenes, M.R., Franklin, B.A., Lamonte, M.J., Lee, I.M., et al., 2011. American College of sports medicine position stand. Quantity and quality of exercise for developing and maintaining cardiorespiratory, musculoskeletal, and neuromotor fitness in apparently healthy adults: guidance for prescribing exercise. Med. Sci. Sports Exerc. 43 (7), 1334–1359.

Greenhaff, P.L., Hultman, E., 1999. The biomechanical basis of exercise. In: Maughan, R.J. (Ed.), Basic and Applied Sciences for Sports Medicine. Butterworth Heinemann, Oxford.

Haff, G.G., Triplett, N.T. (Eds.), 2015. Essentials of Strength Training and Conditioning, fourth ed. Human Kinetics, Champaign, IL.

Hawkes, D.H., Alizadehkhaiyat, O., Kemp, G.J., Fisher, A.C., Roebuck, M.M., Frostick, S.P., 2015. Electromyographic assessment of muscle fatigue in massive rotator cuff tear. J. Electromyogr. Kinesiol. 25 (1), 93–99.

Hollis, M., Fletcher-Cook, P., 1999. Practical Exercise Therapy, fourth ed. Blackwell Science, Oxford.

Jones, D.A., Round, J.M., 1990. Skeletal Muscle in Health and Disease. Manchester University Press, Manchester.

Lakomy, H.K.A., 1999. The biomechanics of human movement. In: Maughan, R.J. (Ed.), Basic and Applied Sciences for Sports Medicine. Butterworth Heinemann, Oxford.

Lieber, R.L., 2010. Skeletal Muscle Structure, Function and Plasticity. The Physiological Basis of Rehabilitation, third ed. Lippincott Williams & Williams, Philadelphia, PA.

MacDougall, J.D., Elder, G.C., Sale, D.G., Moroz, J.R., Sutton, J.R., 1980. Effects of strength training and immobilization on human muscle fibres. Eur. J. Appl. Physiol. Occup. Physiol. 43 (1), 25–34.

MacQueen, I.J., 1954. Recent advances in the techniques of progressive resistance exercise. Br. Med. J. 2 (4898), 1193–1198.

MacQueen, I.J., 1956. The application of progressive resistance exercise in physiotherapy. Physiotherapy 42 (4), 83–93.

Maughan, R.J., Gleeson, M., 2004. The Biomechanical Basis of Sports Performance. Oxford University Press, Oxford.

McArdle, W.D., Katch, F.I., Katch, V.L., 2015. Exercise Physiology. Lippincott Williams & Wilkins, Philadelphia.

McLean, S.M., Burton, M., Bradley, L., Littlewood, C., 2010. Interventions for enhancing adherence with physiotherapy: a systematic review. Man. Ther. 15 (6), 514–521.

Narici, M., 1999. Human skeletal muscle architecture studied in vivo by non-invasive imaging techniques: functional significance and applications. J. Electromyogr. Kinesiol. 9 (2), 97–103.

Oberg, E., 2007. Physical activity prescription: our best medicine. Integrative Medicine 6 (5), 18–23.

Padulo, J., Guillaume, L., Ardigò, L.P., Chamari, K., 2013. Concentric and eccentric: muscle contraction or exercise? J. Hum. Kinet. 37 (1), 5–6.

Petrof, B.J., 1998. The molecular basis of activity-induced muscle injury in duchenne muscular dystrophy. Mol. Cell. Biochem. 179 (1–2), 111–124.

Triplett, N.T., 2015. Structure and function of body systems. In: Haff, G.G., Triplett, N.T. (Eds.), Essentials of Strength Training and Conditioning, fourth ed. Human Kinetics, Champaign, IL.

Watham, D., Roll, F., 2000. Training methods and modes. In: Baechle, T.R., Earle, R.W. (Eds.), Essentials of Strength Training and Conditioning. Human Kinetics, Champaign, IL.

Wilmore, J.H., Costill, D.L., 2004. Physiology of Sport and Exercise, third ed. Human Kinetics, Champaign, IL.

Zinovieff, A.N., 1951. Heavy resistance exercise. Br. J. Phys. Med. 14 (6), 129–133.

7

Joint Mobility

Andy Kerr

LEARNING OUTCOMES

At the end of this chapter, you should be able to:
1. Describe the structure and function of joints.
2. Classify joint movement.
3. List factors that restrict and assist normal joint range of movement.
4. Discuss causes of abnormally restricted joint range of movement.
5. Provide a rationale for the use of different therapeutic techniques to increase joint mobility.

INTRODUCTION

The body can be considered to be composed of segments divided between the axial and appendicular skeleton. There are many models that describe this segmental arrangement; the one that is used in this book divides the body into eight segments. The head and neck and the trunk make up the two segments of the axial skeleton. The other six segments form the appendicular skeleton and are equally divided between the upper and lower limbs; the upper limb consists of arm, forearm, and wrist and hand, while the lower limb consists of the thigh, leg, and foot and ankle. All movements involve relative motion between and across these bony segments, be they in the appendicular or axial skeleton.

Junctions between these segments are provided by the joints (juncture, articulations or arthroses), which are classified into three groups:

1. **Fibrous or fixed** (synarthroses) joints, which really have no movement at all, for example joints between the plates in the skull, but some, for example the tibiofibular joint, have a small range of movement (ROM).
2. **Cartilaginous** (amphiarthroses) joints, which have limited movement, for example intervertebral discs.
3. **Synovial** (diarthroses) joints, which under normal circumstances move pretty freely, for example the knee joint, (see Fig. 7.1).

The embryological development of the joints begins very early; by week 7 of gestation there is already a sort of knee joint template in place. This initial template is made of cartilaginous tissue, not bone, but gradually this is replaced by bone through a process called mineralisation. The ends of bones (joint surfaces), however, are left as cartilage. Although the exact mechanism of joint formation in the embryo is still unknown, it seems that movement is a big factor; the absence of movement (lots of reasons for this) will result in malformed joints; this is discussed more in Chapter 10.

The combination of the bones that form the rigid core of the segments, the muscles that produce the force to cause (and control) the movement and the joints about which the movement occurs is described together as the musculoskeletal system. It is vital that this musculoskeletal system is intact for functional movement to occur. The role of the muscles producing and controlling movement was described in detail in Chapter 6 and specific muscles will be discussed again within the case studies at the end of this book, but the central component of this system, the synovial joints (the bit that moves), will be described below.

The major characteristics of a synovial joint include the surface of the opposing bones, which are covered in articular cartilage. These bony ends are joined together via ligaments, and the whole joint complex, which may or may not include the ligaments, is surrounded by an extensive synovium-lined fibrous joint capsule. The viscous synovial fluid secreted by this synovial membrane not only provides the articular cartilage with nutrition but acts with it to decrease the coefficient of friction within the joint to a level that is low enough to reduce the possibility of joint surface destruction. Intracapsular structures are usually covered by synovium. The dynamic stability of the joint is provided by the surrounding muscles, which help the ligaments and capsule to keep the joint congruent. See Fig. 7.1. Intra-articular discs, or menisci, may be found within the synovial joint, helping congruity (and therefore stability) and acting as shock absorbers. Labra and fat pads may also be found within the joints, having the function of increasing joint surface area (and possibly stability) and shock absorption, respectively.

There are a large number of different types of synovial joint, classified according to their shape—for example plane, saddle, hinge, pivot, ball and socket, condylar and ellipsoid (Palastanga et al., 2006)—but movement at all of these joints can be considered as either physiological or accessory. A physiological movement is the movement that the joint performs under voluntary control of the muscles or is performed passively by an external force but still within the available range of the joint. Accessory movements are those movements of the joints that a person cannot perform actively but that can be performed on that person by an external force. They are an integral part of the physiological movement that cannot be isolated and performed actively by muscular effort.

Although there may seem to be a large number of directions in which joints may move, a system of description has been devised to make the visual analysis of movement more simple. From the anatomical position (standing upright with the upper limbs at the sides and palms and head facing forwards), movements can be described as occurring in three planes and around three axes (Fig. 7.2).

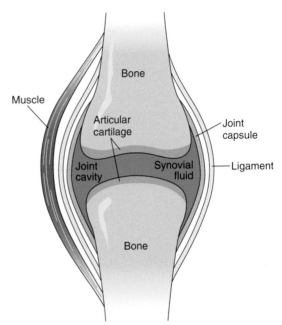

Fig. 7.1 Diagram of a Synovial Joint.

The frontal (or coronal) plane splits the body into front and back halves, the sagittal plane splits the body into right and left halves, and the transverse plane splits the body into top and bottom halves. Movement through these planes take place around three axes. The axes are perpendicular to the plane of movement. Therefore there are two horizontal axes and one vertical axis. The sagittal axis is at 90 degrees to the frontal plane and therefore allows movements within that frontal plane. These movements consist of abduction, adduction, deviation (e.g. radial deviation) and lateral flexion (e.g. lateral trunk flexion). The frontal axis allows movements of the segments within the sagittal plane and consists of the movements of flexion and extension. Both frontal and sagittal are horizontal axes. The vertical axis is at 90 degrees to the horizontal plane, and movements around this axis give rotatory motion (e.g. internal hip rotation).

The actual movements performed can be described in terms of the degrees of freedom the joint allows. A uniaxial joint will possess only one degree of freedom, that is rotation about one axis. An example of this is flexion and extension at the elbow. A biaxial joint has two degrees of freedom; for example, the radiocarpal joint has flexion and extension at the wrist about one axis and ulnar and radial deviation about the other axis. The movement available at a multiaxial joint can be described as having three degrees of freedom. This type of movement can be observed at the shoulder, where flexion/extension, abduction/adduction and internal/external rotation all take place (Activity Box 7.1).

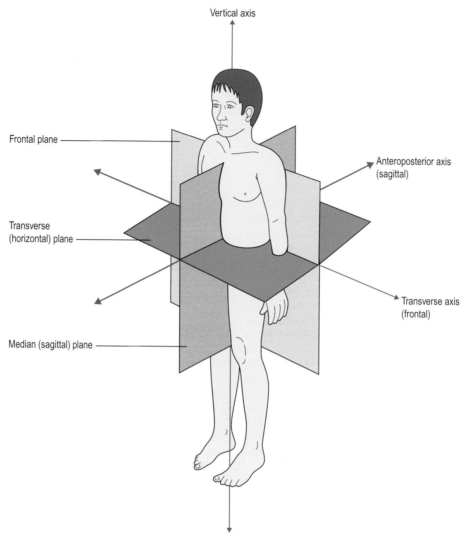

Fig. 7.2 Planes and Axes.

ACTIVITY BOX 7.1

Movements of the body segments are described in terms of their planes and axes. For example the knee joint moves in the sagittal plane about a frontal axis for flexion and extension and in the frontal plane about a sagittal axis for abduction and adduction. Now describe the axes and planes for the elbow, the shoulder, the hip and the wrist.

An alternative system for describing joint movement is with the Cartesian system, which allows any permutation of movement to be described in the three planes. It has, as shown in Fig. 7.3, three directions:

1. Anteroposterior (the x direction).
2. Mediolateral (the z direction).
3. Superior–inferior (the y direction).

It is worth noting that this axis convention may differ depending on the country you are moving in. For example, in the United States, the z direction is superior–inferior, the y is anteroposterior and the x is mediolateral.

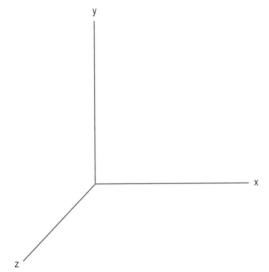

Fig. 7.3 The Cartesian Coordinate System.

RANGE OF MOVEMENT

With the number and combination of uniaxial, biaxial and multiaxial joints, the body may adopt manifold positions, which might be functional or just fun. When these positions or movements are analysed, the components are broken down for each individual joint with the ROM of that joint being described. This movement may not be the maximum movement that the joint is capable of achieving, that is its full ROM, but only a functional component of it.

Movements of the joints are dependent on many factors, and the description of these factors is largely dependent on the professional training of the observer. One such discipline is arthrokinematics. This is the intimate mechanics of the joints and is dependent, for its description, largely on the shape of the joint surfaces. Most of the synovial joints are complex in their formation, having more than one axis within the joint. These joints, being ovoid in shape with different axes for the same joint, have the ability to bring about different movements. This means that, although joints have roughly reciprocally shaped surfaces, the maximum congruity of the articular surfaces occurs at specific positions within the ROM and does not necessarily equate with the end of range of the physiological movement. The position of maximum congruity is called the close-packed position and is the position of greatest joint stability. At this close-packed position, not only is there most joint surface contact but the ligaments are typically taut. The loose-packed position, conversely, is where contact between the joint surfaces is at its least; muscle, ligaments and capsule are usually lax, and therefore the joint is in its least stable position.

Physiological movements always contain a combination of physiological and accessory movements. For example, side flexion of the cervical spine, which, if examined closely, will be seen to involve a combination of both side flexion and rotation. By studying the arthrokinematics of the joint, it can be shown that there is a combination of accessory-type movements occurring during physiological joint movements. These accessory movements are considered to be of three types: spin, roll and glide, see Fig. 7.4. A roll refers to one surface rolling over another, like a ball rolling over a surface. An example of roll is seen when the femoral condyles roll over the fixed tibial plateaus during the knee extension movement when standing up from a chair. Gliding is a translatory movement, one fixed point sliding over the other joint surface. A glide usually takes place in an anteroposterior or mediolateral direction, and this type of movement is again seen when the femur slides forwards on a fixed tibia at the knee joint. Spin is like a top spinning, a rotational motion. These movements are illustrated in Fig. 7.4. Accessory movements enable the ROM to be increased at the joint and maximise the congruency of the joint surfaces to improve stability (Norkin and Levangie, 2005). Descriptions of these movements and their combinations for specific joints can be found in many anatomical texts. So, it can be seen that movement at joints is not the straightforward unidimensional process it might appear at first.

Movement is caused by a force acting on the bony segment. This force may be an internal force, the isotonic work of the muscle, or an external force, the force of gravity for example. When the joint is moved by the force of muscle contraction, either concentrically or eccentrically, the range of joint movement may be described in terms of the excursion (or lengthening) of the muscle. This excursion consists of the full range of the muscle, that is, the inner, middle and outer range, each being roughly a third of the full ROM. The inner range is where the muscle is at its shortest, the middle range is the middle third of the muscle excursion, and the outer range is where the muscle is at its longest. This is graphically illustrated in Fig. 7.5.

The actual range, through which the joint moves, either actively or passively, is measured in degrees of a circle. ROM is usually measured clinically with a goniometer, which is essentially a protractor with a moving arm. This gives an acceptable objective measurement that may be used conveniently when analysing joint motion as part of movement analysis or used as an objective marker when assessing patients; see Chapter 11 for a fuller discussion of measurement issues.

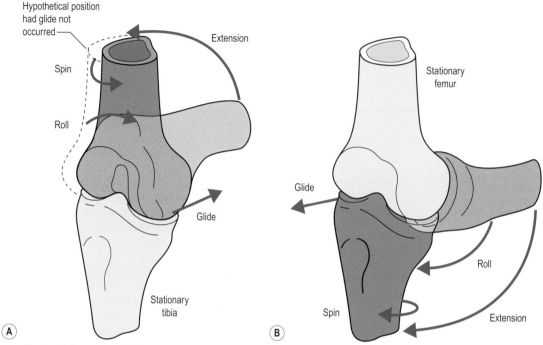

Fig. 7.4 Diagrammatic Representation of Roll, Spin and Glide at the Knee. (A) With stationary tibia and (B) with stationary femur.

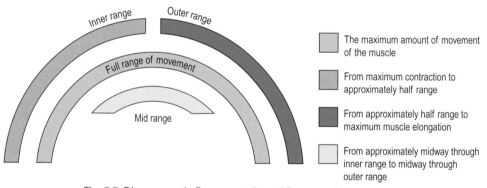

Fig. 7.5 Diagrammatic Representation of Ranges of Movement.

Try Activity Box 7.2 it will be useful to reinforce your understanding of the above text. It will deepen your understanding if you could do this task twice, once now and then after reading the sit-to-stand case study in Chapter 17.

FACTORS INVOLVED IN ASSISTING AND RESTRICTING RANGE OF MOVEMENT

Anatomical, physiological and arthrokinematic factors combine to allow a normal joint range as well as restrict or limit a joint.

ACTIVITY BOX 7.2

Work in small groups (2-3) to observe the sit to stand movement. One person performs the activity while the others observe the movement closely. Try to estimate the ROM at the hip, knee and ankle and identify the muscles that are working to produce the movement. Describe the ROM of the muscle (inner, middle, outer) and the type of muscle contraction (eccentric, concentric, isometric) throughout the activity.

Normal Range

Normal ROM is permitted by the following:

- Shape of the bone ends (articular surface).
- Articular cartilage.
- Capsule supporting the synovial membrane.
- Elastic ligaments.
- Intact neuromuscular and musculoskeletal system.
- Muscle strength.

The reciprocal convex and concave shapes of the joint surfaces—combined with the accessory movements of roll, spin and glide—provide a greater surface area over which the two bone ends can move. Articular cartilage, present on the articulating surfaces of the bone ends, has the dual function of providing a smooth surface over which the bone ends can glide and affording the joint protection from wear and tear. Both the functions of the articular cartilage are enhanced by the presence of synovial fluid within the joint. The fluid layer over the two joint surfaces will reduce the amount of friction between the bone ends when movements occur and act as a form of shock absorber to reduce the potentially injurious effects of repetitive impact, particularly in weight-bearing joints. Synovial fluid produced by the synovial membrane also provides the joint with some of its nutrition. Most of the capsule surrounding joints is lax, thus permitting a large ROM by the joint.

Many joints have additional structures within them; examples of these are the menisci in the knee or the glenoidal labrum within the shoulder. Both these structures, and others like them, can act as a mechanism for increasing the joint surface, increasing congruity and stability within the joint. Occasionally, the ligaments surrounding the joints contain a higher proportion of elastic fibres than usual, in addition to the usual collagen. This provides the joint with a greater degree of flexibility as well as the ability to restore itself to its default posture with only minimal muscular effort. An example of this is the ligamentum flavum, which connects adjacent laminae of the spine. It permits separation of these laminae in flexion and ensures that the end range is not reached abruptly. It then assists in returning the spine to the erect position after flexion has occurred (Standring, 2005).

Normal Joint Constraint in an Intact (Healthy) System

Joint mobility is normally constrained by:

- Shape of the articular surface and congruency with adjacent surface.
- Limit of a ligament's extensibility.
- Limit of a tendon and muscle's extensibility.
- Apposition of soft tissue.
- Negative pressure within the joint space.

The main factors that normally limit joint mobility are the shape of the joints and the type of structures that run over them. Articular surface contact could mean that the joint is in the close-packed position, as in the elbow, where the joint is actually prevented from extending beyond approximately 180 degrees by the olecranon of the ulna butting up against the olecranon fossa in the humerus. Flexion of the elbow, on the other hand, is limited by the bulk of the biceps brachii pressing against the forearm, this being an example of soft tissue apposition.

Most ligaments, and all tendons, are primarily composed of white fibrous collagen. One of the properties of collagen is that it is fairly stiff; it does not deform/stretch easily. Stretching (deformation) of ligaments can only really be achieved by strong forces. Therefore within normal activities, if the ligaments or tendons are at their maximum length, no more joint movement is possible. This is illustrated by McMahon et al. (1998), who point out that the inferior band of the inferior glenohumeral ligament is the primary restraint to anterior stability following a shoulder dislocation. When considering normal movement, Branch et al. (1995) point out that the anterior and posterior components of the glenohumeral capsuloligamentous complex limit the external and internal rotation of the glenohumeral joint, respectively.

It must be remembered, as O'Brien et al. (1995) describe, that differing positions of joints will mean different structures will limit movement. This point is taken a stage further by Warner et al. (1992), who showed that glenohumeral compression through muscle contraction provides stability against inferior translation of the humeral head, and this effect is more important to stability than intercapsular pressure or ligament tension. This agrees with Wuelker et al. (1998), who found that the rotator cuff force significantly contributes to stabilisation of the glenohumeral joint during arm motion.

The structure of muscle, on the other hand, offers the opportunity for more stretch, as it crosses the joint, and thus affords greater mobility, but it still has limited extensibility. The limitation that muscle offers to joint mobility is seen particularly in muscles that stretch over two joints (bi-articular muscles), such as the hamstrings which cross both the hip and knee joints. If the hip is flexed then the amount of knee extension will be limited, as the muscle is already near its maximum possible length. If the hip is extended, then the hamstrings are no longer near the limit of their potential length and will therefore allow for a greater range of knee extension. This is sometimes called passive joint insufficiency.

It is important that the person analysing the movement (particularly if they are a therapist hoping to increase joint flexibility) becomes aware of the normal joint limitations

FURTHER INFORMATION 7.1   The Evidence for Therapeutic Stretching

Stretching tissues (muscles, tendons, skin etc.) has been a mainstay in the practice of physiotherapists, masseurs, sports therapists (and many more) for as long as these professions have existed. We have all been taught how to stretch in school and the immediate effect on flexibility is evident to all. What is more contentious is the claim that stretching before participating in sport can prevent injury. This has been debated by many authors, with no clear consensus. There is even some thought that stretching could increase the risk of injury by making the tissue more compliant and therefore less strong, and perhaps even interfere with athletic performance. Some of the debate stems from a lack of clarity around what a stretch is and whether it should go to the end of the range or just to a comfortable range we don't know (i.e. how vigorous the stretch should be). Of course there is also the issue of what kind of sport is involved and whether you need as much joint mobility as possible; for example in gymnastics a stretch might have to be vigorous, but not so much (arguably) for rugby. Certainly these days, end-of-range stretches are not generally performed by professional sportspeople in sports such as football or rugby. What is your experience? What do you think, does it prevent injury?

I have copied a couple of references below which deal with this issue. They are worth a read.

McHugh, M.P., Cosgrave, C.H., 2010. To stretch or not to stretch: the role of stretching in injury prevention and performance. Scand. J. Med. Sci. Sports 20 (2), 169–181.
Leppänen, M., Aaltonen, S., Parkkari, J., Heinonen, A., Kujala, U.M., 2014. Interventions to prevent sports related injuries: a systematic review and meta-analysis of randomised controlled trials. Sports Med. 44 (4), 473–486.

and can recognise these by both visual analysis and recognising how the joint feels at the end of passive range. This is referred to as the *end feel* of the joint and will be different according to the circumstance of the particular joint. For example, the feel of a bony end block, as in the elbow extension, is quite different from that of soft tissue apposition, as in full flexion of the elbow. There is also the springy end feel when the joint movement has been ended by tendon and/or ligamentous restriction. It is only by recognising the normal end feel of joints that therapists become skilled at recognising pathological joint changes, so get practising (Further Information 7.1). (Try Activity Box 7.3.)

ACTIVITY BOX 7.3

Work with a partner and move the major joints of the body passively to their physiological limits. Identify (by end feel if possible) what is preventing further movement; sometimes it helps to close your eyes, and remember what the end range feels like. Move to a different partner and perform the same passive movements. See if you can detect any differences and similarities. Discuss your findings with your colleagues; can you identify the structure(s) that limits the movement?

Abnormal Limitation

Joint range really becomes an issue when there is an abnormal limitation, which is why you need to become acquainted with normal joint ranges. Abnormal limitation of joint range is usually brought about by either injury to, or disease of, its structure, surface or surrounding soft tissue (in particular the muscles producing the movement).

The following factors can be regarded as potential causes of a loss of joint mobility:

- destruction of bone and cartilage
- bone fracture
- foreign body in joint
- tearing or displacement of intracapsular structures
- adhesions or scar tissue
- muscle atrophy or hypertrophy
- muscle tear, rupture or denervation
- pain
- psychological factors
- oedema
- neurological impairment

Destruction of Bone and Cartilage

Any disease that destroys the articular cartilage, such as osteoarthritis, will impair the functioning of the joint and thus the movement will be limited. This may be for two reasons. Either the disrupted surface will physically prevent the movement due to eroded worn surfaces, or the individual splints (self-limits the movement) the joint themselves to reduce the pain produced when the two inflamed surfaces articulate with each other. Either singly or in combination, these factors may actually prevent movement altogether.

Fracture

A fracture near to or within the joint will also prevent movement via mechanical obstruction or pain. The same applies to fragments of cartilage or bone, which may become loose in the joint space and interfere with the normal articulation, for example a piece of cartilage from a meniscal tear in the knee.

Tearing or Displacement of Intracapsular Structures

Field et al. (1997) demonstrated that recurrent anterior unidirectional shoulder instability is most commonly associated with an avulsion (pulling out) of the glenoidal attachment of the labroligamentous complex (known as a Bankart lesion). This would limit the ROM available. Tearing of the meniscus of the knee is a common example of this type of injury, which can lead to a hard block (or lock) in movement.

Soft Tissue Lesions

If there has been an injury to the soft tissue surrounding or within the joint, then repair to that tissue usually takes place by the formation of fibrous or scar tissue, which does not have the same extensibility as the tissue it is replacing. Fibrous adhesions may also form; these can bind structures together (including the joint surface themselves), and hence restrict movement.

Injury or Immobilisation

If immobilisation of soft tissue occurs, there are biomechanical, biochemical and physiological changes that take place within 1 week. These changes are magnified in the presence of trauma or oedema (Cowin and Doty, 2007). These structural changes are a result of stress deprivation, which causes the matrix of the tissue to be remodelled to its new resting length while being held immobile (Hardy and Woodall, 1998). The net result of this will be a decrease in the ROM. If muscle tissue is held in a shortened position there will be absorption of the sarcomeres (muscle cells), causing a consequent change in length. This shortening in length is termed *adaptive shortening* and will limit joint movement, particularly if it occurs in the bi-articular muscles.

Muscular Changes and Pathology

The joint itself may be intact, but if the muscles that produce the movement have a dysfunction, then the net result is a decrease in active ROM. If the muscle is atrophied to a large degree, then it would not create sufficient force to move the joint through its full range. Conversely, if there was a large amount of muscle hypertrophy, ROM would also be decreased because of the increased amount of soft tissue apposition.

Neurological Impairment

The muscle itself may be intact, but its neural control may be impaired. This impairment could be from total denervation (i.e. the electrical impulses do not reach the muscle), causing flaccidity of the muscle, to disturbed signals from the motor cortex in the brain, for example following a stroke. Local spinal reflexes (if uninhibited) may also have the effect of limiting movement by causing the muscle to be in spasm (uncontrolled muscle activity).

Pain

The body's response to pain is usually to keep the part still (typically in a loose pack position which minimises the pressure within the joint) and avoid movement. This may only be short term, but if the pain becomes chronic, then adaptive shortening is likely to occur. The pain may disappear, but the movement and postural pattern that the brain adopted may continue. Other psychological problems, such as depression, lack of motivation or reduced self-confidence, may also be responsible for the subject restricting joint movement. This may also be transient and cause no physical limitation of movement, but if the condition persists, then adaptive shortening may occur.

Hypertrophy

When a muscle is overdeveloped, for example in a bodybuilder or sportsperson, soft tissue apposition may cause a decrease in ROM.

Ageing

The effects of ageing on the musculoskeletal system will be outlined for you in Chapter 10 but it is worth mentioning them here in relation to joint mobility. There are several reasons for losing joint mobility with age. Many of these are linked to specific diseases such as diabetes (Abate et al., 2010) and osteoarthritis (Johnson and Hunter, 2014) but there are also the effects of ageing itself. Muscle strength declines, reducing active range; connective tissues such as tendons and skin become less elastic, reducing passive range; and the articular cartilage reduces in thickness and smoothness (Lotz and Loeser, 2012), making it less easy for the joint surfaces to glide (as well as increasing the risk of injury).

Hypermobility

It is important to remember that what has so far been discussed describes a decrease in movement, what you might call *hypomobility*, but the opposite is also possible. This is termed *hypermobility* when the ROM exceeds that of the expected physiological range. This could be caused by pathological change either at the joint or elsewhere within the musculoskeletal or neuromuscular systems. It may, however, be a natural phenomenon caused mainly by laxity of ligaments or a congenital joint deformity, and it can also result from a deliberate attempt to stretch the joint range well beyond that which is functionally acceptable, for example with a gymnast or ballet dancer. As Lewit (1993) states, this may be an advantage to these sportspeople, but with increased mobility there may be a decrease in stability, with the disadvantage of possible problems in the future. Exercises focussed on strengthening the dynamic joint stabilisers (muscles) have been shown to be effective in children with hypermobility syndrome (Kerr et al., 2000). There is also the possibility of subluxation of the joint occurring during movement, which could result in neurological damage. If the joint is hypermobile, there is also the possibility that the joint will articulate on bone that is not designed for this function, and therefore there is a great risk of degenerative changes occurring at the joint surfaces (Further Information 7.2).

Effects of Decreased Range of Movement

The effects of a decreased range of joint movement will obviously depend on how much the range is decreased and the importance that joint plays in functional activity. Limited flexion at the knee, for example, will have a major effect on essential functional activities such as toileting and walking. Myles et al. (2002) measured the knee movement of people after a joint replacement and found a flexion range of at least 80 degrees was necessary to carry out tasks such as going up and down stairs and getting in and out of a bath. Limitation of ROM at one of the metatarsals, however, may have little major effect on any functional activity, even gait. The human body is very adaptable, and a decrease in the range of one joint can be compensated by movement at another joint.

Treatment

Before treatment can be given for any decrease in ROM, it is obvious from the above that the cause of the decrease will have to be ascertained. It has been shown that the cause may be in the joint structure (surface or intracapsular), the structures surrounding or running over the joint (ligaments or tendons) or the neuromuscular system that produces the movements. So, to establish the pathological changes that have occurred, it is vital that the therapist performs a full and detailed assessment. Once the cause is known, the therapist can choose a method of treatment whose physiological effects alter the pathological changes that have occurred to limit joint movement. The one thing they cannot do, however, is alter the anatomy.

Once the assessment has been made, it is important to know the physiological effects of the possible treatment options and match them with the effects they will have on the pathological changes. This is the rationale of the treatment.

Limitation of movement, from whatever cause, impairs function of the joint and the muscles producing the movement. Measures that increase the ROM must also include methods that strengthen the muscles in their new, lengthened position. The degree of ROM gained must be able to be controlled, and the stability of the joint maintained, or further injury may result.

It is important that details of the anatomy and arthrokinematics are understood as well as the pathology of the joint, as these have an effect on the rationale of treatment choice when there is a pathological reduction in joint range.

Many studies have looked at actual joint ranges of physiological ROM and presented tables of values (Norkin and White, 2003). It is accepted, however, that each ROM is specific to each individual, and discrepancies may even exist when comparing contralateral sides of the same individual. Two of the factors that have an effect on ROM are age and gender. Younger children appear to have a greater amount of hip flexion, abduction, lateral rotation and ankle dorsiflexion than an adult does. Elbow movements are also greater than those of an adult, while there is less hip extension, knee extension and ankle plantar flexion. Older age groups seem to have a general decrease across all joints. Connective tissue may become stiffer, but lack of activity through full range may be a major cause (Robergs and Keteyian, 2003). Gender appears to have different effects on different joints depending on which movement that joint is performing (Norkin and White, 2003).

There are many ways to increase ROM. The most obvious is the use of movement itself. The main classifications of

---

FURTHER INFORMATION 7.2 Test for Hypermobility

The following test is called the nine-point Beighton score and is used to assess for joint hypermobility syndrome in adults and children. One point is given for each side of the body for the first four manoeuvres listed below, such that the hypermobility score is a maximum of nine if all are positive.

1. Passive dorsiflexion of the fifth metacarpophalangeal joint to ≥90 degrees (1 point for left; 1 point for right).
2. Opposition of the thumb to the anterior aspect of the same forearm (1 point for left; 1 point for right).
3. Hyperextension of the elbow to ≥10 degrees (1 point for left; 1 point for right).
4. Hyperextension of the knee, in supine lying, to ≥10 degrees (1 point for left; 1 point for right).
5. Placing of hands flat on the floor in standing without bending the knees (1 point).

A score of 4 or more on the test is an important aspect for diagnosing joint hypermobility.

For more information (and diagrams in case you didn't follow the instructions) see Ross, J., Grahame, R., 2011. Joint hypermobility syndrome. B.M.J. 342, c7167. doi: https://doi.org/10.1136/bmj.c7167

the therapeutic movements are described below. (Try Activity Box 7.4.)

TYPES OF THERAPEUTIC MOVEMENT OF JOINTS

Movement is the main method for increasing joint range. A therapist may use the different ways a joint moves as a basis for different approaches. There are two main types of movement:

1. Passive movement.
2. Active movement.

Passive movement is defined as those movements produced entirely by an external force, that is, with no voluntary muscle work. These can be subdivided into:

- Relaxed passive movements.
- Passive stretching.
- Accessory movements.
- Passive joint manipulations.

Active movements are those movements within the unrestricted range of a joint produced by an active contraction of the muscles crossing the joint. These can be subdivided into:

- Active assisted exercise.
- Free active exercise.

Passive Movement

Relaxed Passive Movements

These are movements performed within the normal joint range by an external force and involve no muscle work of the particular joint, or joints, at which the movement takes place. These movements can be performed in three ways:

1. Manual relaxed passive movements are movements performed by another person, usually the therapist, within the normal range.
2. Auto-assisted passive movements are performed within the normal range by the patients themselves, that is using their unaffected limbs.
3. Mechanical relaxed passive movements are performed by a machine but still occur within the normal range. For example, the continuous passive motion devices used to help people recover after a knee replacement. These devices do not have convincing clinical evidence and

are therefore not routinely used in practice anymore (Harvey et al., 2014). There may yet be a role here for the emerging technology of therapeutic robots; watch this space.

Manual relaxed passive movements. Relaxed passive movement has been a core physiotherapy skill for many years. Like many established rehabilitation treatments there is little evidence of its clinical effectiveness; however it remains an acceptable and widely used treatment (Stockley et al., 2010).

Indications. Manual relaxed passive movements are indicated when the patient is unable to perform an active full-range movement. The reasons for this inability may include unconsciousness, weak or denervated muscle, spinal injury, pain, neurological disease or enforced rest.

Potential outcomes

- Maintain ROM.
- Prevent soft tissue adaptive shortening.
- Maintain integrity of soft tissue and muscle elasticity.
- Increase venous circulation.
- Increase synovial fluid production and therefore joint cartilage nutrition.
- Increase kinaesthetic awareness.
- Maintain functional movement patterns.
- Reduce pain.
- Provided the sensation of movement to the patient; this may be important psychologically and can be a pleasant sensation.

Maintaining range of movement and preventing contractures. If muscle is not moved through its full range, it will adapt to the demands being placed on it. The actin and myosin protein filaments (the contractile element) will be reabsorbed and thus the area for cross-bridge formation will be decreased. This will cause muscle weakness and the inability to perform the movement. The muscles will adapt to the new position and become shortened; that is, they will adaptively shorten. The noncontractile elements within the muscle, the connective tissue, will add to this effect by altering the collagen turnover rate, which is the balance of collagen production and destruction (Cowin and Doty, 2007). If more collagen is produced, as in immobilisation, it increases the stiffness of the muscle and decreases its propensity to stretch. If no movement takes place, then the muscle will adapt to the new position and thus contractures will occur.

Other soft tissues, such as ligaments and tendons, will also be similarly affected. As they have a greater proportion of collagen, the increase and change in consistency will also lead to stiffness and eventually to contractures.

Maintaining integrity of soft tissue and muscle elasticity. By placing stresses on these tissues, the collagen turnover rate is normalised and the elasticity of the tissues maintained. Early controlled motion is therefore vital to prevent the negative effects of immobilisation and maintain normal viscoelasticity and homeostasis of the connective tissue. Passive movements will not, however, increase the strength of the muscle, as this requires the greater physiological demand of active and resisted work.

Increase venous circulation. If a limb, particularly the lower limb, is not moved, venous congestion may occur. This is because the muscle pump does not work to aid venous return. Pooling of the blood occurs and is increased through dilation of the vessels caused by the physical pressure of the blood on the veins and the possible lack of sympathetic tone. This decrease in flow can lead to an increased risk of deep vein thrombosis. Passive movements can help reduce this. This is achieved by physically compressing the veins by the limb being moved, and one-way flow is achieved via the valves within the veins themselves. Lymph is also encouraged to move. Compression of the tissues through movement will also increase the hydrostatic pressure and thus encourage tissue perfusion and fluid reabsorption. This may be useful in reducing oedema.

Joint cartilage nutrition. If the synovial fluid is swept over the articular cartilage during the passive movement, it will provide nutrition and help prevent deterioration of the surface. Production and absorption of the synovial fluid by the synovial membrane are stimulated by joint movement. This is quite an important effect and is lost if the joint is immobile for any length of time. If the immobility is caused by injury, then movement is of greater importance, as one of the consequences of injury is inflammation and repair by fibrosis, which in itself will increase the risk of adhesions forming within the joint. Therefore with passive movement, this risk will be decreased.

Kinaesthetic awareness. To perform coordinated, energy-efficient and safe movement, it is important for the central nervous system to receive information about the position and movement of the joints and soft tissue. This information is supplied by sensors (proprioceptors) in the many structures in and surrounding the joints. This kinaesthetic awareness may be impaired if there is a long period of immobilisation. The function of these sensors and integrity of the pathways may be maintained by performing passive movements; it can often simply provide a pleasant sensation of movement.

Reduce pain. Passive movements can reduce local musculoskeletal pain through a neural mechanism that inhibits activity of parts of the brain related to the perception of pain (Nielsen et al., 2009). Stimulation of proprioceptors through movement may also reduce pain, as it is understood through the Gate Control Theory of Pain, where nonpainful stimulation (e.g. movement, touch and heat) blocks the painful sensation; see Moayedi and Davis (2013) for a recent update on pain theories. The removal of inflammatory waste products and chemical irritants from the area, through increased circulation, may also be facilitated by passive movement.

Contraindications

- Immediately post injury, as this may increase the inflammatory process and cause further damage.
- Early fractures, when movement may cause disruption of the fracture site.
- When pain may be beyond the patient's tolerance.
- Muscle or ligament incomplete tears when further damage may occur.
- If circulation is potentially compromised.

Principles of application. Passive movements may be performed either in the anatomical planes or in functional patterns. The choice and type of movement will depend on the findings of the assessment and the aims of the treatment. The same basic principles of application need to be considered whichever movement is chosen, as follows:

- The segment should be comfortable, supported and localised to the specific joints.
- The patient should be comfortable, warm and supported.
- Handholds should support the segment and protect the joint.
- The motion should be smooth, controlled and rhythmical.
- Speed and duration should be appropriate for the desired effects.
- Range should be the maximum available without stretching or causing pain.
- Segments should be positioned so that muscles that stretch over two or more joints are not restricting joint range.

Auto-relaxed passive movements. Although the rationale is the same, the method of application must be modified. Patients who have to perform their own passive movements are usually those with a long-term problem. People with spinal injuries, for example, must retain their joint range and muscle length if they are to perform the functions necessary for daily living (Bromley, 2006).

Mechanical relaxed passive movements. Unlike manual or auto-passive movements, which, by their nature, have to be carried out intermittently, mechanical passive movements may be carried out continuously. Mechanical devices for producing continuous passive movement were first used by Salter in 1970 (McCarthy et al., 1993). Although their designs and protocols of use may differ, they all have essentially the same function.

The rationale is the same as for any relaxed passive movement, but the use of continuous passive movement devices was particularly popular following surgery (Kisner and Colby, 2007) with the aim of increasing ROM, decreasing pain and facilitating wound healing by helping to reduce swelling. However, a more recent Cochrane review found little evidence that they were effective, so they are no longer used routinely after joint surgery (Harvey et al., 2014).

Passive Stretching

Passive stretching differs from relaxed passive movement in that it takes the movement beyond the usual range. This available range may be limited because of disease or injury. Stretching may also take the joint beyond the normal physiological range. Whereas relaxed passive movements maintain the length of soft tissue and hence joint range, stretching should result in an increase in the length of the soft tissue structures crossing over the joint, with the consequent increase in joint range. Passive stretching is not the only method of increasing joint range via the soft tissues. This can also be attained via active stretching, which will be discussed further on.

Stretching of biological material. Most biological materials are viscoelastic. This means that they have a mixture of viscous and elastic properties. Viscosity is a property of a fluid that is a measure of its resistance to flow; essentially it is a function of the friction between the molecules. Honey has a higher viscosity (resistance to flow) than water, or to put it another way honey pours more slowly from the jar. In many materials, this viscosity can be decreased by agitating it (e.g. stretching it or warming it). Think of how you get the last bits out of a bottle of tomato sauce, lots of shaking and banging and eventually it flows more easily on to your plate. This ability of a material to flow more easily after it has been 'shaken about' is called *thixotropy* and is an important consideration in stretching which we will discuss a little later.

Elasticity is the ability of a solid to return to its original shape and properties after a distorting (change in shape/length) stress has been removed. This is discussed in more detail in Chapter 5. Connective tissue (bone, skin, tendon etc.) is viscoelastic so will resist being stretched but will 'flow' over time at a rate that depends on its makeup; when the stretch is removed, the tissue is able (to a variable degree) to recover its original shape and strength. The amount of force being applied in a stretch is called *stress* and the change in length of the tissue is called *strain*. The relationship between stress and strain is an important engineering concept and one that also applies to biological materials under stretch. A useful way of describing the relationship between stress and strain is to plot a graph of the stress versus strain and discuss the resulting curves.

Loading and unloading paths. For uniformly elastic materials (think of an elastic band or a piece of theraband), kinetic energy (E_k) from the stretching movement is changed into potential energy (E_p) which is stored within the fibres of the tissue. When the stress/load is released, it is this potential energy that returns the material to its

original length and shape. This is represented graphically in Fig. 7.6.

For viscoelastic materials, some of the strain energy is stored as potential and some is dissipated as heat as the fibres glide past each producing heat through friction. Therefore once the applied load is removed, there is not enough stored energy to regain the normal configuration. This is shown in Fig. 7.6.

Within the enclosed area in the graph (Fig. 7.7) is shown the hysteresis loop, this represents the energy dissipated (lost) as heat when the material is stretched and the stress released, allowing a return to the nonstressed condition. Therefore continual loading and unloading will produce heat. The amount of hysteresis (heat produced) is dependent on the strain rate (how fast the force is applied). This loss of energy does not allow the material to return to its original state; hence, permanent deformation has taken place.

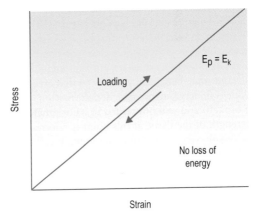

Fig. 7.6 Loading and Unloading Paths (Where $E_k = E_p$).

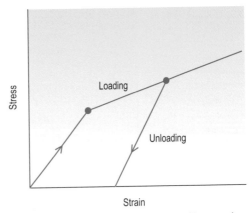

Fig. 7.7 Elastic Materials Exhibiting Hysteresis.

When considering biological tissue, it is important to know the micro- and macrostructure of the tissue concerned. Not many biological tissues are pure, most are a composite (mixture) of materials. This may mean that they have fibres in an aqueous matrix (which therefore makes them viscoelastic), or that they have a combination of different fibres, or both. Orientation of the composite fibres is also of importance. If the fibres are arranged in parallel and the stress is applied in the direction of the fibres, then the material will be strong and possibly stiff (a measure of the resistance to stress). If there is irregular orientation of the fibres, then there will be less strength but what strength there is will be multidirectional.

The stress–strain curve for a 'general' biological tissue can be seen in Fig. 7.8. Although not presenting the graph of any particular tissue, it shows the characteristics that are common to most biological tissues.

The toe region of the graph (Fig. 7.8) represents the straightening of the wavy collagen. It represents no change in the structure of the tissue under stress. The elastic range is the area under the graph where the tissue will return to its original length once the tension is released (between elastic region and elastic limit); this is called Hooke's Law. The elastic limit, or yield point, is that point beyond which the tissue does not return to its original length when the stress is removed. Plastic range refers to that area in which the tissue is undergoing permanent deformation (fibres are being broken) and will not return to its original position. The strength of the tissue at this point is referred to as its yield strength, whereas the ultimate strength is the greatest load the tissue can sustain before strain occurs without further stress. There is a point, which is usually greater than the ultimate strength, at which necking occurs. Necking is when considerable weakening occurs and strain continues to increase even if the stress or loading is greatly reduced or even removed. At the point of failure of the tissue, it has reached its breaking strength; that is, the load at the time the tissue fails and rupture occurs.

Another property of tissue that is important when considering stretching is its stiffness, which is a measure of the resistance offered by the tissue to deformation. The stiffness of a tissue is often rate- and speed-dependent. The ductility of the tissue is its capacity to absorb plastic deformation before failure occurs. If the tissue has an increase in strain with a constant stress, then this increase in length is referred to as creep. This phenomenon is often used in serial splinting, when the tissue is held in a cast under constant load; over time the tissue undergoes further lengthening. The resilience of material is its ability to recover quickly from its deformation, whereas damping refers to the slow return to shape (Soderberg, 1997). Let's now consider some of the main materials that make up the musculoskeletal system.

Bone. Bone is nonhomogeneous, a mixture of materials; therefore it will vary in its response to stress. It is a composite of dense compact bone and cancellous spongy bone. During loading, compact bone is seen to be stiff, with a high ultimate strength and a large modulus of elasticity. It can resist rapidly applied loads better than loads that are applied slowly. These properties are shown in Fig. 7.9, in which the different amounts of stress needed to produce the same amount of strain and ultimate failure are shown for loads in the longitudinal and transverse directions. The graphs of fast and slow loading also illustrate the time-dependent response of the bone to stress (see Fig. 7.9). Cancellous bone, on the other hand, is more compliant; hence, it has greater shock-absorbing capacity.

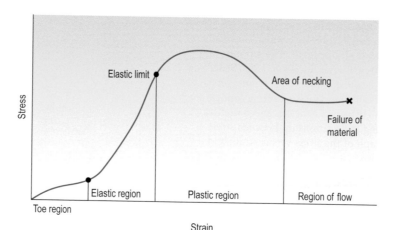

Fig. 7.8 Typical Stress–Strain Curve for Biological Material.

Soft tissues. Most soft tissues found in the musculo-skeletal system are a composite material of mainly type 1 collagen, elastin and the aqueous ground substance. The collagen is composed of crimped fibrils (see Fig 7.10) that are aggregated into fibres, and its prime function is to withstand axial tension.

On stretching, the crimps straighten out and the collagen then stores the potential energy that will returns the fibril to the original position (Fig. 7.10). As the collagen is surrounded by fluid (gel-like ground substance), it also possesses fluid properties of creep and hysteresis.

Elastin is highly elastic even at high-stress strains; that is, it possesses a low modulus of elasticity, whereas that for collagen is high. The importance of these properties is illustrated in Fig. 7.11, which shows the stress–strain curves for the ligamentum flavum (70% elastin) and the anterior cruciate ligament (90% collagen).

Tendons. Fibrous connective tissue is mainly composed of collagen and ground substance, functioning primarily as a passive transmitter of the force produced by muscle contraction. Compared with muscle, the tendon is stiffer, has higher tensile strength and can endure larger stresses (Cribb and Scott, 1995). The tendon can support a large stress with only a small strain and thus makes muscle contraction more efficient, as not much of the muscle action is wasted on movement of the tendon. This facilitates greater apposition of the bones. The properties of a tendon are dependent on the type and proportion of its fibres, as shown in Fig. 7.12. The resultant strain of a tendon is also time-dependent and the tissue exhibits a hysteresis loop, showing that deformation of the tendon will be permanent. This can be seen from Fig. 7.13. Tendons have a low shear modulus, which means they do not stretch easily when a shear force (forces you

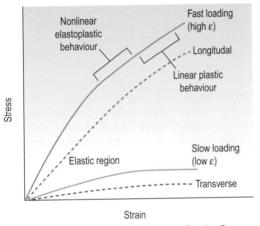

Fig. 7.9 Strain Rate–Dependent Stress–Strain Curves for Cortical Bone Under Longitudinal Stress *(Continuous Line)* and Direction-Dependent Stress *(Dotted Line)*.

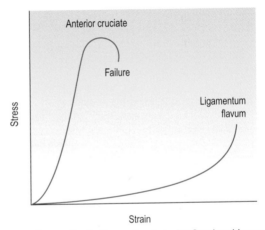

Fig. 7.11 Stress–Strain Curves for Anterior Cruciate Ligament and Ligamentum Flavum.

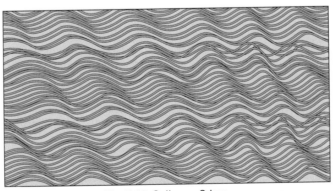

Fig. 7.10 Collagen Crimp.

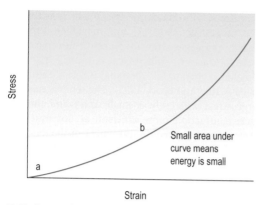

Fig. 7.12 Stress–Strain Curve for a Typical Tendon. *a*, Low strain (elastic fibres dominate and crimping straightens); *b*, stiffer (viscoelastic matrix takes over).

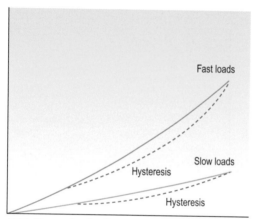

Fig. 7.13 Stress–Strain Curve Showing Rate Dependency and Hysteresis for the Tendon.

experience when sliding over a surface) and can, therefore, harness the pulling force of the muscle very well.

Ligaments. Most ligaments contain a greater proportion of elastin than tendons and therefore have higher flexibility and lower strength and stiffness than tendons. Sometimes, however, ligaments have greater strength if resistance is applied quickly.

Muscle. Muscles vary in their reaction to stress, depending on which muscle is being studied and the age of that muscle. The structure of the muscle with its attendant tendon also has a role in the strain that occurs when stress is applied to the muscle–tendon–bone complex (Soderberg, 1997).

Muscle, however, is an active tissue, and the force produced within the muscle is caused by its contraction. Active tension is developed in the muscle as a result of cross-bridge formation, and passive tension is developed as a result of the

stress placed on the connective tissue elements of the muscle when it is stretched past its resting length. Active tension is decreased, however, as the cross-bridges are pulled apart. Therefore as muscle lengthens, passive tension increases. (See Chapter 6 for more details of muscle action.)

Articular cartilage. Cartilage has a high fluid content, so it has greater ability to flow and is more variable in its properties due to the clever evolution of multiple layers of collagen fibres, which are orientated in different directions. In the top layer the fibres lie parallel to the joint surface to help cope with the shear (sliding) forces. In the deeper parts of the tissue the fibres become more vertical to resist compressive forces.

Factors that can affect the stress–strain response of tissue

Immobilisation. During immobilisation, there will be a decrease in the collagen turnover rate with a consequent weak bonding between the new, nonstressed fibres. There will also be adhesion formation, with consequently greater cross-linking between fibres, and ground substance will not retain its viscous properties (less water content). Without the presence of stress to instruct the way the collagen fibres are lined up, the orientation of the fibres will become haphazard, reducing the strength of the tissue. Even a decrease in normal activity will result in a decrease in the size and amount of collagen fibres, leading to weaker tissues.

Effects of age. One of the natural consequences of the ageing process is the decrease in tensile strength and elastic modulus (elasticity) of all soft tissues. This leads to a decrease in the ability to quickly adapt to an applied force, with the increased chance of overuse injury, fatigue and trauma (Svensson et al., 2016). The effects of ageing are discussed in more detail in Chapter 10.

Effects of drugs. Corticosteroid injections are sometimes used to treat tendon injuries, particularly chronic injuries related to overuse. They are, however, known to reduce the tensile strength (ability to resist lengthening forces) of collagen, so care should be taken when stretching an individual with a history of multiple corticosteroid injections (Haraldsson et al., 2006).

In fact, all the above effects must be taken into consideration when stretching is performed.

As has been described, stretching of collagen is caused mainly by plastic deformation, as the material is fairly inelastic. Connective tissue will reorganise itself in response to a sustained stretch provided the stress is not too great or applied for too long (Cowin and Doty, 2007). Therefore any stretch that does occur will be fairly permanent. It can be seen, then, that care must be taken not to reach the necking phase, as this would compromise the integrity of the tissue being stretched and affect its function. This could lead to a decrease in stability and a greater risk of further injury to the joint.

To summarise, the effects of stretching are to:

- increase joint ROM.
- increase soft tissue length.
- relieve muscle spasm.
- increase tissue compliance in preparation for an athletic event. Note that stretching may improve compliance but this can be at the expense of tissue strength. Stretching before gymnastics may be advisable but not perhaps for other sports (see Further Information 7.1).

Performing a stretch. Passive stretching can, like passive movements, be performed as manual, auto- or mechanical stretching. In manual (or auto-) stretching, the therapist (or patient) produces the sustained stretch at the end of range with the patient relaxed. It is generally accepted that the stretch should be held for 15 to 60 seconds and repeated several times (Young and Behm, 2002). When stretching a muscle tendon complex, it is important that the sarcomeres have an opportunity to *give* before the tendon can be stretched. Sarcomere *give* occurs when the force applied to the muscle is sufficient to separate the actin and myosin filaments so that the noncontractile components of the complex can be stretched. Mechanical stretching involves a low stress being applied by a machine, or perhaps an orthotic (splint) over a prolonged period, sometimes days and weeks.

The above discussion refers to static stretching, which is defined as a slow sustained stretch at the end of range. This should be held, as stated, 15 and 60 seconds, but it is possible that a patient will be unable to tolerate a stretch held for even 15 seconds, and therefore the duration may have to be built up from a few seconds. This type of passive stretching is in contrast to ballistic stretching, which is defined as small end-of-range bounces. Despite having been used for many years, ballistic stretching remains contentious; there is some evidence of an increased injury risk (Vujnovich and Dawson, 1994); however it is considered to be an effective technique which should be used with skill and care, with the right patients/clients (Konrad and Tilp, 2014).

As well as static and ballistic stretching, there are techniques that are based on physiological principles such as a maximal muscle relaxation following a maximal contraction. These are known as proprioceptive neuromuscular facilitation techniques, or PNF for short (see Activity Box 7.5 for further information and an activity you can do to compare the effectiveness of the techniques).

Accessory Movements

Accessory movements are those movements of the joints that a person cannot perform actively but that can be performed on that person by an external force. Although these movements form an integral part of the normal physiological movement and occur throughout the ROM, they cannot be physically isolated by patients themselves. However, if the accessory movement was being performed by the physiotherapist, the patient would be able to stop the movement from taking place. These movements take the form of glides (medially, laterally or longitudinally), compressions, distractions or rotations.

Anatomists group accessory movements into two categories: type 1 are those that cannot be performed unless resistance is provided to the active movement, and type 2 are movements that can be produced only when the subject's muscles are relaxed (Standring, 2005). The latter are the type used for therapeutic purposes. Accessory movements are used to increase the ROM at joints and to decrease any pain that is present. These benefits are in addition to those of passive movements. The mechanism for decreasing pain depends, of course, on the cause of that pain. If the pain is caused by the decrease in ROM, then the rationale of treatment will be the same as that for increasing the range. If not, then the usual effect of small-amplitude movements, applied rhythmically to the joints, is to inhibit the afferent impulse traffic from articular receptors, thus blocking the pain; this mechanism is believed to work through the pain gate theory (Moayedi and Davis, 2013).

Twomey (1992) suggests that articular cartilage facilitates the ROM of joints. If there is joint immobility, the articular cartilage will degenerate more quickly, as it requires movement and loading to ensure adequate nutrition. This nutrition is facilitated by the synovial fluid, which is swept over the joint surface. As the stimulation of the synovial membrane declines, the amount of synovial fluid produced is decreased, becoming thicker with decreased osmolarity. Accessory movements assist in the maintenance of synovial production and, by the small oscillatory movements they make, produce the washing effect of the synovial fluid over the joint surfaces. Twomey (1992) also suggests that movement is important for the nutrition of all collagenous tissue as well as the prevention of adaptive shortening. Small-amplitude movements at the end of range will elongate connective tissue, ligaments, joint capsule and other periarticular fascia via the processes described in the previous section dealing with stretching (*Performing a stretch*). End range movements may also break down any intraarticular adhesions (tissue forming between the two articular surfaces) that could form through joint immobilisation.

Manipulation

Joint manipulations differ from all other types of therapeutic movement, because the patient has no control over the procedure. These movements are potentially dangerous and should therefore be performed only by skilled professionals

ACTIVITY BOX 7.5   What Kind of Stretching Works Best?

As we have discussed, the evidence for stretching to prevent injuries is not clear but we do know that stretching can increase the range of motion available at a joint by increasing the length (although perhaps only temporarily) of the soft tissues. There are different types of stretching techniques that work on different mechanisms so let's do a wee experiment to see which one is most effective for an immediate change in range and which, if any, has a lasting effect.

In a group of three people choose one person to be the measurer (they will need either a goniometer or a tape measure), one person to perform the stretching technique and the last person will be the one having their tissue stretched (tip: don't choose someone who is very flexible or who has had a relevant injury).

We will tackle the hamstring muscle as it is a muscle that often needs stretching (that's another thing to think about).

First task is to measure something that will tell us about the length of the hamstring muscle. Taking it out of the body and putting it on a table is out of the question, so we need an indirect method. One way is to record the popliteal angle (angle between thigh and lower leg measured in the popliteal fossa). This is usually done in supine lying with the hip placed in 90 degrees of flexion, or you could measure the distance (with a tape measure) between tip of the fingers and the toes during a reaching movement with knees held straight.

Decide whether it will be an active test (the person moves their leg) or a passive test (the measurer moves their leg). This is yet another factor to consider; main thing is to be consistent.

Take three measurements from both sides and calculate the average, for each side. Next a warm-up is probably a good idea to prepare the tissue for stretching. Two to five minutes of light jogging on the spot should suffice.

Ok, now apply one of the stretching techniques to the left side and then a different one to the right side.

1. **Static hold**. Three repetitions. Each stretch should be held at the limit of the range for at least 30 s. Remember to bend the knee of the leg not being stretched.

2. **Hold relax technique**. The muscle is placed in a near end-range position. In this case by lying on the back with the hip at 90 degrees and the knee straightened as far as it will go. The muscle to be stretched (hamstrings) develops a large (maximum if possible) isometric contraction. That is, the person being stretched should try to flex their knee and this is resisted by the 'physio', so that no joint movement occurs. After 10–15 s of this contraction the individual is asked to relax and the 'physio' moves their knee into a little more extension. This is believed to work through stimulation of the Golgi tendon organ which reflexively relaxes the muscle when too much tension is sensed within the tendon (it's a protective reflex). Be sure to control the stretching movement.

3. **Dynamic stretching**. This is probably best done by the individual themselves. Move to the end of joint range; now perform repetitive stretches, each one only a second or two long, for around 30 s total. It has been described as bouncing if that helps you to visualise this stretch.

Once the stretching has been completed, record the popliteal angle as before (or fingertips to toes).

Wait for 30 min (a seated position is probably best) and measure the range of motion again.

- Which technique had the best results, and which lasted the longest?
- Reflect on how these stretching techniques might be working.

---

with much experience in the mobilisation of joints. Manipulations are small-amplitude, forceful, high velocity thrusting movements that take the joint past the available physiological range. Manipulations are performed very quickly before the subject has time to prevent the movement from taking place. Lewit (1993) describes manipulation as a technique for treating end-range blocking of joints. Displaced intraarticular material may be one reason for the restriction of movement. Joint misalignment may be another. This blocking or restriction of movement, he claims, has two effects: one is the restriction of the subject's functional movement; the other is the effect on the accessory movement or joint play. Restrictions caused by meniscal or other material within the joint are termed *loose bodies*.

Lack of movement of a joint may lead to adaptive shortening of the soft tissue structures surrounding it: capsule, ligaments, tendons or muscles, for example. This secondary consequence will in itself cause a restriction of movement and possibly pain when movement is attempted. Thus a vicious circle is set up. The initial immobility may be a consequence of pain. If the pain is caused by trauma to the joint, then the problem may be compounded by the presence of adhesions within and around the joint that are the natural consequence of the inflammatory process.

Shortened soft tissue structures may also be manipulated to physically break the structures. Creating this level of tissue damage to obtain greater joint flexibility may be performed under a general anaesthetic; this is called an MUA (manipulation under anaesthetic).

Effects. The primary effect of manipulating the joint is to restore its mobility. A secondary effect may be to decrease pain, if the pain was a direct result of abnormal tension on structures caused by incorrect functioning of the joint.

These effects are brought about in a variety of ways. As the joint is manipulated, space is created between the surfaces. The movement of the surfaces, together with the greater space created, possibly causes any physical obstruction between the joint surfaces to be moved clear. Joint surfaces may then be realigned, causing the correct afferent information to be sent to the spinal cord. Fibrous adhesions resulting from the inflammatory exudate, the organisation of the synovial fluid, or the adaptive shortening of any soft tissue structure will be physically torn. This takes the structure through the plastic phase and very rapidly past the breaking point. The intended consequence of this procedure is to free the joint to perform its full functional excursion.

Contraindications for the above technique are the same as those for relaxed passive movements.

Thixotropy You may recall the word thixotropy; I mentioned it a few pages ago. This is the ability of a material/substance to alter its viscosity (resistance to flow) when it is agitated/moved about. Think of shaking a ketchup bottle to get the last bits of sauce to start moving. This is a property of connective tissue that can be exploited to gain more range, or at least do it more comfortably, for example gentle movements of a joint before you stretch it. It really is just the warm-up. But remember this simple step before you try to gain more range; agitate the tissues with gentle movements and if this is not possible, then simply warm them up; it has the same thixotropic effect.

Active Movement

Active movements can be thought of as movements of the joint within the unrestricted range that are produced by the muscles that pass over that joint. The movements may be active assisted or free active. Therapeutically, these movements are performed as exercise.

Active assisted exercise is exercise carried out when the prime movers of a joint are not strong enough to perform the full ROM. The forces that need to be overcome are friction, gravity and the effects of the mechanical disadvantage of lever length. Assistance may be given by any external force, but it is important that the external force provides assistance only so that the movement is simply augmented and does not become a passive movement. The external force has to be applied in the direction of the muscular action but not necessarily at the same point.

External assistance may be:
- Manual assistance.
- Mechanical assistance.
- Auto-assistance.
- Electrical stimulation, for example functional electrical stimulation (FES).

Manual assisted exercise is when the subject's muscular effort is assisted by the therapist. The therapist changes the assistance as the muscle progresses through its ROM, compensating for such factors as angle of pull and length–tension relationships. The amount of assistance may also be changed as the muscle strength increases.

Mechanical assistance may be provided by a variety of apparatus. Isokinetic equipment has the facility for active assisted movement provided the trigger forces are set low enough. The most useful mechanical assistance is sling suspension, in which the assistance is given in two ways. First, the resisting force of friction is reduced by physically lifting the segment clear of its resting surface, which also helps to counteract the force of gravity by supporting the segment. Second, depending on the point of fixation of the sling suspension, gravity may be used to assist the movement, provided the desired movement occurs on the downward arc of the curve produced by the segment within the sling suspension.

Auto-assisted exercise may be performed by the subject using the same principles as those of manual assistance. More common, however, is for the assistance to be a combined form of auto- and mechanical assistance. This is seen in the use of bicycle pedals for lower limb mobility or pulleys for upper limb mobility.

Electrical Stimulation

The use of electrical stimulation to activate a muscle contraction and move a joint has been around for centuries. Even the ancient Egyptians used electrical eels to stimulate flaccid muscle. The modern-day equivalent is called FES which is typically used within a functional movement, for example walking. The electrical stimulation is timed to contract the muscle at a specific point (e.g. when the heel comes off the ground) to assist in the movement.

Free active exercise differs from assisted exercise in that the movement is carried out by the subject, with no assistance or resistance to the movement except that of the force of gravity. There are many ways in which free active movements can be performed:
- Rhythmical: this uses momentum to help perform the movement taking place in one plane but in opposite directions.
- Pendular: these are movements performed in an arc and are useful for improving mobility as, on the down-curve of the arc, the movement is assisted by gravity.

Single or Patterned

Depending on the aims of the intended movement, the choice of single or patterned movements is made. As a general rule, single movements are used to demonstrate or restore actions, whereas patterned movements are used for functional activities. The use of biceps brachii to flex the elbow as a pure movement is an example of a single movement. Reaching out to pick up an object (food) and taking it to the mouth also involves flexion of the elbow, but this movement also uses other joint movements in a functional pattern (the feeding pattern), for example supination and pronation of the forearm. These movements may also be classed by their effect:

- Localised: designed to produce a local or specific effect, such as mobilising a particular joint or strengthening a particular muscle.
- General: gives a widespread effect over many joints or muscles; running, for example.

Exercise affects all the systems of the body and is covered elsewhere in this book and many other textbooks. What must be remembered, however, is that the effects produced cannot be isolated to one particular system or even one effect within that system. Exercise, for example, will maintain muscle length and joint range, but it may also alter the strength (aerobic and anaerobic capacity) of that muscle and have a more widespread effect on the cardiovascular system.

One of the major local effects of exercise is the increased rate of protein synthesis, thus producing more actin and myosin as a response and facilitating an increase in muscle length. Connective tissue also responds to increased exercise by becoming stronger in order to cope with the increase

in function that is required of that muscle (Cowin and Doty, 2007).

If active exercise is performed regularly and through the available physiological range, it has all the effects of passive exercise that were previously explained, including maintaining joint range, increasing joint nutrition and decreasing pain. Active movement has the advantage of strengthening muscles to some extent, thus providing stability for the joint with its increased range. Another advantage of performing active movements is that, if they are performed in a rhythmical manner, they may promote relaxation of the muscles surrounding the joint. If this happens, then the joint range may well be increased, especially if the restriction was caused by muscle spasm.

CONCLUSION

Movement occurring at joints depends on a variety of anatomical and biomechanical factors that can assist and/or limit the available ROM. How movements are classified and described will depend on which discipline is being studied. For this text, movements are classified as either active or passive, with subdivisions of each. Restriction of movement, caused by pathological changes, can be successfully managed by the therapist using different forms of movement. This is achieved once the rationale of the chosen method is known and correctly applied to the fully assessed patient.

The preceding descriptions by no means represent an exhaustive survey of the therapeutic modalities available to improve joint range and muscle length. They are, however, representative of the basic principles of the techniques that are used based on normal joint movement.

SELF-ASSESSMENT QUESTIONS

1. Fibrous joints (synarthroses) have
   a. No movement.
   b. Some limited movement.
   c. Pretty free movement.
2. Synovial fluid
   a. Nourishes the cartilage.
   b. Reduces friction.
   c. Stores white blood cells.
   d. Act as a force dampener.
3. True or false?
   Accessory movements occur as part of a normal physiological movement but cannot be performed in isolation.
4. And adduction movements occur in the
   a. Sagittal plane about a frontal axis.
   b. Transverse plane about a sagittal axis.

   c. Frontal plane about a sagittal axis.
   d. Sagittal plane about a transverse axis.
5. The knee is a(an)
   a. Ellipsoid joint.
   b. Condylar joint.
   c. Simple joint.
   d. Hinge joint.
6. A joint's close-packed position is
   a. When the articular surfaces rub against each other.
   b. The position of maximum congruency between the surfaces.
   c. The end of physiological range.
   d. Usually painful.

7. Which of the following movements is not (usually) an accessory joint movement?
   a. Spin
   b. Roll
   c. Rub
   d. Glide

8. The apposition of _____ tissue is one of the normal constraints to joint movement.
   a. Bony
   b. Soft
   c. Articular
   d. Viscous

9. Manual passive movements are indicated when a patient
   a. Is unable to actively perform the movement themselves.
   b. Has too much pain.
   c. Has active inflammation in a joint.
   d. Is uncooperative.

10. Contractures are
    a. Short burst muscle contractions.
    b. Adaptive shortening of the muscle.
    c. Muscle spasms.
    d. Impossible to resolve.

REFERENCES

Abate, M., et al., 2010. Limited joint mobility in diabetes and ageing: recent advances in pathogenesis and therapy. Int. J. Immunopathol. Pharmacol. 23 (4), 997–1003.

Branch, T.P., Lawton, R.L., Iobst, C.A., Hutton, W.C., 1995. The role of glenohumeral capsular ligaments in internal and external rotation of the humerus. Am. J. Sports Med. 23 (5), 632–637.

Bromley, I., 2006. Tetraplegia and Paraplegia: A Guide for Physiotherapists, fifth ed. Churchill Livingstone, Edinburgh.

Cowin, S.C., Doty, S.B., 2007. Tissue Mechanics. Springer Science & Business Media, New York.

Cribb, A.M., Scott, J.E., 1995. Tendon response to tensile stress: an ultrastructural investigation of collagen: proteoglycan interactions in stressed tendon. J. Anat. 187 (Pt 2), 423–428.

Field, L.D., Bokor, D.J., Savoie, F.H., 1997. Humeral and glenoid detachment of the anterior inferior glenohumeral ligament: a cause of anterior shoulder instability. J. Shoulder Elbow Surg. 6 (1), 6–10.

Haraldsson, B.T., Langberg, H., Aagaard, P., Zuurmond, A.M., van El, B., Degroot, J., et al., 2006. Corticosteroids reduce the tensile strength of isolated collagen fascicles. Am. J. Sports Med. 34 (12), 1992–1997.

Hardy, M., Woodall, W., 1998. Therapeutic effects of heat, cold and stretch on connective tissue. J. Hand Ther. 11 (2), 148–156.

Harvey, L.A., Brosseau, L., Herbert, R.D., 2014. Continuous passive motion following total knee arthroplasty in people with arthritis. Cochrane Database Syst. Rev. (2), CD004260.

Johnson, V.L., Hunter, D.J., 2014. The epidemiology of osteoarthritis. Best Pract. Res. Clin. Rheumatol. 28 (1), 5–15.

Kerr, A., Macmillan, C.E., Uttley, W.S., Luqmani, R.A., 2000. Physiotherapy for children with hypermobility syndrome. Physiotherapy 86 (6), 313–317.

Kisner, C., Colby, L., 2007. Therapeutic Exercise, Foundations and Techniques, second ed. FA Davis, Philadelphia.

Konrad, A., Tilp, M., 2014. Effects of ballistic stretching training on the properties of human muscle and tendon structures. J. Appl. Physiol. 117 (1), 29–35.

Lewit, K., 1993. Manipulative Therapy in Rehabilitation of the Locomotor System, second ed. Butterworth-Heinemann, Oxford.

Lotz, M., Loeser, R.F., 2012. Effects of aging on articular cartilage homeostasis. Bone 51 (2), 241–248.

McCarthy, M., Yates, C., Anderson, M., Yates-McCarthy, J., 1993. The effects of immediate continuous passive movement on pain during the inflammatory phase of soft tissue healing following anterior cruciate ligament reconstruction. J. Sport Phys. Ther 17 (2), 96–101.

McMahon, P.J., Tibone, J.E., Cawley, P.W., et al., 1998. The anterior band of the inferior glenohumeral ligament: biomechanical properties from tensile testing in the position of apprehension. J. Shoulder Elbow Surg. 7 (5), 467–471.

Moayedi, M., Davis, K.D., 2013. Theories of pain: from specificity to gate control. J. Neurophysiol. 109 (1), 5–12.

Myles, C.M., Rowe, P.J., Walker, C.R., Nutton, R.W., 2002. Knee joint functional range of movement prior to and following total knee arthroplasty measured using flexible electrogoniometry. Gait Posture 16 (1), 46–54.

Nielsen, M.M., Mortensen, A., Sørensen, J.K., Simonsen, O., Graven-Nielsen, T., 2009. Reduction of experimental muscle pain by passive physiological movements. Man. Ther. 14 (1), 101–109.

Norkin, C., Levangie, P., 2005. Joint Structure and Function: A Comprehensive Analysis, fourth ed. FA Davis, Philadelphia.

Norkin, C., White, J., 2003. Measurement of Joint Motion: A Guide to Goniometry, third ed. FA Davis, Philadelphia.

O'Brien, S.J., Schwarts, R.S., Warren, R.F., Torzilli, P.A., 1995. Capsular restraints to anterior–posterior motion of the abducted shoulder: a biomechanical study. J. Shoulder Elbow Surg. 4 (4), 298–308.

Palastanga, N., Soames, R., Palastanga, D., 2006. Anatomy and Human Movement Pocket Book. Churchill Livingstone, Elsevier, Edinburgh.

Robergs, R.A., Keteyian, S.J., 2003. Fundamentals of Exercise Physiology for Fitness Performance and Health, second ed. McGraw-Hill, Boston.

Soderberg, G.L., 1997. Kinesiology—Application to Pathological Motion, second ed. Williams & Wilkins, Baltimore.

Standring, S., 2005. Gray's Anatomy, Thirty-Ninth Ed. Elsevier, Edinburgh.

Stockley, R.C., Hughes, J., Morrison, J., Rooney, J., 2010. An investigation of the use of passive movements in intensive care by UK physiotherapists. Physiotherapy 96 (3), 228–233.

Svensson, R.B., Heinemeier, K.M., Couppé, C., Kjaer, M., Magnusson, S.P., 2016. Effect of aging and exercise on the tendon. J. Appl. Physiol. 121 (6), 1237–1246.

Twomey, L.T., 1992. A rationale for the treatment of back pain and joint pain by manual therapy. Phys. Ther. 72 (12), 885–892.

Vujnovich, A.L., Dawson, N.J., 1994. The effect of therapeutic muscle stretch on neural processing. J. Orthop. Sports Phys. Ther. 20 (3), 145–153.

Warner, J.J., Deng, X.H., Warren, R.F., Torzilli, P.A., 1992. Static capsuloligamentous restraints to superior–inferior translation of the glenohumeral joint. Am. J. Sports Med. 20 (6), 675–685.

Wuelker, N., Korell, M., Thren, K., 1998. Dynamic glenohumeral joint stability. J. Shoulder Elbow Surg. 7 (1), 43–52.

Young, W.B., Behm, D., 2002. Should static stretching be used during a warm-up for strength and power activities? Strength Cond. J. 24 (6), 33–37.

Posture and Balance

Clare Kell and Andy Kerr

LEARNING OUTCOMES

After reading this chapter, you will be able to:
1. Describe the features of an ideal posture and the way it adapts through life.
2. Explain the mechanisms used to maintain a functional posture.
3. List the systems involved in maintaining a posture: including sensory, control and effector/output.
4. Provide an insight on posture and balance problems and the way they are treated.

INTRODUCTION

Posture has been variously defined as: an attitude or position of the body (Cech and Martin, 2002); the maintenance for a period of time of a position in space as a prelude or background to movement (Bray et al., 1999); or the intrinsic mechanisms of the human body that counteract gravity (Basmajian, 1965). In many cases, although not stated in the definition, authors proceed to discuss the upright standing position, giving the misleading impression that posture is only really related to this position, perhaps because it is regarded as the most challenging posture. However, as we will describe in this chapter, posture relates to all possible positions—lying, sitting, kneeling, crouching, standing etc.

In this chapter the term posture refers to the alignment of body segments to position the body for engagement in functional activity and be responsive to both expected and unexpected perturbations (disturbances in balance). Such a definition acknowledges the active (albeit subconscious) nature of posture and its maintenance.

In this chapter we will introduce the requirements and challenges of a bipedal standing posture, before describing, in more detail, standing, sitting and lying postures. The chapter will proceed with an in-depth discussion about the intrinsic and extrinsic requirements, as well as the sensory, control and effector systems essential for the maintenance of posture and balance. Please try the self-assessment questions at the end to make sure you have retained the essential bits of information. Throughout the chapter we have added practical activities; please try these as well because they will help you to gain a practical, working knowledge to apply in your professional practice.

HUMAN POSTURE

Adaptations to Bipedalism

The evolution of bipedalism has conferred great benefits to humans, not least the freedom to use the upper limbs for survival skills such as hunting and gathering food (Niemitz, 2010). However, there are also clear disadvantages such as generally slower mobility (just try and outrun your average quadruped), reduced stability from the combination of a higher centre of mass (CoM) and a much smaller base of support (BoS) (see Chapter 3 for a biomechanical description) and pressure being distributed over two not four feet. We are still coping with these disadvantages today; for example, falls are a major issue for health care, but we have made some evolutionary adaptations to help us cope. With the body's weight now being transmitted through a reduced area of support (the spine, legs and feet), the bipedal human has gradually improved its musculoskeletal system, most evidently in the spine and foot, for dealing with this doubling of load.

Adaptations of the Spine

The increased size of the vertebral bodies themselves, particularly in the lumbar spine (Lewin, 2009), is perhaps the most obvious adaptation to the increased forces created by an upright posture, but the whole structure shows clear signs of adaptation.

The modern human spine is a biomechanically efficient structure designed as an S shape (Fig. 8.1) so that the curves can both support the column (and appendages) and provide a spring-like response to loading. This elasticated rod, with its combination of curves and arches, effectively distributes the body's weight while offering both support and flexibility to the body as a whole (Oxland, 2016). The strength and elasticity are not just created by the bony anatomy; the highly elastic ligamentum flavum, made of 80% elastin fibres (Bogduk 2005), helps the spine to keep its curves and recoil after loading, and the activity of antagonist muscle pairs, which cross the vertebrae, also act as springs to stabilise the column and distribute force. However, such a many-linked chain brings its own problems. For example, humans are beleaguered with the problem of postural low back pain due to the loading through this part of the body; quadrupeds are unlikely to experience this.

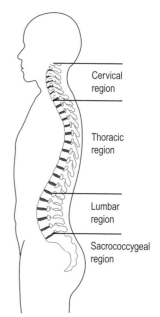

Fig. 8.1 The Curves of the Vertebral Column.

Adaptations of the Foot

Because the foot is the human's contact point with the ground (at least when upright), a basic knowledge of foot anatomy and biomechanics is important to understand human posture. Bipedal stance requires the foot to be both rigid, for weight support and propulsion, and compliant (relatively) so that it can adapt to different surfaces. The human foot is another highly evolved part of modern humans that is distinguished from our primate cousins in having permanent arches (Rolian et al., 2010). As with the spine, the foot has three arches (medial longitudinal, lateral longitudinal and transverse); these combine with the interlocking bones, ligaments and muscles to provide great strength and flexibility. In quiet standing, thick pieces of connective tissue (e.g. plantar aponeurosis and spring ligament) support the bones forming these arches to minimise muscular effort. At the end of the stance phase of gait (preswing), the extension of the toes tightens the longitudinal arches (windlass effect) to stiffen the foot, creating a rigid lever for effective propulsion (push-off). The foot's flexibility is provided by a mobile forefoot and subtalar joint, which has many degrees of freedom. This flexibility allows the foot to shape itself to the surface. It is truly a remarkable structure but, like the spine, is not without its problems, which is why we need experts like podiatrists to help us.

There are many other evolutionary adaptations that can be traced back to the start of bipedalism 3 million years ago such as our Achilles tendon (Malvankar and Khan, 2011); we would encourage you to explore this interesting area, but, for the moment, we need to move on. In the next section we will look at the development of standing posture before taking a look at the 'ideal' postures in standing, sitting and lying.

Development of the S-Shaped Spine Across the Lifespan

Cech and Martin (2002) described postural and functional development throughout life, the salient points of which we will now summarise. At birth, the newborn infant spine is characterised by two concave forward-facing curves (kyphosis) in the thoracic and pelvic regions. The latter curve is facilitated by the sacrum, being composed of individual sacral bones at this stage. At about 3 to 4 months of age, as the infant tries to raise his or her head from the prone lying position, gravitational interaction causes the convex forward development of the cervical spine (lordosis). The final curve, the convex forward lumbar curve (lordosis), begins to form as the baby gains sitting balance (around 4 months). Standing and walking (around 13 months) further increase the lumbar lordosis by tilting the pelvis anteriorly, which helps the toddler to generate forward (and unfortunately downward) acceleration.

At this stage the child's feet are still pretty flat, without an obvious arch (look at a toddler's footprints in the sand compared with your own); however, they do have proportionally larger feet which helps with the stability problem a little. The location of the CoM is different from adulthood, being higher (around T12 compared with S2) and further forward, in response to the baby's proportionately larger head and organs (e.g. liver). A relatively high CoM creates an even greater challenge for stability, which is commonly countered in toddlerhood with a wide BoS (see chapter 10); however, falls are a frequent learning experience at this age, despite the large feet. Cech and Martin suggest the foot arches and spinal curves begin to take adult form around the age of 6 years. However, it must be remembered that the child has many more years of growth in front of them, when the spine's development can be challenged and adapted in response to environmental stressors. Nissinen et al. (1993) highlight the specific vulnerability of the spine during puberty. With rapid growth over a short period, there is the possibility of abnormal growth or altered alignment. These issues of spinal structure related to function are essential to both postural assessment and management and will be dealt with later in the chapter.

By the age of 22 years, when growth has generally stopped (Nissinen et al., 2000), the spinal curves and location of the body's CoM within it will have matured. Ignoring for the moment all the factors (social, anatomical, environmental and pathological) that can influence an individual's posture, the position of upright stance will generally remain unchanged

until a point in later life when ageing results in a changing interaction between physical ability and gravitational pull. Decreased muscle and bone mass, along with diminished motor control and intervertebral disc degeneration, combine to change the standing posture, drawing it more into flexion (lowering the CoM) and reversing those curves developed during infancy (Le Huec et al., 2011). Therefore there is a tendency for the ageing population to display a stooped standing posture with reduced cervical spine curve and a flattened lumbar lordosis (Fig. 8.2). This posture is known to reduce mobility and increase the risk of falling (Katzman et al., 2010). In the feet the reduced elasticity in the structures supporting the longitudinal arches mean they are less able to support the weight of the body and the feet tend to drop into a flatter posture with the resulting decrease in biomechanical efficiency for walking and risk of pain from weight bearing on structures not used to this type of loading.

Before we move on to more detailed descriptions of posture, it is time for a practical activity; try Activity Box 8.1.

'Ideal' Alignment of Segments

The word *ideal* is, in many ways, unhelpful because it suggests a form of perfection against which we are all measured and towards which we are all trying to strive. Throughout this chapter, when reference is made to the term *ideal*, you are advised to see it as a term used simply to explore biomechanical systems. The ideal, or what is sometimes called a neutral posture, is therefore simply a reference frame from which real human posture can be described and understood; it is a

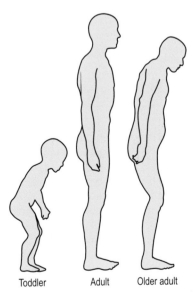

Fig. 8.2 The Curves of the Vertebral Column Across the Lifespan.

Toddler   Adult   Older adult

useful reference frame for clinical practice. Recognising that this chapter focuses on the physical influences on human posture and balance, readers are encouraged to include their understanding of the social, psychological and environmental influences on and consequences for a specific individual's postural alignment; to help you do this, try Activity Box 8.2.

With these caveats, an ideal posture can be described as one that aligns the body segments so that the linear and rotational forces (moments) generated by gravity and counterbalanced by muscle action are minimised at each point in the chain (Han et al., 2011). The hallmark of such a posture would be that it requires minimal energy to maintain. Consequently, one person's posture is not identical

to another's; individual variations in anatomy will mean this minimal energy posture is likely to vary between people. Caution is therefore advised when categorising postures as poor or nonideal, as there may be good anatomical reasons for someone's posture: it may be *his or her* ideal minimal energy posture even if it looks wrong to you. A careful history, including the environment and culture within which the individual exists, and physical examination, should be undertaken. Pearsall and Reid (1992) concluded their research with the observation that the most striking finding from their work was the postural variability between subjects; they suggested each subject was displaying a posture that optimally compensated for their specific anthropometric differences.

Upright Stance

The line of gravity (LoG) is a useful tool to use when assessing an individual's posture. Imagine a plumb line (a vertical line directed, by gravity, to the centre of the Earth) running through each vertically stacked segment of the body (head, trunk, pelvis, legs, feet). You could even fashion your own LoG using a weight on the end of a piece of string, although the scientific method would be to use a forceplate and x-rays. The popular opinion (e.g. Pearsall and Reid, 1992) is that this LoG passes (ideally) through the following points in the sagittal plane:

* The mastoid process or tragus of the ear.
* Just anterior to the shoulder joint.
* Just posterior, or through, the hip joint.
* Just anterior, or through, the knee joint.
* Just anterior to the ankle joint.

The research (Le Huec et al., 2011) suggests that this relationship between the imagined (or measured) LoG and the joints generates small moments (turning forces) that tend to keep both knee and hip joints in slight extension and the ankle in dorsiflexion while standing.

Viewed from behind (posterior view, Fig. 8.3A), the observer would expect to see the following anatomical landmarks symmetrically aligned with the horizontal: ear lobes, scapulae, waist creases, posterior iliac spines (dimples), buttock creases and knee creases. With bare feet placed anteriorly and separated by the width of the hips, the Achilles tendons would follow a perpendicular line to the floor; you may see a curve indicating a valgus (concave curve) or varus (convex curve) hind foot. The spinous processes would follow a direct line from head to floor, without deviation to the left or right that could indicate a scoliosis (curve in spine).

A front, or anterior, view (see Fig. 8.3B) is good for noting central alignment (e.g. centrality of the chin above the sternum, a central and relaxed umbilicus, upward-facing anterior iliac spines and anterior-facing patellae). The observer would also notice a symmetric distribution

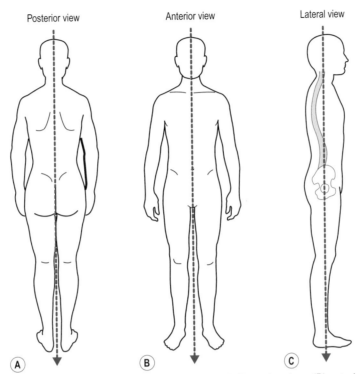

Fig. 8.3 The 'Ideal' Alignment of Segments in Standing. (A) Posterior view, (B) anterior view and (C) lateral view.

of weight through the feet. If you could run your hands around the edge of the feet, you would feel that they were equally accepting their load, turning neither inwards nor outwards; the longitudinal arches would be identical and about 2 to 3 cm off the ground (this will vary). You may even wish to measure the height of the arch (Activity Box 8.3).

Observing the ideal upright stance posture from either side (lateral view, see Fig. 8.3C) would show the head evenly balanced on the neck, with no excessive chin protrusion or retraction. The spinal curves would demonstrate an open S shape such that the rib cage is anteriorly facing and the abdomen would be flat but relaxed. A side view would show only one cheekbone, one shoulder, one scapula, one nipple, one buttock and one knee; if two of anything can be seen, segmental rotation may be occurring, but check that you are viewing the body at 90 degrees. To clearly assess segmental rotation, the posture should be observed from all sides.

Sitting

The height of the CoM is, of course, lower in sitting than standing, but it is actually higher within the body and further forward thanks to the forward position of the legs. The BoS

ACTIVITY BOX 8.3   Measuring the Height of the Arch With Navicular Drop Height

Measuring the height of the arch (navicular drop height) is a good way to objectively measure the degree of pronation. Get a partner, and try yourself.

In a standing position, mark the navicular tuberosity (you may wish to refer to your anatomy books, but it is the nobbly bit that sticks out on the inside of your foot, below the malleolus and a little further along the foot) and measure the height to the ground (tape measure); normal values are approximately 5 cm. Now ask your partner to relax his or her feet; the navicular tuberosity should drop a little (approximately 1 cm), but if there is excessive pronation this will drop by more than 1 cm. Compare left and right and then each other: any differences?

Further Reading

Vinicombe, A., Raspovic, A., Menz, H.B., 2001. Reliability of navicular displacement measurement as a clinical indicator of foot posture. J. Am. Podiatr. Med. Assoc. 91 (5), 262–268.

increases substantially as it now includes the chair. Much less load is now being placed on the lower extremities. In general terms, this posture requires less energy to maintain than upright stance, being inherently more stable. However, a major change is the angle of the pelvis on the lumbar spine, as the former is tilted backwards to allow the ischial tuberosities to be the focus of weight transference to the base (Oxland, 2016). The resultant flexion of the lumbar spine results in greater loading on the intervertebral discs (lumbar spine in particular) and stretching of the posterior structures of that vertebral segment. It may be counterintuitive, but sitting has been measured to create greater forces in the spine than standing (Table 8.1).

Prolonged sitting postures can therefore have a detrimental effect on the lumbar spine. Unfortunately, we are spending more and more of our time in sitting, which is undoubtedly a major factor in the increasing incidence of low back pain. Supporting the lumbar spine with an appropriately measured and placed lumbar roll can dramatically reduce lumbar vertebral loading by altering the angle of the pelvis. There are also different chair designs that aim to achieve the same effect on the pelvis angle. (Please also see Chapter 16 for more thorough exploration of sitting.)

Ideally, the sitting posture should be supported by a chair whose backrest is high enough to support the upper thoracic spine (Fig. 8.4) and that inclines slightly forwards so that the lumbar spine is encouraged to stay extended (Oxland, 2016). The person's bottom should be placed to the back of the seat, with up to two-thirds of their thighs supported on the chair base to avoid compression of the posterior knee structures. Ideally, the chair height should be adaptable so that the knees and ankles will be at right angles as the feet are placed hip distance apart on the floor (Activity Box 8.4).

Lying

Lying is a very stable posture, a low CoM placed well within a large BoS. In this position, humans achieve equilibrium with minimal energy expenditure, which is probably why we spend around half our lives in this position, sleeping, watching TV, relaxing. The length of time spent in this posture means it is important to understand what is happening to the alignment of our segments in this position because it could still be the cause of posturally related problems.

First, the lying position is composed of three distinct segmental orientations: supine (face up), prone (face down) and side lying. Each of these postures offers different contact points to the supporting surface and therefore exposes different areas to gravitational influence. The ideal supine position is one that mirrors the segmental alignment of upright stance (see Fig. 8.3). This position can be achieved only when the supporting surface is adaptable enough to permit indentation of the backward-protruding structures (e.g. the occiput, scapulae, thoracic spinous processes, sacral spines, ischial tuberosities and heels) (Fig. 8.5A). Too hard a surface will lead to these areas succumbing to pressure injuries (see Fig. 8.5B), and too soft a support will result in mass spinal flexion (see Fig. 8.5C). Pillows should be kept to a minimum (unless required for medical reasons) to avoid malaligning adjacent segments in the chain.

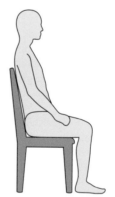

Fig. 8.4 The 'Ideal' Alignment of Segments in Sitting.

TABLE 8.1 **Mechanical Forces Experienced at the L4/L5 Intervertebral Disc**	
Posture	Mechanical Load at L4/L5 Intervertebral Disc: Newtons (N)
Prone lying	144 N
Side lying	240 N
Upright standing	800 N
Upright sitting	996 N

From Sato, K., Kikuchi, S., Yonezawa, T., 1999. In vivo intradiscal pressure measurement in healthy individuals and in patients with ongoing back problems. Spine 24 (23), 2468–2474.

ACTIVITY BOX 8.4   **Sitting Posture Observations**

Observe your colleagues or the people sitting around you. How are they sitting? What factors could you change? How are you sitting at the moment? How long can you remain in this position?

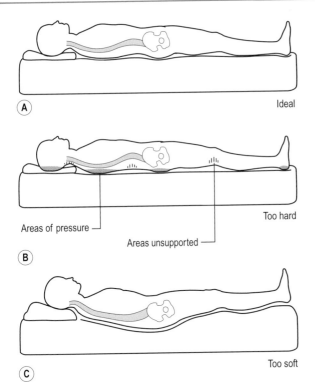

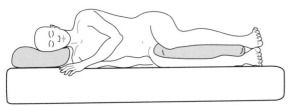

Fig. 8.5 Possible mattress influences on segmental alignment in supine lying: (A) the 'ideal' alignment, (B) the possible effects of a very firm mattress and (C) the possible effects of a very soft mattress.

Fig. 8.6 The 'Ideal' Alignment of Segments in Side Lying.

Because of the necessity to rotate the cervical spine to breathe, and the accompanying hyperextension of the lumbar spine, the prone position is not generally advised for long periods, but it can be a useful antidote to a day spent in flexed sitting postures.

The ideal side-lying posture again aims to mimic upright stance alignment. However, the influence of gravity in this position necessitates support from external structures, most commonly pillows (Fig. 8.6). For the reasons outlined previously, the supporting surface should allow indentation of prominent bony structures but not be too soft

to encourage side flexion. In side lying, the cervical and lumbar curves require support because of their hanging free between the wider head and pelvis. However, as with supine lying, the use of external support must be targeted to the individual, supporting not exaggerating existing curves. If a pillow under the head is required, it should be accompanied by, or include, an extra support for the neck. The best option is to place a roll to support the neck; the worst is to use a pillow that forces the head into side flexion and by morning supports only the ear! Similarly, a small roll may be needed to support the lumbar spine at the waist. Finally, in the side-lying position, gravity draws the top leg towards the bottom, and the ideal hip distance separation of the lower limbs is lost, with resulting side flexion and rotation of the lumbar spine. To counteract this rotation, it is advisable to lie with a pillow positioned between the knees. The previous description provides the ideal posture for segmental alignment, reduction of joint moments and a mechanically stress-free sleep. While seemingly overpadded, this support is used widely throughout patient care environments.

Summary

This section has reviewed the ideal segmental alignment in three frequently described resting postures. You are reminded that the *ideal* is used as a frame of reference for postural assessment purposes and not as a guide to therapeutic outcome; the latter depends on an individual's functional environment. Postural analysis should be conducted in *each* position listed previously, as poor alignments will emerge or become unmasked when gravitational and stability influences are changed. The most obvious change is seen when moving from standing to sitting, the posterior tilting of the pelvis causing the lumbar spine to flex and experience high levels of pressure.

Requirements for Achieving the 'Ideal' Posture

A quick observation of family and friends will show you that very few people demonstrate the ideal posture we have described. Why is this? Why do some people develop 'problem' or 'symptomatic' postures and not others?

The maintenance of any posture requires the following: an integrated system for detecting the posture, checking whether it is really what is wanted and then bringing about any necessary change; effective and efficient muscles that can be appropriately recruited and then maintain the activity required; soft tissue structures of the appropriate length and flexibility to restrain and permit movement as designed; a psychological state that is motivated to engage with postural control; and an environment that permits postural alteration (e.g. women might have problems trying to stand upright with high-heeled shoes and short, tight skirts!).

Postural Alignment in the Real World

Several detailed studies have observed childhood postures in upright stance and observed those children until growth has stopped. Of interest to our discussion is the percentage of children who, while completely asymptomatic, display asymmetrical spinal postures. Juskeliene et al. (1996) found asymmetry in 46.9% of 6- to 7-year-olds, and Nissinen et al. (1989) reported spinal asymmetry in 21% of 10 year olds. At 13 years old, the Nissinen population exhibited all sorts of postural combinations that were more common in girls than in boys (Nissinen et al., 1993), but when growth had stopped (age 22 years), equal numbers of boys and girls had asymptomatic, asymmetrical postures, with the most common presentation being a right scoliosis (Nissinen et al., 2000). So what sort of things could be causing these asymmetries?

Factors Influencing Segmental Alignment
In Childhood and Adolescence

Juskeliene et al. (1996) reported that increased rates of asymmetry were found in two groups of children: those who had frequent childhood illnesses (defined in this study as having four or more acute illnesses in a year) and those who undertook little physical activity. The least asymmetry was found in the most active children. The researchers concluded by stressing the importance of muscle health and strength in the development of growing spinal alignment.

Their study of participants over a long period (from age 11 to 22 years) has enabled Nissinen and colleagues to make the following observations:

- Left-handedness is a powerful determinant of hyperkyphosis (excessive thoracic kyphosis curve), probably resulting from sitting at desks designed for right-handed students (Nissinen et al., 1995)
- Puberty is a 'dangerous' time for spinal development, because of the imbalance between bone growth spurt and growth and development of the supporting and controlling soft tissue structures. Post puberty, twice as many girls as boys had developed a scoliosis, probably because their sitting height (height while sitting at a desk) had increased faster than the boys had, and they were still all using the same standard class desks (Nissinen et al., 1993).
- Thoracic kyphosis is more prominent in males, whereas females are more lordotic (Poussa et al., 2005).
- Finally, around the age of 22 (i.e. during the slowing down phases of bone growth), hyperkyphosis was more prevalent among men than in women (Poussa et al., 2005).

The key messages from this extensive longitudinal study suggest that we should be concerned about the environments in which children spend a considerable part of their day, and also acknowledge that postural development continues well past puberty and into young adulthood.

Gillespie (2002) reviewed the impact on childhood spinal development of computer (desktops and laptops) and electronic games (handheld and computer or screen-based) use. Reporting staggering numbers of hours spent by children and young people in these activities, Gillespie noted that 'children and adolescents are increasingly engaged in activities that simulate work demands known to cause repetitive strain injury in working adults'. During such activities, Gillespie (2002) suggests that young people are in deep concentration while adopting postures that are not suited to their needs (e.g. using environments where desk and chair heights are fixed, where there is a tendency for sharing computers but with only one mouse and keyboard, and where there is the tendency for children to use desktop computers at home set up for their parents—although she does make the astute observation that many units are not in fact set up appropriately for the adults using them either!).

Drawing on this work, Gillespie et al. (2006) explored the impact of computer and electronic game use on self-reported episodes of musculoskeletal pain and/or discomfort. Their study suggests that girls were more likely than boys to report symptoms, but in general, there was no overt link between hours spent engaged in these activities and reported episodes of musculoskeletal discomfort. However, Gillespie et al. (2006) did note that discomfort was reported most when the young person was at risk of being overweight or needed vision correction.

However, concluding on a positive note, Gillespie (2002) suggests that, unlike adults, children, when uncomfortable, are happy to climb on to tables or chairs, lie on the floor, etc. and in so doing may be reducing the actual negative influence that they experience; she suggests that perhaps adults could learn from the unselfconscious attitudes of children! Fig. 8.7 depicts the ideal computer station posture, with the screen height and angle adjusted so that a comfortable head position is maintained; does this reflect the position you adopt? (Try Activity Box 8.5.)

In Adulthood

If reduced physical activity and the adoption of sustained sitting postures are risk factors for children adopting postural asymmetry and back pain, what factors influence adult posture?

Grieco (1986) considered this issue while reviewing the likely impact on the spine from taking millions of years to become *Homo erectus* ('the upright man') and the relatively recent development of *Homo sedens* ('the seated man') in the execution of many of today's employment tasks. Grieco

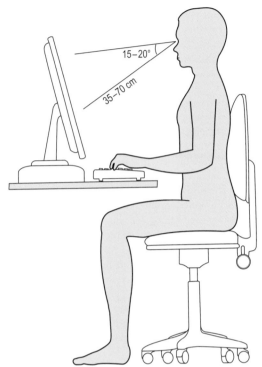

Fig. 8.7 The 'Ideal' Computer Station Posture.

15–20°

35–70 cm

ACTIVITY BOX 8.5 How Much Do You Sit and Lie?

A prolonged sitting posture is evidently bad for your back. This sedentary position (along with lying) has also been statistically associated with diseases such as diabetes and heart disease (Chastin et al., 2015). How much time do you spend in these positions?

Keep a diary for 7 days (or use a Fitbit or similar) to record your activity and postures over 7 days, 24 h/day.

Once you have this information, reflect on what you might do to change, provided you think you need to. To give you a reference, Jans et al. (2007) recorded sitting postures lasting between a third and half of the working day.

reviewed the positions and ergonomics of workstations and working patterns and made the following observations:

- Enforced posture should be considered a risk factor (to soft tissue and spinal injury) on the same level as the lifting of weights and vibration.
- Ischaemia (reduced blood flow) in the paravertebral muscles occurs with prolonged isometric muscle contraction, as seen in the maintenance of unsupported postures

(and that can be any posture: i.e. sitting, standing but not lying).

- The problem, in terms of spinal injury, is one of a fixed posture, not the loading of the spine at any one time; vertebral disc nourishment occurs via a pump or sponge mechanism, i.e. as a result of changing pressure resulting from change in posture.
- Ergonomic chairs may decrease the loading on the spine in general, but because the occupier is more comfortable, they do not move around as much, and then the fixed posture becomes the problem.
- All employees should be educated in the use of ergonomically sound devices and have 10-min 'postural pauses' built into their work pattern on an at least 50-minute basis.

In conclusion, Grieco (1986) suggested that adults are susceptible to the same postural stresses as children but this time in their pursuit of employment. Postural education is a key factor in his argument to resolve these issues. Despite our knowledge of the dangers of a seated posture, we continue to adopt this position for prolonged periods in our working and leisure lives. It seems education and exercise have, so far, had little impact on our sitting behaviour (Chau et al., 2010). What do you think? How can we reduce sitting time?

Other causes of fixed postures. We must not forget that there are many adults in our population who—for reasons of loneliness, weakness, illness etc.—remain static or confined to one posture for substantial periods. Prolonged sitting, for whatever reason, will lead to the functional adaptation of a reduced lumbar spine lordosis, an increased thoracic kyphosis and reduced range of movement at the hips and knees into extension (Cech and Martin, 2002). As the ideal thoracic alignment is designed to encourage maximal efficiency of lung function, people with static postures, especially with a thoracic hyperkyphosis, are at risk of developing pathologies associated with poor ventilation (e.g. reduced lung capacity and tidal volumes, leading to chest infections, and reduced efficiency of the thoracic venous pump, causing problems for lower limb venous return and fluid distribution) (Bray et al., 1999). There is also a risk of pressure sores at contact areas such as the ischial tuberosities in sitting or scapula/buttocks in supine lying; these can be life threatening if left untreated. These problems of fixed postures are compounded if the person is elderly and therefore their soft tissues are already reduced in flexibility, strength and ability to recover after injury.

Hormone-related changes. Cutler et al. (1993) analysed the postures of 136 healthy women who were premenopausal and postmenopausal to see if there was a relationship between hormonal levels and postural hyperkyphosis (the so-called dowager's hump attributed to postmenopausal osteoporotic women). The results suggested that there was no real link between degree of kyphosis and age, hormone levels or calcium intake. Again, there appeared to be a weak link with exercise levels: while many women displayed a kyphosis, the more active women were more able to straighten out of the kyphosis posture.

Temporary influences on postural alignment. The classic temporary influences on posture include situations in which weight distribution alters, as in pregnancy and when pain and/or pathological processes alter mood, tolerance levels and general engagement with the environment (Clancy and McVicar, 2002). If the underlying cause of these postures is rectified promptly, no lasting adaptation to the new posture should occur, as a return to functional activity will restrengthen supporting muscles and soft tissues.

Defined Postural Deviations From the 'Ideal'

Postural analysis has historically characterised nonideal postures into six types: (1) scoliosis, (2) kyphosis, (3) hyperlordosis (hollow back), (4) combined kypholordotic posture, (5) swayback and (6) flat back (Fig. 8.8). All refer to deviations from the ideal. You should note that this categorisation system rarely indicates that the defined deviation originated within the spine itself. The following section will briefly describe each of these postural types and discuss how the spinal deviation impacts on the segmental alignment of the whole body; a malalignment in one part of the body will have to be compensated for in another to keep the LoG falling within the BoS and your head straight. Compensations will depend on the patient and context but would include structural realignment and/or increased muscle work in adjoining segments.

Scoliosis (See Fig. 8.8B)

- A static (fixed) or mobile (correctable) lateral curve usually seen in the thoracic and lumbar spinal regions.
- Soft tissues and muscles on the side of the concavity will be shortened, whereas those on the convex side will be longer and potentially weaker.
- Depending on the severity of the scoliosis, a compensatory side flexion may be seen further up the segmental chain.
- If the deviation is caused by a problem lower down (e.g. a difference in leg lengths), the scoliosis may itself be the compensation.

Kyphosis (See Fig. 8.8C)

- Again, this can be static or mobile. Many people adopt this slouched posture over short periods with no lasting effect.
- Always refers to an increased anterior curvature of the thoracic spine.

- A common posture in the older population.
- An increased kyphosis affects the higher segments such that the eyes focus on the ground unless the cervical spine compensates by increasing its lordosis, a position likely to cause muscle tension and joint compressions. Common symptoms of this effect are pain and headaches because the neck is not conditioned to cope with or adapt to this position.
- A long-standing kyphotic posture will result in shortening all musculature on the anterior chest wall (e.g. pectoral muscles) and the lengthening of the erector spinae to compensate.
- Severe kyphosis may result in impaired lung function caused by altered biomechanics for thoracic expansion, i.e. an impaired bucket-handle movement.
- It generally leads to reduced mobility and increases the risk of falling.
- Occasionally, a kyphosis is the result of a compensation for shortened hip flexors.

Hyperlordosis (See Fig. 8.8D)

- The pelvis is held in an anterior tilted posture.
- Seen after (and in late) pregnancy and when abdominal muscles are weak.
- This position leads to an increased lumbar lordosis that shortens both the spinal extensors and the anterior muscles controlling the pelvis: iliopsoas, rectus femoris and tensor fasciae latae (Palastanga et al., 2006).
- The drawing forwards of the pelvis will lengthen and weaken the glutei and abdominal muscles.
- The posture is called *kypholordotic* if it is combined with a compensatory increase in the thoracic kyphosis (see Fig. 8.8E).

Swayback (See Fig. 8.8F)

- Also known as *relaxed*, the characteristic profile of this posture is the slouch.
- Adopting this posture uses the least amount of active muscle work, as the posture is generally maintained by soft tissue and ligament length (e.g. pushing the pelvis forwards so that the hips go into extension allows the pelvis to 'hang' on the anterior ligaments of the hip). Particularly the iliofemoral ligament, which, perhaps unsurprisingly, is the strongest ligament in the body as it resists hip extension in this position.
- This posture is commonly adopted by boys with Duchenne muscular dystrophy, for example.
- Working back up the segments, this anterior shift will need to be compensated for by an increased lumbar lordosis and thoracic kyphosis. The head will usually be held forwards of ideal.

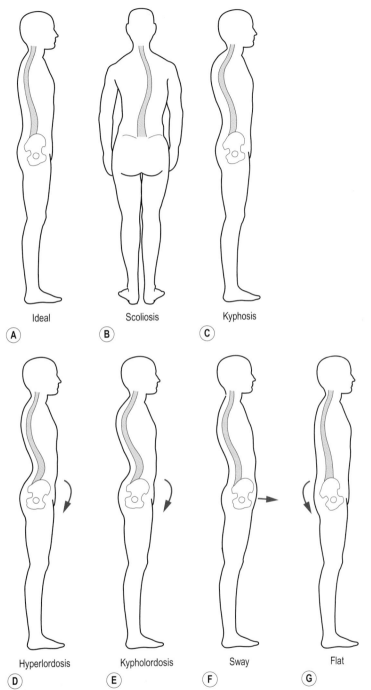

Fig. 8.8 Diagrammatic representations of 'ideal' posture and deviations from it: (A) 'ideal', (B) scoliosis, (C) kyphosis, (D) hyperlordosis, (E) kypholordosis, (F) swayback and (G) flat back.

- Depending on the extent of the pelvic shift, the knees may be locked into extension so that stance is maintained via bony approximation.
- A mixed picture of altered joint and muscle biomechanics is presented by this posture, each deviation requiring careful assessment and consideration of the cause or compensation conundrum.

Flat Back (See Fig. 8.8G)

- The key feature of this posture is a posterior tilting pelvis, which reduces the lumbar lordosis and gives the back its characteristic flat appearance.
- People adopting long-term slouched sitting positions commonly develop this posture.
- A posterior tilting pelvis may result in the person standing in hyperextension at both hips and knees, with lengthened hip flexors.
- Abdominal muscles are likely to be tight and strong, with the erector spinae reciprocally weak and long.
- Further up the segmental chain, the loss of lumbar lordosis will be compensated for by an anteriorly positioned head, which in turn may be compensated for by a slightly increased thoracic kyphosis.

Summary

This section has outlined the common features of a number of postural types, including the 'ideal'. Hopefully this will stand you in good stead for when you come across abnormal postures and people with symptoms caused by their posture, such as postural backache. You should consolidate this knowledge through observation and trying the self-assessment exercise at the end. Please bear in mind that having one of these postures does not automatically give the bearer pain, discomfort or any other problem. Kisner and Colby (2007) detailed examples of when problems may arise for each postural type, but note that most people are symptom free. It is also important to note at this stage that the existence of a pure flat back, for example, is as rare as the ideal alignment. We should also remember that we constantly move in and out of many postures; it is being in a fixed posture that seems to cause the problems. As we know, each person's posture is the result of interaction with their environment. While the given labels are useful for reference and help your practice, postural assessment and intervention can occur only on a case-by-case basis.

MAINTAINING A FUNCTIONAL POSTURE

Introduction

Now that normal posture has been defined and the influences that affect segmental alignment described, the chapter will now consider balance (postural control). Despite the potential instability of a relatively high CoM above a small BoS, humans are usually able to maintain their posture and control the alignment of all segments so that functional movements are stable. In a nutshell, human postural control (balance) requires information from and integration between the systems responsible for visual, vestibular and somatosensory input and motor output. Despite the enormity of the task, we are only fleetingly aware of the systems' ongoing efforts to move and support our body in relation to gravity. Lackner and DiZio (2000) describe the perception of effortlessly standing on one foot, our bodies seemingly unaware of the huge forces that are being transmitted and balanced through our supporting segments; it is only when we are ill or fatigued that we feel every newton of load!

This section of the chapter will review the components of the balance system and discuss how they are integrated to produce the background for functional activity. The chapter adopts the systems theory approach to motor control, described by Shumway-Cook and Woollacott (2016). The section will conclude with a discussion about the factors that influence normal balance and consideration of the impact of abnormal control on effective and efficient movement. (Try Activity Box 8.6.)

Definitions

For clarity, we will begin by defining some terms. First postural control is the 'act of maintaining, achieving or restoring a state of balance during any posture or activity' (Pollock et al., 2000). For this reason, it is used interchangeably with the

---

ACTIVITY BOX 8.6   Feeling Balanced?

Get into a standing position (if you can), and make sure you can hold onto something in case you wobble. Stand still, and look at your body position. You can start where you like, but the pelvis is often a good start point. Is it tilted forward (bum sticking out)? What about your legs—is the left the same as the right, are either more rotated? Go through your whole body, and look at the way each part is positioned. Now lift one leg off the ground, and feel how your body reacts. Do you use your arms? Which part of you is working hardest?

Now try the same thing with your eyes closed (remember to have something secure nearby to hold if you feel wobbly).

What is the difference? Are you working harder to maintain stability, LoG within BoS?

This activity should have given you some clues to the systems (and strategies) involved in maintaining standing balance.

term balance. Lee (1988) and Williams et al. (1994) describe a system as a device or set of elements that transform input into a single or a selection of desired outputs. To function, a system requires inputs, the ability to create outputs, and a means for the two to communicate together. In this context, the term *control system* refers to an ability of the system to set and then achieve its output; for example when reaching for an object, our postural control (balance) system is able to decide and then execute the right amount of compensatory postural reactions (outputs) to maintain stability during the reaching movement.

Regulation refers, in this instance, to the ability of the system to do more than simply control for an output in a given situation. Regulation is the ability of the system to maintain the correct output, i.e. in response to feedback gained from what is actually happening and in anticipation of what is to come. It is this ability of the postural control system to anticipate, regulate and react responsively to its environment that gives the human an exceptional array of highly skilled functional activities.

How Does Balance Work?

To answer this question, this section will consider the first two steps in postural control (balance): (1) posture and movement sensation (inputs) and (2) integration of these inputs. We will look at the final step, movement and posture output, in more detail in 'Postural control synergies used for standing' later in the chapter.

Posture and Movement Sensation

For any system to produce an effective product, it must receive good, up-to-date and relevant input data. Such is the intensity and diversity of the information required to frame functional movement that three sensory systems are used for input: the vestibular system, the visual system and the somatosensory (big word that just means sensations from the body; soma means body) system.

Vestibular system. Located in the inner ear are two sensory systems that send information down the eighth cranial nerve, the vestibulocochlear nerve. The cochlear portion of the cranial nerve carries information from the cochlear portion of the inner ear; this is concerned with auditory stimulation—this is what we hear. Although not directly related to balance, overstimulation or unexpected stimulation of this system can affect postural control, as we shall see later. The vestibular system comprises the other part of the inner ear complex and is responsible for our awareness of head orientation with respect to gravity and the head's linear and angular acceleration (i.e. any change in velocity and direction of the head). In this respect, they act like both a spirit level and an accelerometer (a device that measures acceleration; you have one in your smartphone).

While this is not the text for detailed physiological discussion, it is important at this point to note that the sensory receptors of the vestibular system are constantly firing and that it is the change in firing rate and pattern that are detected and interpreted by the interpretation centre for this system, the vestibular nuclei of the brainstem. The vestibular nuclei collect and redistribute information to other movement interpretation centres (e.g. the cerebellum, reticular formation, thalamus and cerebral cortex) but can also affect system output directly, e.g. the vestibuloocular reflex helps to stabilise eye movement when the head is moving (e.g. eyes move to right when the head moves to left). This reflex is very useful for hunting or reading when moving. Collectively, the nuclei will influence the antigravity muscles of the neck, trunk and limbs via the vestibuloocular and vestibulospinal tracts.

Visual system. The visual system provides the most amount of information for balance, as you probably discovered in Activity Box 8.6. The eyes provide the sense of sight, which plays an essential role in giving us information about where our bodies are in space. This is sometimes referred to as visual proprioception. Visual proprioception is perceived in the brain, providing a constantly updated map of the body's position in space, the relationship between one body part and another and the motion of our body. It is understood that information from the eyes passes to the superior colliculi (roof of the midbrain), where sensory maps compute how close to the body and how close to the midline of the body the movement is occurring. Information from the superior colliculi (visual system) passes to three main regions:

1. Regions of the brainstem that control eye movements.
2. The tectospinal tract that helps control neck and head movement.
3. The tectopontine tract that, through connections with the cerebellum, processes eye–head control.

In this way, the visual system is controlling output so that the postural control (balance) system can be sure about head position and movement in space with respect to surrounding objects (Shumway-Cook and Woollacott, 2016). Eye-tracking technology is beginning to reveal just how much our eyes are involved in balance particularly when moving, e.g. the input needed to plan avoidance trajectories in healthy and impaired individuals (Stuart et al., 2017).

Somatosensory system (the body sensors). The awareness of joint position (proprioception) is provided by information from the unmyelinated Ruffini fibres in the joints themselves, the muscle spindles of muscles passing over the joints and the effector motor command signals. In the hands and feet, where precise joint proprioception is crucial, a fourth input, from the cutaneous mechanoreceptors (sensitive to pressure), adds to the information pool. While we are able to think about the position of our limbs, proprioception is an essentially subconscious level sense.

When you were standing with your eyes closed (see Activity Box 8.6) you were relying on these proprioceptors as well as the vestibular system. It is thought that information from the somatosensory receptors listed here passes directly to the motor neurons controlling postural stability at spinal level. In this way, sensory information can modulate movement that results from commands originating in higher centres of the nervous system (Shumway-Cook and Woollacott, 2016). Such a direct communication system enables quick response times and is used to good effect when the sensors detect the likelihood of a fall. For example, if a person is standing, the pressure receptors in the feet will detect the perturbation and respond by effecting actions to widen the BoS (induce a stepping reaction) and/or lower the CoM. We use this response every time we shift our CoM over one leg (as in walking); detecting increased pressure under one foot, the somatosensory system responds by increasing extensor motor tone on the supporting side and simultaneously increasing flexor tone on the opposite side. Both these actions working together have the effect of transferring the CoM over the new BoS (the supporting limb). Try it quickly now. Stand with your feet apart, imagine the LoG equidistant between your feet and a little in front of your ankles and just allow your body to lean a little further forward; you will start to feel a response to this balance problem with increased activity in your calf muscles.

When Do We Need the Input?

Many authors have described the type of information that needs to be inputted to the postural control system. A summary of the described follows:

To form an output, it is important to know where you are at the start. Input data must therefore describe the *initial conditions*. We learn patterns of common postures and movements, but we can be caught out when something changes (e.g. when we have a leg in plaster). To avoid frequent falls every time something changes, information is needed about alterations to both the internal and external environments that would challenge our balance so that we can refine our solutions. These *challenges to balance* are also called perturbations and are described as being mechanical in origin if they occur as a result of external or self-generated forces, or sensory if they are the result of an unexpected sensory input (e.g. an object moving quickly into our visual field or a loud crash occurring). Such is the complexity of the information received that the brain is able to determine the strength, duration, frequency and direction of the perturbation. (Try Activity Box 8.7.)

Sensory Integration

How the nervous system integrates and responds effectively and efficiently to the wealth of incoming sensory data about

postural and environmental positioning is the focus of much research. Although there is some disagreement about specific sensory integration processes, it is widely agreed that all three forms of sensory input (visual, vestibular and somatosensory) are used to maintain an upright posture.

But how does the nervous system work out which inputs to favour, which to downplay, etc.? Shumway-Cook and Woollacott (2016) draw on more than three decades of research to suggest that the possible processes behind the sensory integration needed to effect postural control align with the following two theories.

Intermodal theory of sensory organisation. Shumway-Cook and Woollacott suggest all three sensory inputs contribute equally at all times and it is their interaction (i.e. the relationship between the three senses at any one moment) that provides the information essential for establishing postural orientation.

Sensory weighting theory. Instead of all three senses contributing equally, the central nervous system modifies the weight or importance of each input depending on its perceived accuracy. For example, when we are wearing footwear that is impeding (or overloading) our foot somatosensory receptors, the input from this sense will be downplayed and input from visual and vestibular sources upgraded. Researchers supporting this theory suggest that the advantage of such a weighting system is that we can maintain stability in a variety of environments. This theory may also explain the different postural control strategies witnessed to come into play during different tasks and between people of different ages and in different environments.

Whichever (if either) theory is correct, all researchers and practitioners agree that the sensory processing needed to effect postural control is highly complex and task dependent.

Regulation and Anticipatory Control

Once a movement has begun, the sensory systems cannot relax. The postural control system requires ongoing information *(feedback)* about the effect of the planned response (see Chapter 15 for more information on feedback). Sensory inputs inform higher centres about the achieved or expected output, and then an error signal representing the difference between actual and desired output is detected. The response is a modification of the output signal (muscle contraction). We are normally unaware of this process because feedback involving all the subsystems occurs at an automatic level. If you are sitting at a desk reading this, reach out for your pencil/mobile phone. You have the basic movement pattern ready, but your eyes and proprioceptors are giving constant feedback to optimise the movement accuracy so that you reach the target efficiently.

Of course, no system is perfect, and relying on a feedback system has its problems. The process just described has many steps to produce a movement, and for feedback to be effective the whole process has to be completed repeatedly as the movement or correction continues in a constant loop of movement monitoring and correction. Loop delay, or the time it takes to make a correction, is one of the big problems with feedback systems. Nerve conduction problems or difficulties with central processing may delay this feedback loop. Some individuals will therefore move with a high risk of error and thus have difficulty producing efficient, effective movement.

To combat some of these problems, we also have another mechanism for making adjustments: anticipatory control (Shumway-Cook and Woollacott, 2016). Anticipatory control is a process in which signals for postural compensation and modification are sent before sensory information is required (even before the main movement begins); it is a sign that a movement is well known, the expected problems have all been learnt and a strategy developed through repetition. Sometimes this is useful in a sports context because the movements need to happen too fast to be delayed by a feedback loop (e.g. the ability of a tennis player to return a serve of more than 100 mph). This is why it is sometimes also called feedforward control (Kanekar and Aruin, 2015).

Anticipatory control occurs during most of our regular daily activities (e.g. writing and stepping), reducing movement execution times considerably and therefore increasing the efficiency of the task effected. Kanekar and Aruin (2015) report that anticipatory control is effected by muscle synergies and that these synergies are the same as those used by the postural control feedback systems. Building on these results, researchers have now confirmed that postural muscle synergies are preselected in advance of planned action when that action is serial (one movement after another), expected and/or practised. The process for this central preselection is known as *central set* (Shumway-Cook and Woollacott, 2016) and is thought to be responsible for both our rapid postural responses in known environments and the skill with which postural control responses are modulated during practiced

activities. The central set therefore reduces the risk of our overrecruiting or underrecruiting postural control–related muscles, thus increasing our postural efficiency. Although the processes of anticipatory control set out previously appear to reflect current research consensus, there is much less agreement about where within the central nervous system these processes are coordinated (Activity Box 8.8). (More information is provided in Chapters 9 and 15.)

Conclusion

This section has reviewed the systems used to maintain balance while the body is performing functional activities. We have seen that movement requires the dynamic and ongoing interplay of vision, proprioception, contact cues, efferent control and internal (previously learned) models. Such multisensory input is essential for body orientation, the apparent stability of our surroundings and ultimately movement control. Finally, it must be acknowledged that not all postural control occurs at a purely subconscious level. Increasing attention levels may be likely when postural/movement tasks occur with secondary tasks; this is called dual tasking and is a useful model for understanding where the attention is directed. In addition, there is a plethora of literature exploring the normal consequences of the human

---

ACTIVITY BOX 8.8 Conscious or Unconscious Control

Think about the following situation. You are walking down the stairs in a busy building, holding your books in front of you (so you cannot see your feet) and chatting to your companions; all is fine and you arrive safely at the bottom. How does the difficulty of the activity (walking down the stairs) change when you start to worry about where your feet are? Now what is going on? Several things are happening here. First, you are adding in extra communication loops and increasing the time delay from sensory input to motor output, but second, to see your feet you are probably going to have to lean forwards to see the steps—what does this do to your CoM? What do you think is happening in your vestibular system when you look down at the step? How does your visual system cope with sensing the height you could fall? What happens if a step is suddenly a different height from the rest?

Is it a good idea to make patients' balance responses conscious? Or should we try to build up segmental, automatic control by staging the complexity and difficulty (in terms of segments needing to be controlled against gravity) of the activities we ask them to practise?

ageing process and the ensuing increase in conscious balance control (see Lacour et al., 2008). Thinking about your balance is not wrong, but it does slow down your response times (Jacobs and Horak, 2007), making you vulnerable, especially in standing. Elderly people who may be consciously thinking about their balance more frequently than most are thus particularly at risk of falls while dual-tasking (Lacour et al., 2008).

Postural Control Synergies in Standing

In relaxed standing, the body is constantly undergoing small adjustments in position; this is called postural sway and is probably caused by respiration, blood movement and need to avoid prolonged pressure. Small perturbations to stable postures, such as upright quiet standing, can be accommodated without any central control because of the intrinsic elastic properties of muscle. Together with reflexive loops (stretch reflex), muscles behave in a similar manner to a spring. During small perturbations, muscle acts as a stretching spring to resist the disturbance. In upright standing, with the CoM projected anterior to the ankle joints, it is the calf muscles that play an important role in accommodating small perturbations, particularly in the anterior/posterior direction. However, the body in standing is vulnerable to large and potentially multidirectional perturbations. To meet these challenges, the human body has developed an efficient but complex suite of responses. While we know this latter to be a fact from our personal experience of balancing, research is still evolving to help us unpick the system's complexity. What follows therefore is part of a developing field of research. You are advised to explore the recent original texts if this is a specific area of interest for you and your practice.

Managing Anteroposterior Challenges

In standing, the body uses three main strategies to combat threats to balance and stability in the anteroposterior directions: (1) the ankle strategy, (2) the hip strategy and (3) the stepping strategy. The process of balance management is subconscious and reduces response times by treating effector muscles as groups or *muscle synergies*. A synergy describes the functional coupling of groups of muscles that are constrained to work together as a unit (Shumway-Cook and Woollacott, 2016). Sending one signal to a synergy will therefore get a wide-ranging, set response—'cutting out the middleman'—reducing response times and increasing effectiveness.

Ankle Strategy

The ankle strategy is used when the foot is fully supported on the contact surface so that the dorsiflexors and plantar flexors about the ankle joint can exert their influence through *reverse action* (i.e. if we sway backwards, the anterior tibialis

muscles will contract to bring us back to midline, pulling the body over the foot). Similarly, a forward sway will cause the gastrocnemius to become active (because the perturbation is now greater than can be accommodated by intrinsic properties alone) and draw the CoM forwards over the BoS (Cech and Martin, 2002). The ankle strategy is like an *inverted pendulum* with body mass rotating over the fixed point on the ground (feet) via the ankles; it is effective for correcting small perturbations when standing on a firm surface (so active when you stand quietly) and obviously requires intact joint range and muscle strength about the ankle (Shumway-Cook and Woollacott, 2016). See Fig. 8.9; the positive and negative symbols indicate the relative activity of the plantar flexors (gastrocnemius/soleus) and dorsiflexors (tibialis anterior mainly).

Hip Strategy

When the perturbations are greater than a small sway, when the disturbance is quickly applied or when the foot is on a small contact surface, the body uses another strategy: the hip strategy. Using the large muscles of the hip and knee together, the hip strategy is better able to control the CoM and prevent a fall (Shumway-Cook and Woollacott, 2016). The controlling joint (hip) is after all close to the CoM. The hip strategy is evoked in preference to the ankle strategy for all perturbations that come from a mediolateral direction. The ankle is rather limited in this direction compared to the multiple degrees of freedom offered by the hip joints.

Stepping Strategy

The third strategy, the stepping strategy, has been referred to previously and is evoked when the perturbation is strong enough to really threaten stability. In this instance, a gross movement (e.g. a step or hop) is required to change the BoS so that the CoM can still fall within it and stability can be regained.

Managing Perturbations From Other Directions

Because of the limited mediolateral movements possible at the ankle and knee joints, these joints do not play a large or initial role in the adjustments needed to maintain mediolateral stability (Shumway-Cook and Woollacott, 2016). The primary mediolateral control of balance therefore occurs about the hip and trunk. As a consequence, the initiation of muscle activity from a mediolateral perturbation occurs in a proximal to distal direction.

Of course, balance challenges can come from multiple directions, not just in one. In this case the balance system's response draws on the complexity of muscle synergies (i.e. the notion that one muscle may be part of several synergies) (Shumway-Cook and Woollacott, 2016), in essence a mixture of the previous strategies.

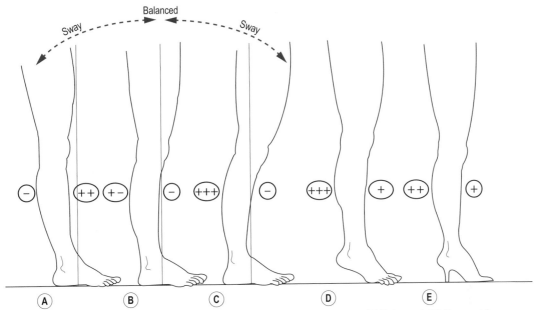

Fig. 8.9 Muscular activity in leg muscles in five states: (A) Backward sway, (B) Balanced, (C) Forward Sway, (D) Rising on toes, (E) Wearing heeled footwear.

Measurement of Balance

Clinical measures of balance are widely used in practice to assess someone's risk of falling (Activity Box 8.9). Tests like single leg standing and clinical scales such as the Berg Balance Scale are widely used, but reactive balance (i.e. introducing a perturbation and assessing the response) are not so well used, despite these kinds of tests having greater potential to reveal impaired balance (Sibley et al., 2011). Technology can be used to provide more objective measurements. Body-worn sensors (e.g. accelerometers and gyroscopes) have the capacity to collect balance data over long periods of time and during activities of daily living (Hubble et al., 2015). A forceplate (see Chapter 2) has also been well used to measure balance. A forceplate measures force, including the location of the force being applied to the ground; this is called the centre of pressure (CoP). This can tell us where the overall body force (combination of gravity and muscle action) is located (see Chapter 2). In Fig. 8.10, we can see a typical CoP signal during quiet stance; the system captures and plots the CoP location at rates of 1000 times a second (depending on the forceplate), and if you join the dots up, you get the spaghetti plot illustrated in Fig. 8.10. You can measure the width and length of this pile of spaghetti to give you an objective measure of standing balance. The speed of CoP movement might also be interesting for dynamic balance. This is the same type of technology used in the

ACTIVITY BOX 8.9   Romberg Test

The simplest and probably most widely used test for balance (in standing) is called the Romberg test and is based on the three strategies described previously. Why not try it with your partner?

Ask him or her to stand in his or her bare feet, feet together, arms comfortably by his or her side.

Stand beside him or her for safety.

Observe his or her movement.

Now ask him or her to close his or her eyes and again observe the movement, and this time record how long he or she can maintain this position (within reason). You may observe the ankle strategy, but it should be controlled.

You can add a little push from the back to see if he or she responds appropriately with a stepping reaction. Or to the side where you might observe the hip strategy.

There is also the sharpened Romberg where the feet are positioned deliberately to reduce the BoS and make the test more challenging. A description with video clips is available from https://www.physio-pedia.com/Romberg _Test (accessed on 02.03.18).

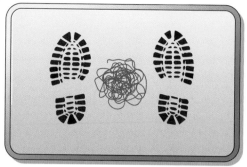

Fig. 8.10 Using Centre of Pressure Measurement to Assess Standing Balance.

ACTIVITY BOX 8.10

How do you think the changes seen with ageing will be noticed in terms of balance? How might coexisting multipathology (e.g. cataracts and arthritis) challenge postural control? What are the possible consequences on movement speed, energy efficiency, etc.?

Wii balance board; not surprisingly, then, this has been used to test and train balance (Clark et al., 2010).

Summary

We will summarise the previous section with a list of requirements for effective balance control.

Requirements for an integrated postural control response.

- Intact sensory system: sensors, nerves and communication pathways. Particularly the three main balance sensors (visual, vestibular and proprioception)
- Intact central nervous system: conduction pathways, internal communication networks and framework for pattern reference or learned response patterns relevant to individual shape and body symmetry or alignment.
- Intact musculoskeletal system: effector pathways including nerves, neuromuscular junctions, strength and endurance of muscles and range of movement about effector joints.
- Psychological engagement with surroundings: remember that the reticular formation is responsible for coordinating postural muscle tone activity in response to levels of higher centre arousal.
- An external environment that allows accurate postural changes to be made when perturbations occur.

Factors That Affect Postural Control

Obviously, anything that impairs the functioning of the systems listed previously will affect postural control responses, but there are some common situations that will challenge balance responses.

Ageing

The effects of the ageing process on the postural control systems of healthy people can be summarised as follows:

- Body sway increases with age. Only about a third of older adults are able to maintain balance using the ankle strategy.
- The sensory systems decline as part of the ageing process, but the visual system fares better than the others, becoming

increasingly important as sensation and muscle strength reduce in the lower limbs and the vestibular system declines.

- Both nerve conduction speeds and central processing in the brainstem slow with age. The reduced conduction speed will cause longer delays in the ankle strategy than the hip strategy due to the relatively longer distance.
- The higher attentional demands required during postural control in older people mean there is less capacity to perform other tasks such as talking, thinking or manipulation.

In practice, these challenges result in people having to give more conscious attention to their posture during everyday activities, leaving little room for error or capacity to respond to sudden change in circumstances (e.g. loud noises or sudden movements) (Lacour et al., 2008). You don't have to be of retirement age to experience the effects of ageing on balance. Poulain and Giraudet (2008) explored the balance responses of a range of individuals and suggested that participants aged between 44 and 60 years were becoming more reliant on their visual sensory input, thus becoming very unsteady in darkened environments. Large numbers of our population will therefore find their postural control difficult, resulting in increased conscious control, slower response times and a reduced repertoire of correction responses. However, it is important to note that avoiding obesity and staying physically active are important factors in maintaining the sensory integration needed for effective and efficient postural control (Prioli et al., 2005) (Activity Box 8.10).

Effects of Coexisting Multisystem Activity

Many studies have been conducted to look at the effects of adding activities (dual and multitasking) to people trying to maintain increasingly difficult postures. As balance regulation requires increasing amounts of information-processing capacity (attention), greater demand is made of the available higher centre resources, in turn reducing the capacity for coexisting activity (e.g. memory and comprehension activities). We have already explored the possible challenges for even healthy elderly people in this regard (Lacour et al., 2008).

Effects of High or Low Levels of Exercise

Prolonged exercise (e.g. a 25-km run or an Ironman Triathlon) has been shown to reduce postural control when participants stop the exercise. This reduction relates to the sensory receptors (proprioceptors mainly) adjusting their levels of sensitivity in response to the exercise and consequently needing to recalibrate on exercise cessation; muscular fatigues is also undoubtedly a factor (Paillard, 2012). Cohen et al. (2012) reported a large decrease in performance of balance tests after a long duration space flight. The reduced stimulation from gravity experienced in space desensitises the proprioceptors and vestibular system; a long period of recalibration is therefore required, but the effects are reversible. It is interesting that when astronauts return to land they have a tendency to use the hip strategy far more frequently than ankle strategies, a bit like older people.

One of the effects of prolonged low activity levels may be an increase in body weight. The effect of obesity on postural control has stimulated much research activity, with results suggesting that obesity negatively affects postural responses, especially if perturbations come from mediolateral directions (Goulding et al., 2003). While not ignoring the influence of probable coexisting poor muscle endurance, this research suggests obese people have intact proprioceptive and sensory systems but have adapted different responses. Building on these studies D'Hondt et al. (2008) explored the fine motor control of obese children in standing and found their motor function was poorer than their nonobese peers. This observation suggests some underlying coordination difficulties and is currently challenging the earlier belief that postural control in obese people results from an altered muscle/body weight ratio (increasing body inertia so that more force generation is required for both the perturbation and the appropriate correction to occur).

Summary

In this section, we have thought about the systems required to make postural control efficient and effective and discussed some normal conditions under which predicted responses are challenged. Obviously, however, there are innumerable instances when internal and/or external events can unexpectedly prevent normal balance responses occurring (e.g. a limb amputation or lesions of the central nervous system).

RELEVANCE TO PRACTICE

The final section of this chapter is chiefly concerned with therapeutic practice. We will review the possible precursors to abnormal, symptomatic posture and balance and offer some examples of therapeutic interventions.

Symptomatic Postural Alignment
Identifying Causes for Symptomatic Postures

Earlier in the chapter, we described the ongoing interaction between the internal muscle and soft tissue forces and the external forces of gravity, friction and inertia to create stability during static and dynamic postures. The task for the therapist is to identify the symptom's primary source and discuss with the patient the likely cause(s). We have discussed the importance of taking the patient through a detailed postural assessment in, and between, each of the three main resting postures to note how the patient's current posture deviates from the stated ideal. Causes of postural deviation may include muscles that are too weak, an imbalance between muscles, soft tissues that are too short or too long and joint movements impeded by swelling or hampered by actual or anticipated pain.

Relieving the Symptoms and Preventing Recurrence

It is essential that people suffering with symptomatic postures be given the opportunity to rest in positions of ease, in which their postures are supported, reducing the effort needed for their maintenance. Intervention should target symptom control and prevention through detailed ergonomic review, appropriate muscle strengthening and joint flexibility exercises, as well retraining the patient toward a more ideal posture through education and feedback. Postural rehabilitation is a long-duration activity requiring high patient motivation and patient–therapist interaction and support. At all times, therapists must be aware of the individual needs of the patient and the context and environment in which that patient operates, helping to make therapeutic intervention relevant whenever possible.

Balance Reeducation
Identifying the Causes

If a patient with a recent amputation or spinal cord injury is referred for balance reeducation, then the reasons for balance problems may seem apparent, but therapists must also consider the influence of coexisting pathologies (e.g. visual impairment, altered vestibular processing and general system ageing). Whatever the cause of the balance problem, it is essential that the musculoskeletal system is prepared so that it is in the best condition possible to respond to demands made on it by the central nervous system. For example, sensory endings cannot provide adequate information when surrounded by oedema, nor can the muscle function as required if its connective tissue has shortened. So balance reeducation will involve strengthening muscles, stretching tissues and possibly reducing inflammation.

The central part of balance reeducation, as you might imagine, involves challenging the balance system within a safe learning environment. Balance assessments such as the Berg Balance Scale will help you decide where the main problems lie and therefore where to focus training. For example is it simply the maintenance of a static posture (seated or standing) or perhaps the balance problems are revealed when walking or executing a turning. The therapy challenge is then to develop a tailored rehabilitation program.

The following points reflect the range of questions that should be considered by the therapist when developing such a programme.

Some questions to ask:

- Is there a need to enhance existing sensory stimulation levels? A mirror might help (but might also confuse). Perhaps you could enhance visual attention by asking them to focus on something (e.g. a dot on the wall) and minimise distractions (e.g. by ensuring the department is not too noisy). Would vibration or tactile stimulation help align segments and improve left/right symmetry? Touch is often used by therapists to draw attention to an area for improvement, such as a forward protruding head.
- Should feedback be provided? This could be performance time (e.g. one-legged standing time) or it could be a visual display of their postural sway (e.g. using the Wii or similar). Should feedback be delayed until after the performance (see Chapter 15 for a more detailed discussion on feedback)?
- How good is the patient's segmental control? Should we reduce the difficulty of the starting position by lowering the CoM and increasing the BoS? For example, start the exercise in sitting, then prone kneeling, then standing positions.
- Are they ready to have their balance challenged by expected/unexpected perturbations? What kind or perturbation should be involved? Visual (e.g. a moving object), mechanical (e.g. a wobble board), audio (e.g. listening to music/someone talking), cognitive (e.g. having to do mental arithmetic). You might want to do a combination or try a few and see which one creates the greatest challenge. Of course the patient's preference is also important, and remember perturbations can be as simple as talking to the patient as they stand.
- Does the patient need to give all their attention to the balance task? As we have seen, patients can be encouraged to preparing themselves for a functional activity, using the feedforward control system (anticipation). Directly

thinking about postural control during simple functional activities can interfere with task execution but is essential during more advanced tasks (e.g. a multitasking situation).

This list of prompt questions is incomplete but is intended to help you consider the issues that may impact on the patient's functional activity efficiency and effectiveness.

Balance Training Technology

The use of technology should be encouraged in balance training because not only does it allow more self-practice and provide a greater range of perturbations, but it can also be more fun (and arguably more motivating). Of course, physiotherapists have long used wobble boards to extend balance training, and these can be multiaxial (ball) or single axis depending on the level of challenge required. There have also been balance feedback systems using simple force-sensing technology to display an individual's CoP location (see Fig. 8.10), which can be quickly turned into a game or used to gauge progress. There are now multisensory balance training systems such as the Dynstable (MotekMedical, the Netherlands) which creates mechanical and visual perturbations to help train balance. Fixed to a belt around your waist, your smartphone can also be used to provide balance feedback; you just have to download an app first!

CONCLUSION

This chapter has explored the origins and norms of the upright human posture and the demands that are placed on whole body systems to produce effective functional activities. We have described the 'ideal' postural alignment and discussed the real-life influences that make segmental alignment unique to the individual. We have acknowledged the complexity of postural control (balance), the multisystem integration needed and the frequency of balance problems in the patient and general populations. An understanding of posture and its control is essential for all involved in the rehabilitation of human movement.

SELF-ASSESSMENT QUESTIONS

1. What two functions of the foot has evolution bestowed in modern humans?
   a. A manipulative ability (e.g. to peel a banana)
   b. A rigidity for propulsion
   c. An ability to adapt to varying surfaces
   d. An enhanced capacity to float
2. Which direction is the thoracic spine curved?
   a. Convex
   b. Concave

3. Which of the following statements is incorrect?
   a. The line of gravity is an imaginary line representing the gravitational force vector.
   b. The line of gravity is useful to understand the relative alignment of the body segments.
   c. The line of gravity should pass through the centre of mass.
   d. The line of gravity always lies within the base of support (BoS).

4. In the sagittal plane the LoG 'ideally' passes through
   a. The mastoid process, the scapula, the hip joint (or just behind), the knee joint (or just in front) and the ankle joint (or just in front).
   b. The tragus of the ear, the shoulder (or just in front), the anterior superior iliac spine (or just behind), the knee joint (or just in front) and the ankle joint (or just in front).
   c. The mastoid process, the shoulder (or just in front), the hip joint (or just behind), the knee joint (or just in front) and just in front of the ankle joint.
   d. The mastoid process, the shoulder (or just in front), the hip joint (or just in front), the knee joint (or just in front) and the ankle joint (or just in front).

5. How does the pelvis move when you sit down (from standing) on a standard chair?
   a. Tilts posteriorly
   b. Tilts anteriorly
   c. Stays the same

6. Which standing posture demands the least energy?
   a. Swayback
   b. Kypholordosis
   c. Flat back
   d. Hyperlordosis

7. Which posture creates the most pressure between the lumbar intervertebral discs?
   a. Standing
   b. Lying
   c. Sitting
   d. Prone kneeling

8. Describe the ankle strategy.

9. How can you test someone's balance?

10. List three things associated with ageing that effect balance.

11. What is the difference between feedback and feedforward (anticipatory control)?

12. If you experienced a very large push from behind, which strategy would you probably use to maintain your stability?
    a. Ankle strategy
    b. Hip strategy
    c. Stepping strategy

13. Name the three main sensory inputs used to control balance.

14. Name two technologies which could be used to train balance.

REFERENCES

Basmajian, J.V., 1965. Man's posture. Arch. Phys. Med. Rehabil. 45, 26–36.

Bogduk, N., 2005. Clinical Anatomy of the Lumbar Spine and Sacrum. Elsevier Health Sciences, Sydney.

Bray, J.J., MacKnight, A.D.C., Mills, R.G., 1999. Lecture Notes on Human Physiology, fourth ed. Blackwell Science, Oxford.

Cech, D.J., Martin, S., 2002. Functional Movement Development Across the Life Span, second ed. WB Saunders, Philadelphia.

Cohen, H.S., Kimball, K.T., Mulavara, A.P., Bloomberg, J.J., Paloski, W.H., 2012. Posturography and locomotor tests of dynamic balance after long-duration spaceflight. J. Vestib. Res. 22 (4), 191–196.

Chastin, S.F., Palarea-Albaladejo, J., Dontje, M.L., Skelton, D.A., 2015. Combined effects of time spent in physical activity, sedentary behaviors and sleep on obesity and cardio-metabolic health markers: a novel compositional data analysis approach. PLoS ONE 10 (10), e0139984.

Chau, J.Y., van der Ploeg, H.P., Van Uffelen, J.G., Wong, J., Riphagen, I., Healy, G.N., et al., 2010. Are workplace interventions to reduce sitting effective? A systematic review. Prev. Med. 51 (5), 352–356.

Clancy, J., McVicar, A.J., 2002. Physiology and Anatomy: A Homeostatic Approach, second ed. Arnold, London.

Clark, R.A., Bryant, A.L., Pua, Y., McCrory, P., Bennell, K., Hunt, M., 2010. Validity and reliability of the nintendo wii balance board for assessment of standing balance. Gait Posture 31 (3), 307–310.

Cutler, W.B., Friedmann, E., Genovese-Stone, E., 1993. Prevalence of kyphosis in a healthy sample of pre- and postmenopausal women. Am. J. Phys. Med. Rehabil. 72, 219–225.

D'Hondt, E., Deforche, B., De Boudeaudhujj, I., Lenoir, M., 2008. Childhood obesity affects fine motor skill performance under different postural constraints. Neurosci. Lett. 440, 72–75.

Gillespie, R.M., 2002. The physical impact of computers and electronic game use on children and adolescents, a review of current literature. Work 18, 249–259.

Gillespie, R.M., Nordin, M., Halpern, M., Koenig, K., Warren, N., Kim, M., 2006. Musculoskeletal impact of computer and electronic game use on children and adolescents. Available from: http://www.iea.cc/ECEE/pdfs/art0235.pdf. Accessed February 3, 2018.

Goulding, A., Jones, I.E., Taylor, R.W., Piggot, J.M., Taylor, D., 2003. Dynamic and static tests of balance and postural sway in boys: effects of previous wrist bone fractures and high adiposity. Gait Posture 17, 136–141.

Grieco, A., 1986. Sitting posture: an old problem and a new one. Ergonomics 29 (3), 345–362.

Han, K.S., Rohlmann, A., Yang, S.J., Kim, B.S., Lim, T.H., 2011. Spinal muscles can create compressive follower loads in the lumbar spine in a neutral standing posture. Med. Eng. Phys. 33 (4), 472–478.

Hubble, R.P., Naughton, G.A., Silburn, P.A., Cole, M.H., 2015. Wearable sensor use for assessing standing balance and walking stability in people with Parkinson's disease: a systematic review. PLoS ONE 10 (4), e0123705.

Jacobs, J.V., Horak, F.B., 2007. Cortical control of postural responses. J. Neural Transm. 114, 1339–1348.

Jans, M.P., Proper, K.I., Hildebrandt, V.H., 2007. Sedentary behavior in Dutch workers: differences between occupations and business sectors. Am. J. Prev. Med. 33 (6), 450–454.

Juskeliene, V., Magnus, P., Bakketteig, L.S., Dailidiene, N., Jurkuvenas, V., 1996. Prevalence and risk factors for asymmetric posture in preschool children aged 6–7 years. Int. J. Epidemiol. 25, 1053–1059.

Kanekar, N., Aruin, A.S., 2015. Improvement of anticipatory postural adjustments for balance control: effect of a single training session. J. Electromyogr. Kinesiol. 25 (2), 400–405.

Katzman, W.B., Wanek, L., Shepherd, J.A., Sellmeyer, D.E., 2010. Age-related hyperkyphosis: its causes, consequences, and management. J. Orthop. Sports Phys. Ther. 40 (6), 352–360.

Kisner, C., Colby, L.A., 2007. Therapeutic Exercise: Foundations and Techniques, fifth ed. FA Davis, Philadelphia.

Lackner, J.R., DiZio, P.A., 2000. Aspects of body self-calibration. Trends Cogn. Sci. 4, 279–288.

Lacour, M., Bernard-Demanze, L., Dumitrescu, M., 2008. Posture control, aging, and attention resources: models and posture-analysis methods. Clin. Neurophysiol. 38 (6), 411–421.

Lee, W.A., 1988. A control systems framework for understanding normal and abnormal posture. Am. J. Occup. Ther. 43, 291–301.

Le Huec, J.C., Saddiki, R., Franke, J., Rigal, J., Aunoble, S., 2011. Equilibrium of the human body and the gravity line: the basics. Eur. Spine J. 20 (5), 558–563.

Lewin, R., 2009. Human evolution: an illustrated introduction. John Wiley & Sons, Oxford UK.

Malvankar, S., Khan, W.S., 2011. Evolution of the achilles tendon: the athlete's achilles heel? Foot (Edinb). 21 (4), 193–197.

Niemitz, C., 2010. The evolution of the upright posture and gait—a review and a new synthesis. Naturwissenschaften 97 (3), 241–263.

Nissinen, M., Heliovaara, M., Seitsamo, J., Poussa, M., 1989. Trunk asymmetry and scoliosis. Anthropometric measurements in prepubertal school children. Acta Paediatr. Scand. 78, 747–753.

Nissinen, M., Heliovaara, M., Seitsamo, J., Poussa, M., 1993. Trunk asymmetry, posture, growth and risk of scoliosis. A

three-year follow-up of finnish prepubertal school children. Spine 18, 8–13.

Nissinen, M., Heliovaara, M., Seitsamo, J., Poussa, M., 1995. Left handedness and risk of thoracic hyperkyphosis in prepubertal schoolchildren. Int. J. Epidemiol. 24, 1178–1181.

Nissinen, M., Heliovaara, M., Seitsamo, J., Kononen, M.H., Hurmerinta, K.A., Poussa, M., 2000. Development of trunk asymmetry in a cohort of children ages 11 to 22 years. Spine 25, 570–574.

Oxland, T.R., 2016. Fundamental biomechanics of the spine— what we have learned in the past 25 years and future directions. J. Biomech. 49 (6), 817–832.

Paillard, T., 2012. Effects of general and local fatigue on postural control: a review. Neurosci. Biobehav. Rev. 36 (1), 162–176.

Palastanga, N., Field, D., Soames, R., 2006. Anatomy and Human Movement: Structure and Function, sixth ed. Butterworth-Heinemann, Edinburgh.

Pearsall, D.J., Reid, J.G., 1992. Line of gravity relative to upright vertebral posture. Clin. Biomech. (Bristol, Avon) 7, 80–86.

Pollock, A.S., Durward, B.R., Rowe, P.J., Paul, J.P., 2000. What is balance? Clin. Rehab. 14 (4), 402–406.

Poulain, I., Giraudet, G., 2008. Age-related changes of visual contribution in posture control. Gait Posture 27, 1–7.

Poussa, M.S., Heliovaara, M.M., Seitsamo, J.T., Kononen, M.H., Hurmerinta, K.A., Nissinen, M.J., 2005. Development of spinal posture in a cohort of children from the age of 11 to 22 years. Eur. Spine J. 14, 738–742.

Prioli, A.C., Freitas, P.B., Barela, J.A., 2005. Physical activity and postural control in the elderly: coupling between visual information and body sway. Gerontology 51, 145–148.

Rolian, C., Lieberman, D.E., Hallgrímsson, B., 2010. The coevolution of human hands and feet. Evolution 64 (6), 1558–1568.

Sato, K., Kikuchi, S., Yonezawa, T., 1999. In vivo intradiscal pressure measurement in healthy individuals and in patients with ongoing back problems. Spine 24 (23), 2468–2474.

Shumway-Cook, A., Woollacott, M., 2016. Motor Control: Translating Research Into Clinical Practice, fifth ed. Lippincott Williams & Wilkins, Philadelphia.

Sibley, K.M., Straus, S.E., Inness, E.L., Salbach, N.M., Jaglal, S.B., 2011. Balance assessment practices and use of standardized balance measures among Ontario physical therapists. Phys. Ther. 91 (11), 1583–1591.

Stuart, S., Galna, B., Delicato, L.S., Lord, S., Rochester, L., 2017. Direct and indirect effects of attention and visual function on gait impairment in Parkinson's disease: influence of task and turning. Eur. J. Neurosci. 46 (1), 1703–1716.

Williams, L.R.T., Caswell, P., Wagner, I., Walmsley, A., Handcock, P, 1994. Regulation of standing posture. N. z. J. Phys. 22, 15–18.

Motor Control

Kristen Hollands

OUTLINE

LEARNING OBJECTIVES

After reading this chapter, you will be able to:
1. Define motor control.
2. Outline the roles of the various components of the motor control system in the control of movement.
3. Understand how models of motor control can be used to explain how we move, in particular:
   a. The degrees of freedom problem and motor abundancy.
   b. The closed and open loop control systems and the role of sensory feedback in the control of movement.
4. Understand what a central pattern generator is and how it may account for the features of specific movements such as gait.
5. Apply knowledge and understanding of motor control to the clinical treatment of movement disorders.

INTRODUCTION

The purpose of this chapter is to help you understand the human nervous system and how it participates in the control of movement, that is, motor control. Motor control refers to the process by which the nervous system coordinates muscles and limbs (motors) to achieve a desired movement. This process includes using sensory information to anticipate and refine the movement according to demands of the environment and the desired outcome of the movement. How the nervous system produces coordinated and complex motor behaviour is of interest to both clinicians and researchers. The purpose of this chapter is to provide an overview of the various neural networks involved in the control of movement, and to outline some of the theories that explain how movements are planned, generated and controlled. We will then apply this understanding to specific movements (e.g. walking and reaching) and consider how motor control can help the clinical treatment of movement disorders. Because the field of motor control relies on many disciplines—including biomechanics, neurophysiology, cognitive psychology—you should refer to specific texts to obtain detailed information about these topics (e.g. Kandel et al., 2000; Schmidt and Lee, 2011; Latash, 2008; Shumway-Cook and Wollacott, 2007; Montgomery and Connolly, 2003).

OVERVIEW OF THE MOTOR CONTROL SYSTEM

Consider for a moment how it is that you are able to reach for the paper coffee cup, open your hand the correct amount, apply the right amount of force to grasp the cup without dropping it (but not so much that you crush it) and bring it to your mouth without spilling (Fig. 9.1). How is it that we can walk quickly, if we are in a rush, or take a slow stroll, when relaxed, navigate slippery and/or bumpy surfaces and often achieve this while talking, texting and/ or looking in shop windows—usually (Activity Box 9.1)— without accident? What does it take for the brain, nerves and muscles to plan and control these seemingly simple tasks?

Movement requires activation of the musculoskeletal system (the muscle motors attached to bony levers) in a manner that is appropriate for:

1. Volition and the intended goal of the movement; this includes task constraints such as getting across the road in the time afforded by traffic lights.
2. The ability or constraints of the body itself; this includes posture, emotional/arousal state like fight or flight and/ or any impairments due to disease/injury.

ACTIVITY BOX 9.1 Walking and Texting

Driving while texting has been banned in many countries as it raises the risk of accidents. But what about walking while texting?

Have a read of the following excerpt from a website (https://consumer.healthday.com) reporting on a recent piece of research. Once you have read it think about your own behaviour.

'Texting, and to a lesser extent reading, on your mobile phone affects your ability to walk and balance. This may impact the safety of people who text and walk at the same time,' Siobhan Schabrun, of the University of Queensland in Australia, said in a journal (PLoS One) news release.

She and her colleagues looked at the effects of texting while walking in 26 healthy people. Each person was asked to walk a straight line three times: once without a cellphone; once while reading a text on a cellphone; and once while texting on a cellphone.

Texting, and to a lesser degree reading, changed the body's movement while walking. When writing a text, the participants walked slower, swerved more and moved their necks less than when they walked without texting or while reading.

There was also an effect on head movement while texting or reading a text message that could make balance more difficult, the researchers noted.

In addition, texting or reading on a cellphone may create a safety risk for pedestrians while crossing the road or trying to avoid obstacles, the study authors noted.

Do you look at your phone when you walk?
Would you go down stairs when texting?
Does it slow you down?
How do you avoid bumping into other people who are also walking and texting?

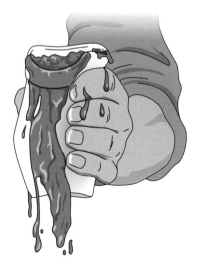

Fig. 9.1 Consider what it takes for the brain, nerves and muscles to control and carry out seemingly simple movements. How do you know with how much force to hold a cup? How do you walk without fully looking where you are going?

3. Environmental conditions through which we will move (i.e. environmental constraints like weight/gravity, slippery surfaces etc.) (Shumway-Cook and Wollacott, 2007).

The instructions or commands for movement are planned in the cortical areas of the brain. Volitional movement is executed by sending signals about the movement plan from the cortex, via the corticospinal pathways, to the brainstem, spinal cord and descending all the way through to motor units in the muscles. The resulting movement is then monitored and adjusted by sensory receptors (all of these elements comprise the motor control system).

Sensory information based on visual, vestibular and somatosensory inputs are combined (in the temporoparietal cortex) to create a body schema that represents the physical state of the body (posture) in relation to the immediate environment (feedback) and the environment through which we are about to move (feedforward). The body schema is then combined with motor commands for the precise movement task (from the premotor and supplementary motor areas) and emotion/arousal state (from the limbic system) to shape and intentionally elicit motor control commands (in the primary motor area, known as M1). Any movement will change body posture relative to the environment and will consequently disrupt balance. For example, consider the abdominal contractions that happen quickly, automatically and BEFORE catching or throwing a medicine ball.

So, posture is adjusted in anticipation of the intended movement to maintain balance. These adjustments are carried along the reticulospinal tract (connecting the brainstem to motor units in the trunk). Motor commands for precise limb control are carried from M1 to the spinal cord and, ultimately, the muscles along the corticospinal tract (Takakusaki, 2013, 2017). The process of making volitional (voluntary) movement, therefore, requires the processing of cognitive information to combine body, task and environmental constraints into a movement plan, and to prepare a stable posture for movement.

We may have awareness of some of these processes (e.g. we may plan with some awareness how much grip force we will use to pick up the coffee cup based on predictions about its weight, or to trip over curbs if our attention is diverted The (Malone and Bastian, 2010) but we are usually unaware of the rest of the automatic movement generation process which typically happens subcortically. Automatic movement processes involve activation of motor neurons (inter-neurons) in the spinal cord that excite or inhibit neuromuscular junctions/motor end plates (the connection points between nerves and muscles), which subsequently achieve activation or relaxation of muscles, as appropriate, for the intended movement. The resulting movement is monitored through muscle, joint and cutaneous sensory receptors describing the status of muscles and movement, that is, length, instantaneous tension, and rate of change of length and tension (Shumway-Cook and Wollacott, 2007). Signals from these sensory receptors transmit information to all levels of the motor control system (spinal cord, cerebellum and cerebral cortex), where they assist in the control of muscle contraction to correct or further shape the movement via an afferent loop of ascending pathways.

Therefore movement control involves various cortical areas blending volition, emotion, feedforward and feedback sensory information to generate a motor plan with descending control over the basal ganglia (movement initiation centre), hypothalamus (emotion), cerebellum (error monitoring), brainstem (postural control) and the spinal cord (activation of muscles) through the corticoreticulospinal pathway (Takakusaki, 2017). This overview of elements of the motor control system and processes may give way to one of the traditional views of motor control, that is, it is purely hierarchical, with a top down (higher brain centres commanding the spinal cord and, in turn, muscles) approach. However, it is important to understand that integration occurs at all levels of control, from the spinal cord up to the cerebral cortex. This integration is necessary to provide the base of postural stability supporting more precise limb movements and for movements to be shaped by sensory feedback (Shumway-Cook and Wollacott, 2007; Kenyon and Blackinton, 2011; Takakusaki, 2017). Indeed, it is the flexible integration of all elements of the motor control system and the fact that movement can be shaped by intention (top-down control) or can be triggered by the environment (bottom-up control; e.g. pain withdrawal reflex) and any combination thereof, which support the huge repertoire of human movement. See Fig. 9.2 for a diagrammatic overview of this integration between sensory, motor and control systems (Activity Box 9.2).

Communication Across Neurons and Transmission of Motor Impulse

From the overview of processes of motor control and the elements of the motor control system described above, it is clear that the transmission of signals with the motor plan, the result of the movement and any corrections needed, is essential to control movement. Communication between the vast numbers of neurons in the human nervous system needs to occur, usually very rapidly. Information within neurons and between neurons is carried by electrical and chemical signals. The rapid transmission of signals, which is vital for human movement, is a function of the action potential. This action potential is achieved by temporary changes of current flow in and out of cells, which then propagate a signal along the nerve axon. A necessary precondition for action potentials is the creation of a membrane potential: the

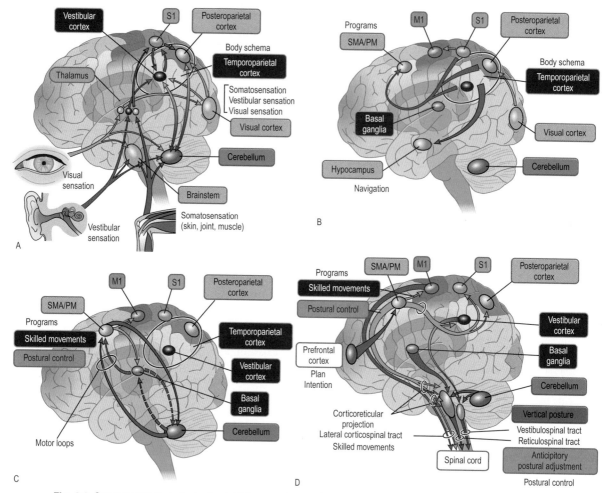

Fig. 9.2 Sensory signals indicate the initial postural state from which movement must be generated (body constraints) and the conditions of the environment ahead, through which we will move (environmental constraints). Somatosensory, vestibular and visual sensations are integrated at the temporoparietal-posterior parietal cortices, where the body schema is generated and updated. Postural adjustments are made in anticipation of the intended movement (task constraints) to protect balance from being disrupted by changes to body orientation relative to the environment. 'Emotional reference' or arousal state (e.g. being in a hurry), from the limbic system, is combined with sensory input to shape volitional and task-specific motor commands. Motor programs of precise movement and postural control are generated in the premotor area *(PM)* and the supplementary motor area *(SMA)*. The volitional process, therefore, requires cognitive information processing to combine body, task and environmental constraints into a cognitive reference for a movement plan. Motor commands for precise limb control are carried by the corticospinal tract arising from the primary motor cortex *(M1)*. The basal ganglia and the cerebellum control volitional and automatic processes by thalamocortical projections and by direct projections to the brainstem, respectively. The brainstem (mid-brain, pons, and medulla) and spinal cord are involved in the automatic processes of activating muscles to generate movement and of monitoring resulting movement through ascending afferent feedback loops. See text for further explanation. (Adapted from Takakusaki, K., 2013. Neurophysiology of gait: from the spinal cord to the frontal lobe. Mov. Disord. 28 (11), 1483–1491, Figs. 1 and 4.)

ACTIVITY BOX 9.2 Automatic and Conscious Movements

This is an observational task. Watch someone perform one (or all) of the following activities:

a. Play a musical instrument
b. Drive a car
c. Play a video game
d. Make a cup of tea

Make a list of their movements, head turning, reaching forward, hand opening/closing etc. Be as detailed as you can, then categorise the movements as either automatic or conscious. For example, if it looks like the movement requires all their attention (e.g. they stop talking or their eyes are focussed on the task) you could say it was conscious, or if the person was able to do other tasks (e.g. talk) at the same time you might say it was automatic. Of course, you don't know for sure, it's just to get you thinking.

SUMMARY BOX 9.1 Important Facts About the Action Potential

- The resting potential creates the excitability of the cell.
- The resting potential is the unequal distribution of ions across the cell membrane, causing a negative charge of −70 mV in the intracellular fluid.
- The action potential emerges if a stimulus is large enough to take the membrane potential above the threshold (−55 mV).
- When the threshold level is reached, voltage-gated Na^+ channels open and Na^+ rushes into the cell, producing the depolarisation period.
- Voltage-gated K^+ channels open to allow K^+ to flow out of the cell and produce the repolarisation period.
- Another action potential cannot be generated during the depolarisation period and during most of the repolarisation period.
- The action potential propagates along the axon, segment by segment, until it reaches the synaptic end bulb at the end of the axon.
- Propagation is more rapid in myelinated axons, where the signal leaps from node to node. Large-diameter axons also propagate signals faster than small-diameter axons.
- Axons of sensory neurons transmitting information about touch, pressure and movement, as well as the axons of motor neurons transmitting movement instructions to the skeletal muscles, are all large and myelinated.

resting potential (Tortora and Derrickson, 2008). Note that no movement is possible if the action potential is completely interrupted, and that movement will be impaired if the signal propagation is abnormal. This may be the case if the myelin sheath that surrounds nerve axons is damaged, such as in multiple sclerosis. Fig. 9.3 shows the concentrations of ions inside and outside the nerve cell during the resting potential. Fig. 9.4 shows the changes in membrane potential during the action potential. The important facts about the action potential are detailed in Summary Box 9.1.

Information transmission from one cell to another occurs at the synapse. The most important components of a synapse are the presynaptic membrane, the synaptic cleft and the postsynaptic membrane (Latash, 2008). An action potential arrives at the presynaptic membrane. This leads to an influx of calcium ions (Ca^{2+}), which, in turn, facilitates the fusion of neurotransmitter vesicles to the membrane for the release of the neurotransmitter into the synaptic cleft. Neurotransmitter molecules diffuse across the synaptic cleft and bind at specialist receptor sites in the postsynaptic neuron. This changes the potential in the postsynaptic neuron as ion channels are opened and the voltage across the cell membrane changes. Depending on the particular type of channel that is being activated, either depolarisation or hyperpolarisation may occur. This explains how an action potential in the presynaptic neuron can cause either excitation or inhibition of the postsynaptic membrane. The opening of sodium ion (Na^+) channels would lead to depolarisation and therefore excitation, whereas the opening of the chloride ion (Cl^-) channels would hyperpolarise the postsynaptic neuron

and lead to inhibition. Fig. 9.5 summarises the events that occur at a synapse.

The Role of Sensation and Afferent Receptors in Motor Control

Receptors

In order to make refinements to the movement, the central nervous system (CNS) needs feedback about the movement to make sure the task is both successful and efficient. It receives this information in the form of the status of muscles, that is, length, instantaneous tension, and rate of change of length and tension (Shumway-Cook and Wollacott, 2007). Muscle spindles detect change in muscle length and the rate of this change, whereas the Golgi tendon organs detect the degree and rate of change of tension. Cutaneous mechanoreceptors detect mechanical distortion of the skin (e.g. stretch and pressure) and therefore provide information about posture in relation to the environment in contact

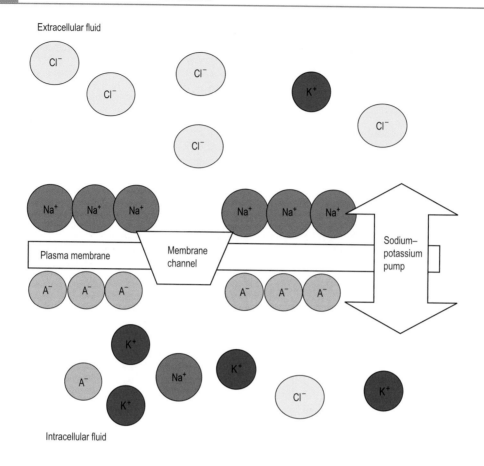

Extracellular fluid

Intracellular fluid

Fig. 9.3 Distribution of ions across the cell membrane during the resting potential.

Ion	Concentration Intracellular Fluid	Concentration in Extracellular Fluid
K$^+$—Potassium	150 mmol/L	5 mmol/L
Na$^+$—Sodium	12 mmol/L	150 mmol/L
Cl$^-$—Chlorine	5 mmol/L	125 mmol/L
A$^-$—Organic anions	150 mmol/L	–

with the body, that is, how the body is leaning over the foot or the nature of the floor beneath the foot. Signals from these sensory receptors transmit information to all levels of the motor control system from the spinal cord and cerebellum to the cerebral cortex. Sensory feedback regarding the ongoing movement assists in the control of muscle contraction allowing correction and further shaping of the movement according to body, task and environmental constraints.

The Muscle Spindle

The muscle spindle has both a static and a dynamic response. The primary and secondary endings respond to the length of the receptor, so impulses transmitted are proportional to the degree of stretch and continue to be transmitted provided the receptor remains stretched. If the spindle receptors shorten, the firing rate decreases. Only the primary endings respond to sudden changes of length by increasing their firing rate, and then only while the length is actually

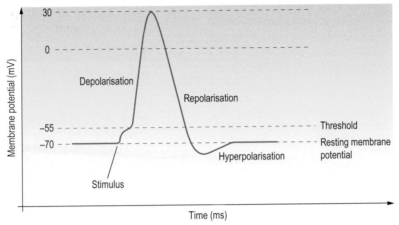

Fig. 9.4 The Action Potential.

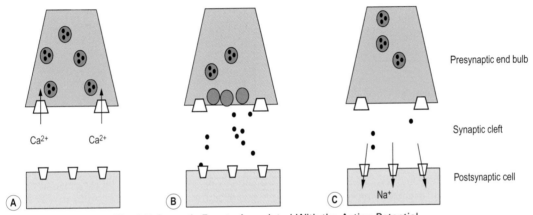

Fig. 9.5 Synaptic Events Associated With the Action Potential.

increasing. Once the length stops increasing, the discharge returns to its original level, although the static response may still be active. If the spindle receptors shorten, then the firing rate decreases.

Control of the static and dynamic response is by the gamma motor neuron. Normally, the muscle spindle emits sensory nerve impulses continuously, with the rate increasing as the spindle is stretched (lengthened) or decreasing as the spindle shortens.

The spinal reflexes associated with the muscle spindle and Golgi tendon organ are the stretch reflex and the tendon reflex, respectively. Stimulation of the stretch reflex leads to a reflex *contraction* of the muscle that has been stretched, whereas the tendon reflex will lead to a reflex *relaxation* of the muscle if there is tension build-up. Both reflexes have a protective function.

The stretch reflex also has the ability to prevent some types of oscillation and jerkiness of body movements, even if the input is jerky, that is, it can help smooth out movement (Hall, 2005) (Activity Box 9.3).

When the motor cortex or other areas of the brain transmit signals to the alpha motor neurons, the gamma motor neurons are nearly always stimulated simultaneously; that is, there is a coactivation of the alpha and gamma systems so that intra- and extrafusal muscle fibres (usually) contract at the same time. This stops the muscle spindle opposing the muscle contraction and maintains a proper damping and load responsiveness of the spindle regardless of the change in muscle length. If the alpha and gamma systems are stimulated simultaneously and the intra- and extrafusal fibres contract equally, then the degree of stimulation of the muscle spindle will not change. If the extrafusal fibres contract less because they are working against a great load, the mismatch will cause a stretch on the spindle, and the resultant stretch reflex will provide extra excitation of the extrafusal fibres to overcome the load (Cohen, 1998).

ACTIVITY BOX 9.3   Stretch Reflex

The stretch reflex (myotatic reflex) occurs when a muscle contracts reflexively (without volitional control) when it is stretched. When the muscle spindle is stretched it sends a sensory signal back to the dorsal horn of the spinal cord; here it makes a single connection (mono-synaptic) to the motor nerve (alpha motor neuron) in the anterior horn, which then causes the muscle to contract. The single connection means it is very fast. This reflex is often tested in a neurological examination to check that all the components are intact or indeed if they have become sensitive (an exaggerated response). Why not try it. With your partner in a sitting position and one leg crossed over the other try to hit (with something that won't injure your partner; you may have access to a tendon hammer for example) the patella tendon.

Did you manage to elicit a contraction in the quadriceps?

Was it the same on both sides?

Was it different when you changed over and you were the guinea pig?

SUMMARY BOX 9.2   Important Facts Associated With Receptors and Reflexes

- Sensory feedback for movement control is mainly provided by receptors inside the muscle and between the muscle and the tendon.
- These receptors are the muscle spindle and the Golgi tendon organ.
- The muscle spindle provides information about muscle length changes.
- The Golgi tendon organ provides information about tension changes.
- Both of these receptors are involved in spinal reflexes.
- The stretch reflex is triggered when a muscle is lengthened (detected by the muscle spindle). It is designed to prevent overstretching of a muscle by causing a reflex contraction of the lengthened muscle.
- The tendon reflex relies on Golgi tendon information and is triggered when tension builds up in the muscle and tendon. It is designed to prevent tearing of a muscle by causing a reflexive relaxation of the muscle.
- Stretch reflex and tension reflex therefore have opposite effects on a muscle.

The gamma efferent system is excited or controlled by areas in the brainstem, with impulses transmitted to that region from the cerebellum, basal ganglia, and cerebral cortex.

Golgi Tendon Organ

The Golgi tendon organ, as a sensory receptor in the muscle tendon, detects relative muscle tension. Therefore it is able to provide the CNS with instantaneous information on the degree of tension of each small segment of each muscle. The Golgi tendon organ is stimulated by increased tension. When the increase in tension is too great, the tendon reflex response is evoked in the same muscle, and this response is entirely inhibitory. The brain dictates a set point of tension beyond which the automatic inhibition of muscle contraction prevents additional tension. Alternatively, if the tension decrease is too low, then the Golgi tendon organ reacts to return the tension to a more normal level. This leads to a loss of inhibition, so allowing the alpha motor neuron to be more active and to increase the muscle tension (Summary Box 9.2).

THEORIES OF MOTOR CONTROL

How Do We Control Movement?

Consider how many different movements you are able to make just in the course of activities of daily living (e.g. reaching for the coffee cup, running for the bus, climbing stairs) and how many of these you actually concentrate on to achieve/control the activity. The ease with which we perform the plethora of skilled movement belies the overwhelming complexity of planning, executing and adapting/correcting movements for different environments, tasks and body conditions. Therefore it can be very easy to overlook how important motor control is in our everyday lives, until it fails. Now that we have an overview of the sensory and neural networks involved in signalling movement plans, this section will cover: what is motor control, why is it important and why does it seem so easy when it is so complicated?!

Considering only the constraints of the body (ignoring, for a moment, the actual task or environmental constraints) reveals how complex a problem the motor control system is faced with when planning and carrying out a movement. For example, imagine, for the sake of simplicity, that movement was achieved purely by using combinations of the >700 muscles in the human body in only 'on' (i.e. contracting) or 'off' (i.e. relaxed) states. This would result in more possible muscle activation patterns than the number of atoms in the universe (Wolpert and Ghahramani, 2000). It is clearly impossible for the motor control system to compute all possible combinations of muscle activation and to select the most metabolically and/or mechanically efficient movement pattern for every given situation. Each possible muscle activation (muscle is on or off) combination is known as one 'degree of freedom' or one way in which the motor system can be arranged to achieve a given movement. The

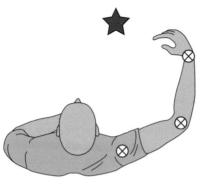

Fig. 9.6 Degrees of Freedom During a Simple Reach to a Target.

ACTIVITY BOX 9.4   Degrees of Freedom

Thought activity: how many ways can you reach for your coffee cup and get it to your mouth? How many different orientations of your shoulder, elbow, wrist and hand apertures can achieve the same functional goal of getting the cup to your mouth? How many different paths can the cup take to get to your mouth? Which of these possible movements is fastest? Which is smoothest? Which protects the content of the cup the most? How do you think you are selecting your preferred movement pattern—is it based on speed, efficiency, safety or does it vary according to whether the contents are hot or how heavy the cup is?

issue of how the motor control system solves the problem of controlling a movement, in the face of the enormous number of potential solutions, is known as the 'degrees of freedom problem' (Bernstein, 1967).

The degrees of freedom problem is amplified if we consider that each individual muscle can be activated to greater or lesser extents (i.e. not just on/off but a sliding scale of muscle tension) and factor in controlling the 100 joints (each, again, with more than two possible states of flexion/extension but also including ad/abduction, pronation/supination). Further, the fact that we have duplication of function between muscles crossing joints adds yet another layer of complexity in controlling movement. Of course, we didn't evolve this motor complexity just to give our brain a daily challenge; the variability (or degrees of freedom) it provides allows what we call motor abundancy—that is, the multiple ways (different combinations of muscle activation and joint configuration) we can achieve the same motor task. Motor abundancy is what allows us to have such a rich and wide repertoire of movement abilities and allows us to adapt movements as the environment changes and if our bodies change, for example, if we had a restriction in knee movement we would quickly adapt a new walking pattern with the same (or similar) result. In Fig. 9.6 there is an example of a simple task, reaching to touch a target (star); the movement all occurs in one plane (transverse plane from above), so the joint movements available are horizontal flexion/extension at the shoulder, flexion/extension of elbow and wrist (the hand is a fingerless blob) abduction/adduction. Think about all the combinations of these three simple joints that could all result in the same task, reaching the target, then add the muscles (range, velocity, motor unit type, slow, fast etc.) and you get an idea of the complexity. Now that you have thought of this simple activity, try a real one in Activity Box 9.4. There must be a simpler solution to controlling movement than planning the activation patterns of

millions of motor units across hundreds of muscles and joints—so what is it?

Support for the idea that simpler movement control solutions must be used is found in the fact that, given all the available motor abundancy, stereotypical features are observable not just within repetitions of a movement but between individuals on the same task (Wolpert and Ghahramani, 2000). All motor control theories attempt to explain how we control coordination (of muscles and joints) and reduce the degrees of freedom problem. Motor control is the study of how sensory information is integrated with intention, in order to plan and execute coordinated muscle forces that generate a desired movement. The field therefore encompasses disciplines of biomechanics, muscle physiology, neurophysiology and cognitive psychology. Motor control theories predict that the brain uses motor programmes or simplified representations of general types of movement (class of actions, e.g. locomotion or reaching), stored in our memory, and containing all the commands required to carry out the intended movement (Schmidt, 2011). In this way one does not need a motor programme for each skill or even to be able to control every possible variable of the movement. Instead, the brain stores a library of movement programmes and these can be modified to yield variations of movement (consider, e.g. the number of styles, some sensible and some silly, in which you can walk!). So, what are the key elements specified in a motor command?

Basic Movements—Open and Closed Loop Control

Everyday movements are usually considered at the task level (such as taking a drink of water from a glass). However, the motor system must, at some stage, make more detailed instructions to muscles to achieve the task. Based on previous experiences, the task in hand and any body or environmental constraints, a movement plan is shaped (Stroeve, 1999) and signals representing that plan are sent from the cortex via the corticospinal pathway to the muscles in a feedforward or open loop manner (i.e. it has only gone in one direction, brain to muscle). Feedforward implies a set of muscle commands that are structured before a movement sequence begins, and that allows the entire movement to be carried out uninfluenced by information about the outcome of the movement or feedback (Latash, 2008). Some, usually fast or ballistic, movements can be achieved in entirety in a feedforward manner (e.g. the throw of a dart). There has been considerable debate about what is coded within individual neurons and populations of neurons involved in storing, shaping and conveying any given motor programme. Given the stereotypical nature of kinematics for specific movement classes (e.g. reach to grasp; van Vliet et al., 2013) proposals are that motor programmes activate muscle groups and specify the movement direction, velocity, acceleration, posture and joint torques (Wolpert and Ghahramani, 2000).

Once the movement has started, sensory receptors will be able to provide feedback about the movement. The motor control networks may then be able to alter the signal about the remaining movement plan (if there is enough time for the sensory input to influence the muscle activation) according to this feedback (this is also known as closed loop control). Feedback corrections or refinement to the movement are achieved via a comparator centre monitoring the outcome of the movement against the original signals for the intended movement (efference copy). Over a period of time, this feedback will, in turn, influence the feedforward signal designed by the control centre and motor learning will have taken place (Schmidt, 2011) (e.g. if you miss the dart board you will change the next throw) (Fig. 9.7).

Using sensory feedback to shape either the feedforward plan, or to refine an ongoing movement via feedback, presents a basic difficulty for the nervous system in forming accurate perceptions about the outside world and the state of the body with respect to the environment. There are two reasons for this difficulty:

1. Transmission of sensory signals from the periphery of the body to the sensorimotor areas of the cortex is relatively slow (taking up to 0.1 seconds). This means the feedback may no longer reflect the state of the movement by the time it is processed and then acted on. While 0.1 seconds may seem a short time, think about how, for example, the body will change during this timeframe when running.

2. Sensory signals may be noisy (providing information not just about the body but also about other nonrelevant details of a busy environment) or only provide partial information (e.g. if you can't see in the dark, then you have to rely only on proprioception to know the posture of the body) (Pruszynski et al., 2011; Wolpert and Ghahramani, 2000).

To overcome these difficulties the motor control system estimates the outcome of an action even before sensory feedback becomes available (this is especially possible for skilled movements in which experience allows accurate prediction) and (when sensation is available and movement time allows) compares the actual feedback to the predicted state to formulate any necessary refinements to the movement. To further facilitate fast and accurate movement planning and refinement, multiple motor responses may be 'made ready' concurrently in anticipation, with inappropriate responses ultimately inhibited, and selected responses activated (Duque et al., 2010). This is how, for example, tennis players can return a service where the ball can travel at 70 m/s, giving you around ~0.3 seconds to process the visual data, make a plan and put it into action (Activity Box 9.5; Summary Box 9.3).

Complex Movements and Central Pattern Generators (A Special Kind of Motor Programme)

Walking requires not just the coordination of a large number of muscles and joints but also the control of posture and the adaptation of stepping patterns in response to the environment. Despite this complexity, we are able to walk while talking and/or looking at other aspects of the environment, indicating control of walking, normally, requires little thought. How are such complex movements achieved so effortlessly? A central, guiding principle in motor control is the idea that movement control is simplified by combining a small number of basic motor programs (neural networks), in different proportions rather than individually controlling each possible movement and/or muscle involved in the movement (Wolpert and Ghahramani, 2000). Walking is

---

ACTIVITY BOX 9.5   Removing Some Sensory Feedback

Try reaching for a cup (empty) in different conditions: with and without vision. Can you manage to get your hand to the cup without continuous vision of where the cup or your hand is? How did your movement change when reaching without sight—was it slower, did you make a few swipes or corrections? Now ask a friend to fill the cup by an unknown amount and reach for it without knowing what weight it may have (you can keep your eyes open this time). How did your planning and movement change? Were you more hesitant or slower? Did you pick up the cup with more/less force than when you knew what weight to expect it to be?

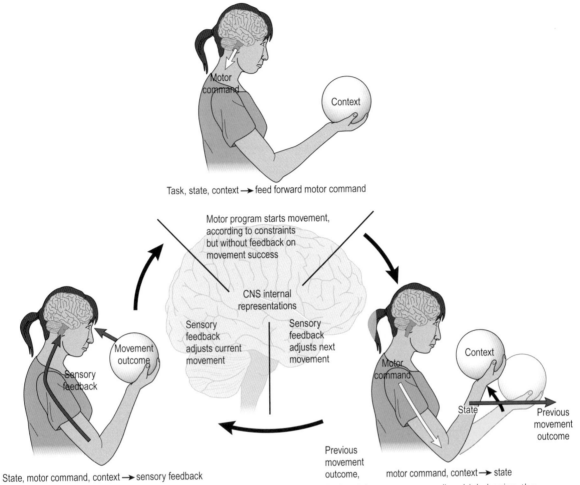

Task, state, context → feed forward motor command

Motor program starts movement, according to constraints but without feedback on movement success

CNS internal representations

Sensory feedback adjusts current movement

Sensory feedback adjusts next movement

Movement outcome

Sensory feedback

Context

Motor command

State

Previous movement outcome

State, motor command, context → sensory feedback

Previous movement outcome, motor command, context → state

Fig. 9.7 At the start of a movement there is a feedforward signal (motor command), which begins the movement in the absence of sensory feedback about how well the movement is achieved (against task, environmental and body constraints). As sensory feedback regarding the movement begins to become available, it may be used to adjust the movement. Finally, once the movement has finished, knowledge of results can influence the shape of the original feedforward motor commands or central nervous system *(CNS)* internal representations of the movement to alter the next time the movement is made. (Adapted from Wolpert, D. M. & Ghahramani, Z. 2000. Computational principles of movement neuroscience. Nat Neurosci, 3 Suppl, 1212-7.)

one such example of a movement controlled by flexibly combining neural networks that contribute each feature of fully functional walking (Activity Box 9.6).

Arguably, the most prominent feature of walking is the alternating rhythm of stance and swing, which is ubiquitously observed in healthy grown adults (with fully developed and functioning neuromusculoskeletal systems), people with sensory deficits (e.g. blind, peripheral neuropathy) and individuals with cortical and spinal cord lesions (and even headless chickens!). The fact that reciprocal flexion and extension can be achieved when cortical and sensory networks are impaired indicates that motor control networks

for stepping must exist subcortically/spinally and must be functional even in the absence of sensory input (i.e. are open loop networks). The particular group of spinal networks that generate rhythmic activity in the absence of inputs from sensory afferents is termed a central pattern generator (CPG) (Grillner et al., 1995; Grillner and Wallen, 1985). Flexor and extensor half-centres, or spinal interneurons, which excite flexor and extensor muscles are combined through mutual inhibition (see Fig. 9.8) (Yuste et al., 2005). In this way a CPG forms a particular kind of motor programme specifying the rhythmic activity of lower limb flexors and extensors, which forms the basis for all forms of locomotion.

But what would gait look like if it was controlled by a CPG that just activates flexion and extension in an alternating fashion without any sensation? How would you prolong a stance phase (or extensor cycle) if you needed to step beyond an obstacle suddenly seen or contacted? Spinal networks do not provide a basis for all the features of gait that we observe in healthy adults, such as the ability to alter the walking rhythm in response to the environment. Nor do these networks, on their own, enable anticipatory regulation of postural control. So, these spinal rhythm generating networks must be combined with other networks to modulate the rhythm through integration with postural control and sensory feedback networks, yielding the full complexity and functionality of walking patterns.

The ability to adapt walking in response to the environment and to anticipate postural control required to provide a stable basis for ongoing locomotor patterns in a range of contexts relies, fundamentally, on sensory feedback. Indeed, physiological studies in both animals and humans support the idea that, although the rhythmic activity of spinal locomotor CPG networks can be triggered and sustained without

---

SUMMARY BOX 9.3 Key Factors Relating to the Nervous System and Movement

- The nervous system initiates and controls all types of movement.
- Movements differ in complexity and characteristics. They can range from a relatively simple contraction of a muscle over one joint to multi-joint and whole-body movements such as those used during walking.
- Voluntary movements are designed from previous experiences and exist as neural networks whose output is delivered to the muscles as a feedforward signal.
- In addition to the feedforward signals, there will also be feedback about movement and the body in relation to the environment, which the brain compares with its expected outcomes and makes any required changes.
- All voluntary movements, including posture, balance and gait, are based on these feedforward and feedback principles.
- The feedback generated through movement experience also provides for the possibility of motor learning (see Chapter 15).

ACTIVITY BOX 9.6 Explaining Gait

Thought activity: Think about how you would describe walking to someone/something who had never seen or heard of this movement before. What are the stereotypical or characteristic features of human bipedal walking? Start with an alternating rhythm of stance and swing (flexion/extension). Now what other ingredients would you add to this—do you need sensation—can you walk without vision/vestibular/somatosensation or brain areas that register and interpret these inputs? (See http://www.miketheheadlesschicken.org/history.) Whatever networks and motor programmes exist to control walking must explain each of the observable, stereotypical features of gait.

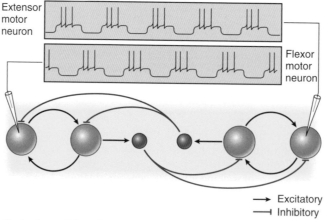

→ Excitatory
⊣ Inhibitory

Fig. 9.8 Schematic illustrations of the spinal central pattern generator *(CPG)* flexor/extensor half-centre with simplified architecture. The half-centre model contains excitatory interneurons that are functionally embedded within inhibitory networks such that when flexors are active extensors are inhibited and vice versa. This circuitry achieves the basic stepping rhythm. (Adapted from Yuste, R., Maclean, J. N., Smith, J. & Lansner, A. 2005. The cortex as a central pattern generator. Nat Rev Neurosci, 6, 477-83.)

feedback, spinal rhythm generation can be modulated by sensory feedback in a phase-dependent manner (Takakusaki, 2013; Rossignol et al., 2006). That is to say that the influence of sensory feedback on the stepping rhythm is different according to the current status of the ongoing step. For example, information from skin receptors of the feet is important in detecting contact with obstacles and in adjusting steps to avoid tripping. The foot is elevated or withdrawn when stimulated during the swing phase (flexing the limb to remove it from contact with an obstacle). But when the same stimulus is applied during the stance phase, the activity of extensor muscles is reinforced to avoid withdrawing the limb on which the body is currently balancing (Rossignol et al., 2006; Takakusaki, 2013). This means that the automatic rhythm of steady-state stepping produced at a spinal level is mediated (upregulated or downregulated) by other networks. The fact that animals and humans with cortical and spinal cord injuries have altered responses to sensory stimulation

and exaggerated muscle tone indicates that supraspinal networks are responsible for processing peripheral sensory input and exerting descending modulation of spinal CPG activity (Takakusaki, 2013; Rossignol et al., 2006). This descending modulation of spinal networks is responsible for initiating compensatory changes when stepping is perturbed (e.g. stumbling corrective reaction) by varying any or all of the amplitude, timing, and force parameters of the ongoing stepping pattern (Wolpert and Ghahramani, 2000).

What about the stepping reflex present at birth? Is this evidence of a central pattern generator for walking? See Chapter 10 for a description of this reflex (Fig. 9.9).

To successfully achieve accurate control of limb movements during community walking (necessary for walking over cluttered and dynamic terrains), posture must be optimised in advance so that stability can be maintained. In other words, feedforward planning will have to include signals to specify posture in anticipation of disturbances to balance that will

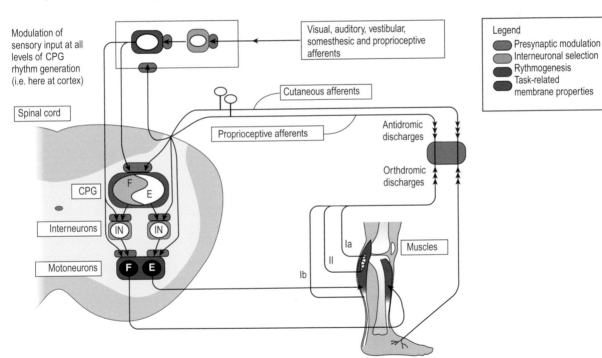

Fig. 9.9 Some Sites for Dynamic Sensorimotor Interactions During Locomotion. Sensory inputs of various modalities reach the spinal cord or the cortex and the gain of responses to sensory stimuli are then modulated at entry and as the signals progress through the central pattern generator *(CPG)* network. This is achieved by opening or closing (light orange) – presynaptic modulation some pathways in different phases of the cycle, otherwise the same input may give rise to excitatory or inhibitory responses in the various phases of the cycle. This is achieved either by inputs processed by those interneurons implicated directly in the pattern generation or through interneurons whose excitability is modulated cyclically by the CPG or the half-centre model. Interneurons enclosed within the *grey* area are considered to be cyclically influenced by the CPG but are not part of the rhythm generation process itself. (Adapted from Rossignol, S., Dubuc, R. & Gossard, J. P. 2006. Dynamic sensorimotor interactions in locomotion. Physiol Rev, 86, 89-154.)

arise as a consequence of walking through different types of terrain (Aruin et al., 2001). Information about body posture from visual, proprioceptive and vestibular sensory systems are integrated in the temporoparietal cortex and are used to update the locomotor programme via the premotor and sensory motor areas, which, in turn, modulate the spinal networks via the corticospinal tract (Takakusaki, 2013, 2017). In this way, networks spread across the spinal cord, brainstem and cortex are flexibly combined to achieve the rhythm of stepping and postural responses that are appropriate for the constraints of the task, environment and body.

THE DAMAGED MOTOR SYSTEM

Ultimately, a better understanding of how movement is controlled dynamically in relation to the environment can lead to improved clinical assessments and treatments (Montgomery and Connolly, 2003; Kenyon and Blackinton, 2011; Shumway-Cook and Wollacott, 2007).

Specifically, an understanding of motor control can be used to guide clinical examination and rehabilitation treatment by:

1. Characterising deficits: describing the aspects of the control process that are affected, (e.g. predicting and planning movement, sensory intactness and the ability to use this feedback, coordination of resulting muscle activation patterns).
2. Predicting ability to benefit from therapy using knowledge of functions served by viable neural control networks and sensory receptors.
3. Guiding the selection of individually targeted rehabilitation programmes based on an understanding of the cause of impairments (van Vliet et al., 2013).

For example, appreciating that a characteristic feature of motor control is motor abundancy and that adaptability of movement is promoted by the descending modulation of spinal networks by sensory motor cortical areas. Therefore clinicians may look for impairments in patients with cortical lesions to present as a limited repertoire of movement patterns and difficulty switching from one movement pattern to another (e.g. Kerr et al., 2017). In contrast, increased variability of gait parameters has been shown to be a hallmark of pathology such as Parkinson disease (PD), which affects subcortical basal ganglia networks. Increased variability may signify an over-reliance on step-by-step control rather than effective prediction and execution of feedforward planning (Peterson and Horak, 2016). In this way, understanding which neural networks are involved in control of any given movement, and how these are affected by a particular condition, provides the opportunity to determine the cause of impairments and then to select treatments targeted at the causes of movement control

deficits; thereby, ultimately yielding greater functional (i.e. compensation) and neurologic (i.e. restitution) recovery. In the case of PD, overactive descending inhibitory drive from the basal ganglia to the spinal locomotor networks (reduced automatic control) results in slow walking (Peterson and Horak, 2016). Treatments that stimulate viable voluntary control networks (e.g. external visual cues) may therefore not only be effective in compensating for movement deficits, but also may increase variability of movement.

Because the networks spread across the spinal cord, brainstem and cortex are flexibly combined to ensure movement patterns are appropriate for the constraints of the task, environment and body, lesions at any level will create particular impairments. Arguably then, the most complete assessment of patients' abilities/impairments and the most effective treatments may be ones in which the adaptability of movement is challenged, and/or those that exploit implicit motor control. For example, treatments for walking rehabilitation that use sensory inputs to elicit changes in the walking pattern (Hollands et al., 2013, & 2015; Nakazawa et al., 2004).

Given your new understanding of the neural pathways involved in controlling walking, and the role of sensation in adjusting movement in response to environment, task and body constraints, consider the theory behind why practising walking in response to visual cues may help people with PD or stroke to improve their walking ability. From Fig. 9.10 you can see that, in PD, the direct pathway between the basal ganglia, the spinal cord and, subsequently, muscles is pathologically overactive and so inhibits automatic motor output. Meanwhile, there is increased volitional control of movement via the motor cortex, which offers a compensatory route around this problem (e.g. a diversion around a road block). This allows an opportunity to use additional sensory inputs (e.g. visual cues) to enhance compensatory volitional/cortical control of movement. This is one example of how understanding the neural networks involved in movement control can help to identify which aspects of movement control might be affected and to predict how best to intervene; for example, using stepping target signals (e.g. a sound or image cue) to elicit a longer step length or faster step in contrast to using explicit feedback (e.g. 'lift your knee higher to take a bigger step' from the therapist). This might work with people with PD because of the primary pathology affecting the basal ganglia and therefore impairing movement automaticity, but would it work as well with stroke survivors with, for example, hemiplegia? Perhaps. However, the variable nature of stroke means a knowledge of exactly which functions are impaired is necessary before the optimal approach can be determined. Is it motor planning? Is it feedback from the body sensors? Is it the feedforward system, for example, insufficient motor drive?

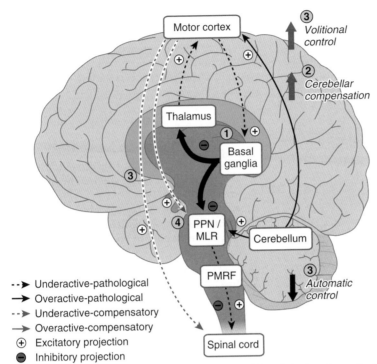

Gait slowness

(1) Overactive inhibitory output from the basal ganglia reduces corticospinal drive and contributes to slowed gait.

(2) Increased cerebellar activity may partially compensate for the overactive basal ganglia inhibition.

Gait variability and asymmetry

(3) Increased volitional (i.e. cortico-spinal), and reduced automatic control of locomotion contributes to variability of gait.

Postural instability

(4) Dysfunctional brainstem activity contributes to postural instability, hypokinesia, and rigidity.

Fig. 9.10 Alterations in overactive inhibitory activity of the basal ganglia *(1)* reduces automatic control via the direct pathway to the brain stem and spinal cord *(4)* in people with Parkinson disease. This contributes to gait slowness and increased postural instability, respectively, and increased cerebellar activity may partially compensate for these alterations *(2)*. Increased volitional control (i.e. cortico-spinal) *(3)* may not only contribute to increased gait variability and asymmetry, but also allow for sensory inputs to assist compensatory cortical control. *MLR*, Mesencephalic locomotor region; *PMRF*, pontomedullary reticular formation; *PPN*, peduncu-lopontine nucleus; *SMA*, supplementary motor area. (Adapted from Peterson, D. S. & Horak, F. B. 2016. Neural Control of Walking in People with Parkinsonism. Physiology (Bethesda), 31, 95-107.)

SUMMARY

Movement is complex. The number of muscles and joints that could participate in a movement task creates manifold solutions. While this provides an amazing amount of flex-ibility in the motor system (abundancy) it also requires a lot of brain work to control it. Humans have simplified this problem, to some extent, by creating a library of movement programmes that are flexibly applied (combined and refined) to a movement task. The central pattern generators are examples of these basic movement programmes, which create rhythmic movements such as the lower limb flexion and extension required during the swing and stance phases of walking. These motor programmes reduce the amount of conscious thought needed to do a lot of movements, leaving you free to get on with the more interesting tasks of texting and window shopping.

The motor control system is comprised of:

1. The CNS: including the primary and secondary motor areas, basal ganglia, brain stem, spinal cord, and all the interconnecting junctions and pathways)
2. The peripheral nervous system: including the efferent motor neurons, sensory receptors (mainly muscle spindle and Golgi tendon organs, eyes, vestibular system sensory receptors) and their interconnecting junctions and pathways
3. The musculoskeletal system (muscles, tendons and bones) that affect the movement.

The feedback system provides integrated information about the environment and the body position during movement and is used as part of a 'closed loop' system to refine movements so that they become accurate and efficient. Movement is possible without feedback; however, in this 'open' system a motor plan is formed and executed from existing motor programmes (developed through previous experiences). This is termed feedforward and is useful when rapid movements are required (i.e. no time to wait for feedback).

Understanding the way movement is controlled will be helpful when you come to assess motor problems in the clinic and to devise appropriate rehabilitation programmes.

This chapter serves as an introduction to the area and you are very much encouraged to explore this fascinating area of motor control through the many available textbooks and scientific journals. Before you move onto the next chapter why not check your understanding by trying the self-assessment exercises.

SELF-ASSESSMENT QUESTIONS

1. Where does transmission of information between neurons occur?
   a. Along the axon
   b. At the synapse
   c. Within the neuron nucleus
   d. Along the myelin sheath
2. The resting potential across a neuron membrane is approximately −70 mV. This is created by the relative (inside and outside the membrane wall) concentration of which ions?
   a. Sodium ions (Na^+)
   b. Potassium ions (K^+)
   c. Chloride ions (Cl^-)
   d. Calcium ion (Ca^{2+})
3. If a threshold is reached an action potential is propagated down the axon from the nucleus to the synapse, which two factors increase how fast the signal is propagated?
   a. Axon size
   b. Number of dendrites
   c. Size of the nucleus
   d. Myelin sheath
4. What does a muscle spindle detect?
   a. Tension in the muscle
   b. Length of the muscle
   c. Rate of tension change
   d. Rate of length change
5. A body schema (the brain's working model of the body position) is built up from inputs from the visual, vestibular and somatosensory systems. What does somatosensory mean?
6. Stimulation of the stretch reflex leads to a reflexive
   a. Contraction of the muscle being stretched.
   b. Relaxation of the muscle being stretched.
   c. Contraction of the opposite muscle.
   d. Contraction of the muscle being stretched and opposite muscle.

7. Opening of sodium ion (Na^+) channels at the postsynaptic membrane will lead to depolarisation and therefore … ?
   a. Excitation of the postsynaptic neuron.
   b. Inhibition of postsynaptic neuron.
   c. Hyperexcitation of the postsynaptic neuron.
   d. Relaxation of the postsynaptic neuron.
8. The degrees of freedom principle refers to what?
   a. The choice of corticospinal tracts available to conduct the motor action potential
   b. The large number of potential solutions to a movement task
   c. The three degrees of movement available at most joints
   d. The selection of isotomic or isometric muscle action
9. Feedforward movements do not require feedback.
   a. True
   b. False
10. Motor programmes or schemas are hard wired into our neural system and cannot be modified.
    a. True
    b. False
11. Central pattern generators control indoor walking.
    a. True
    b. False
12. Which of the following statements would you agree with:
    a. Rehabilitation of functional movements should solely focus on repeating the same movement pattern.
    b. Rehabilitation of functional movements should incorporate variability in movement practice to encourage involvement of the feedback system.

REFERENCES

Aruin, A.S., Ota, T., Latash, M.L., 2001. Anticipatory postural adjustments associated with lateral and rotational perturbations during standing. J. Electromyogr. Kinesiol. 11, 39–51.

Bernstein, N.A., 1967. The Coordination and Regulation of Movements. Pergamon, New York.

Cohen, H., 1998. Neuroscience for Rehabilitation. JB Lippincott, Philadelphia.

Duque, J., Lew, D., Mazzocchio, R., Olivier, E., Ivry, R.B., 2010. Evidence for two concurrent inhibitory mechanisms during response preparation. J. Neurosci. 30, 3793–3802.

Grillner, S., Deliagina, T., Ekeberg, O., El Manira, A., Hill, R.H., Lansner, A., et al., 1995. Neural networks that co-ordinate locomotion and body orientation in lamprey. Trends Neurosci. 18, 270–279.

Grillner, S., Wallen, P., 1985. Central pattern generators for locomotion, with special reference to vertebrates. Annu. Rev. Neurosci. 8, 233–261.

Hall, J.E., 2005. Guyton & Hall Physiology Review. WB Saunders, Philadelphia.

Hollands, K.L., Pelton, T., Wimperis, A., Whitham, D., Jowett, S., Sackley, C., et al., 2013. Visual cue training to improve walking and turning after stroke: a study protocol for a multi-centre, single blind randomised pilot trial. Trials 14, 276. doi:10.1186/1745-6215-14-276.

Hollands, K.L., Pelton, T.A., Wimperis, A., Whitham, D., Tan, W., Jowett, S., et al., 2015. Feasibility and preliminary efficacy of visual cue training to improve adaptability of walking after stroke: multi-centre, single-blind randomised control pilot trial. PLoS ONE 10 (10), e0139261. doi:10.1371/journal.pone.0139261. eCollection 2015.

Kenyon, L.K., Blackinton, M.T., 2011. Applying motor-control theory to physical therapy practice: a case report. Physiother. Can. 63, 345–354.

Kerr, A., Rafferty, Hollands, Barber, Granat, 2017. A technique to record the sedentary to walk movement during free living mobility: a comparison of healthy and stroke populations. Gait Posture 52, 233–236.

Latash, M.L., 2008. Neurophysiological Basis of Movement. Human Kinetics, Leeds.

Malone, L.A., Bastian, A.J., 2010. Thinking about walking: effects of conscious correction versus distraction on locomotor adaptation. J. Neurophysiol. 103, 1954–1962.

Montgomery, P.C., Connolly, B.H., 2003. Clinical Applications for Motor Control. SLACK Incorporated, Thorofare.

Nakazawa, K., Kakihana, W., Kawashima, N., Akai, M., Yano, H., 2004. Induction of locomotor-like EMG activity in paraplegic persons by orthotic gait training. Exp. Brain Res. 157, 117–123.

Peterson, D.S., Horak, F.B., 2016. Neural control of walking in people with Parkinsonism. Physiology (Bethesda) 31, 95–107.

Pruszynski, J.A., Kurtzer, I., Nashed, J.Y., Omrani, M., Brouwer, B., Scott, S.H., 2011. Primary motor cortex underlies multi-joint integration for fast feedback control. Nature 478, 387–390.

Rossignol, S., Dubuc, R., Gossard, J.P., 2006. Dynamic sensorimotor interactions in locomotion. Physiol. Rev. 86, 89–154.

Schmidt, R., Lee, T., 2011. Motor Control and Learning: A Behavioral Emphasis, fifth ed. Human Kinetics, Champaign.

Shumway-Cook, A., Woollacott, M.H., 2007. Motor Control: Translating Research Into Clinical Practice. Lippincott Williams & Wilkins, Philadelphia.

Stroeve, S., 1999. Analysis of the role of proprioceptive information during arm movements using a model of the human arm. Motor Control 3, 158–185.

Takakusaki, K., 2013. Neurophysiology of gait: from the spinal cord to the frontal lobe. Mov. Disord. 28 (11), 1483–1491.

Takakusaki, K., 2017. Functional neuroanatomy for posture and gait control. J. Mov. Disord. 10, 1–17.

Tortora, G.J., Derrickson, B.H., 2008. Principles of Anatomy and Physiology. John Wiley, New York.

Van Vliet, P., Pelton, T.A., Hollands, K.L., Carey, L., Wing, A.M., 2013. Neuroscience findings on coordination of reaching to grasp an object: implications for research. Neurorehabil. Neural Repair 27, 622–635.

Wolpert, D.M., Ghahramani, Z., 2000. Computational principles of movement neuroscience. Nat. Neurosci. 3 (Suppl.), 1212–1217.

Yuste, R., Maclean, J.N., Smith, J., Lansner, A., 2005. The cortex as a central pattern generator. Nat. Rev. Neurosci. 6, 477–483.

10

Development and Decline of Movement

Jennifer Muhaidat and Andy Kerr

OUTLINE

LEARNING OUTCOMES

After reading this chapter, you will be able to:
1. Describe the sequence of movement development in babies and children.
2. Outline the effects that ageing can have on general mobility as well as specific movements.
3. Understand the interaction between physical, cognitive and psychological function in determining the movement behaviour of children and older adults.

4. Explain the effect disease, environment (physical/social) and physical activity can have on the development and decline of movement ability.
5. Understand the role that therapy interventions can have in helping to develop and maintain physical skills throughout the lifespan.

INTRODUCTION

Developing the movement skills necessary for an independent life seems to happen effortlessly and in a predictable sequence. We may not remember these experiences personally but we all recognise the achievement of key milestones, such as sitting and walking, in our younger relatives. Of course, achieving, and then maintaining, these important movement skills is a complex process requiring the integration of all the body systems; inevitably there are people who fail to reach these milestones and people who lose them through

ageing. In the first part of this chapter we will describe the development of physical skills in children and explore some of the influencing factors. In part two we will consider the other end of the life cycle: the loss of movement ability associated with the ageing process.

PART ONE: DEVELOPMENT OF MOVEMENT

Introduction to Child Development

In part one of this chapter we will cover child development, focusing on the acquisition of movement skills. We will describe the typical behaviours involved in gaining head control, manipulation skills, standing and walking, as well as the key milestones for the other physical skills: rolling, sitting etc. This is important knowledge; it is not only critical if you want to work in paediatrics but also useful for understanding adult conditions with impaired movement. Of course, there is more to development than movement skills; cognitive and social development occur at the same time and they all interact with each other. Physical development, for example, is known to impact on cognition through the ability to move around the physical environment and manipulate objects (Sibley and Etnier, 2003). Therefore we will look at some of the key stages in cognitive development.

Before we begin it is worth saying that while most children develop their movement abilities in a similar way, there is considerable variation, which is absolutely normal. Also—and you probably know this already—the ability to develop new skills, and refine old ones, persists through life. It's just that the major steps in movement development are taken during the first few years of life.

Typical Development of Physical Skills

Foetal Movement

Movement begins long before birth. This is most evident when a baby's kicking movements are felt by the mother during the final trimester (24 weeks +) but the foetus starts to move even earlier. Although the heart is considered the first body system to start functioning (around 3 to 4 weeks into gestation), the neuromusculoskeletal system is not far behind. Neuromusculoskeletal is a compound word used to represent the combined musculoskeletal (bones, muscles, tendons etc.) and neural systems (central nervous system, peripheral motor/sensory and sensory organs) that work together to produce movement. By around 7 weeks the baby should be capable and, if healthy, does begin to move. In the beginning this is limited to some general, apparently purposeless, trunk movement, but by 10 weeks the foetus has a wide movement repertoire; gross body movement, twitching, individual head movements, jaw movement, hand-to-face movements and limb stretching (de Vries and Fong, 2006).

This foetal movement is actually critical for the development of the musculoskeletal system (Shea et al., 2015) and is a general indication of the baby's health. An absence of movement can lead to a lack of joint development resulting in conditions such as arthrogryposis (Further Information 10.1).

Movements of the Newborn

Compared to most other mammals we don't have a lot of physical skill at birth. A newborn calf, for example, will be able to stand and take a few steps within the first hour, but for humans it takes around a year before they can do the

---

FURTHER INFORMATION 10.1
Arthrogryposis

Foetal movement is critical to the development of the musculoskeletal system. If, for any reason, this movement does not occur then the muscles and joints will fail to develop normally. The baby is born with muscles that are stiff and shortened fixing the joints into a contracted position which may be either flexed or extended. This condition is called arthrogryposis. The resulting joint contractures can affect almost every part of the body and have a typical pattern; for example, the fingers are usually flexed over the thumb. The more severe cases can prevent the child from achieving physical milestones such as walking. Treatment is based around therapy and sometimes surgery to create functional joint range and exercise to improve muscle strength. Arthrogryposis is therefore the result of foetal akinesia (lack of movement) but the underlying cause(s) are still not fully understood. It could be caused by a malformation in the central nervous system, for example, spina bifida or maternal illness such as rubella.

---

same thing. Although relatively helpless, human newborns do exhibit a range of movements—many of which are related to the primitive reflexes. These are chiefly concerned with survival, which, at this stage, generally means feeding (e.g. the rooting and sucking reflexes) and not falling off your mother (grasp reflex) when you are being carried. Holding on tightly is not so critical for babies these days with a range of manmade transport systems, but back in Neanderthal times it was probably pretty crucial.

The Primitive Reflexes

The primitive reflexes (Table 10.1) are normal reflex actions that are present in the newborn but are gradually inhibited as more mature movement patterns and behaviours become established. Remember that reflexes are automatic, that is, they are out of your voluntary control. The process of developing normal voluntary movement gradually inhibits (suppresses) these reflexes, but they remain with us throughout our life. Injuries to the brain or spinal cord (e.g. a stroke) can release these primitive reflexes again. Consequently, assessing presence and strength of these reflexes is an important way to understand the intactness of the central nervous system (CNS), which comprises the brain and spinal cord. Several of these reflexes do persist normally in later life in a diluted form that we can override to some extent; for example, we all know what happens if someone pops a balloon behind us.

TABLE 10.1   Primitive Reflexes.

Reflex	Stimulus	Response	Should Disappear
Moro	Sudden drop in head position as if falling	Arms shoot out with hands open, legs and head may extend	Around 3–4 months
Startle reflex	Loud noise or rapid movement	Arms shoot out with hands open, legs and head may extend	Around 3–4 months
Rooting	Touch cheek/lips	Head turns towards the tactile sensation	Around 3–4 months
Sucking	Touch roof mouth	Sucking action	2–4 months
Stepping	Stimulation of plantar aspect foot	Rudimentary stepping movement. Unable to support weight	Around 5–6 months
Asymmetrical tonic neck reflex (see Fig. 10.1)	Turning the head to one side	Causes the arm and leg on the side turned to, to extend and the limbs on opposite side to flex. Like a fencing posture	6 months
Symmetrical tonic neck reflex	Flexing the head forward	Arms bend and legs to extend.	Appears briefly around birth then reappears around 6–9 months before finally disappearing by 18 months
'Crawling reflex'	Extending the head	Arms extend and legs flex	
Grip/palmar reflex	Touch palm of hand	Fingers close around stimulus to grasp the object	Around 5–6 months
Galant	Stroke skin on one side of back	Trunk flexes to side stroked	Around 5 months
Swimming	Submerge in water	Rudimentary swimming action	Around 4–6 months
Babinski (plantar reflex)	Sole foot stroked	Extension. Big toe extends and other toes abduct. In healthy adults this response reverses to a flexion response	By 12 months the extension response should have changed to a flexor response

Acquiring Key Movement Skills: The Developmental Milestones

Described below is a generalized process of movement development. Not every child follows the same sequence; many will delay reaching certain milestones and some children will miss out a milestone completely (Further Information 10.2). A delay, or omission, in this process is not likely to be abnormal, just the child following a different developmental trajectory with broadly the same result in the end. The development phases described below do not follow in series (one after the other) but will overlap.

Postural Control Starts With the Eyes

Exploring the environment is done with the eyes first. A newborn baby has the ability to track large objects moving across their field of view, albeit in a crude manner (Von Hofsten and Rosander, 1997). To focus on objects the head has to be steady; therefore the head is the first part of the body the baby gains control over. As an adult, when you walk or run your head is the part of your body that moves the least; this is so the eyes can focus on your environment and probably allow you to run and hunt.

FURTHER INFORMATION 10.2 "Shuffle-Bottom"

Around 9 percent of UK born children develop bottom-shuffling rather than crawling to get around (Robson, 1984). For some reason they have acquired this skill first and once they have a means of getting around they are happy. It has been suggested that these children might achieve walking a little later than children who learn to crawl, possibly because they haven't developed the same strength in their extensor muscles from being in a prone position. The high incidence of bottom shuffling is believed to account for the surnames Bottom-shuffler & Shuffle bottom! (Fox, Palmer and Davies, 2002).

Head Control

Head control is gained gradually over the first 3 months. During this time the head's position is still affected by the primitive reflexes (see Table 10.1) that dominate movement; for example, touching the cheek will cause the head to turn towards the sensation. Gradually, the baby gains independent control of the head's position.

This starts in the prone position. In this position the baby will start to lift their head up against gravity. This may begin with momentary head lifts (head bobbing) and side-to-side turns, which slowly develop into more sustained head holding. The baby then incorporates the arms into the position to prop themselves up so that the movement can be held for longer, allowing a better look around (Fig. 10.2).

In supported sitting (e.g. held in the mother's arms) head control is gradually gained by the baby moving their head incrementally out of the neutral position (i.e. increasing the gravitational moment, see Chapter 2). Gaining this control is a key starting point for hand–eye coordination, which will be critical to developing upper limb functions, such as reach to grasp, which we will cover further on.

When placed in the supine position, during the same period the baby will find it easier to turn their head (e.g. when tracking an object). In this position they don't have to overcome the moments created by gravity. However, in the first 2 to 4 weeks they are kind of stuck in a flexed position. Placed in the supine position, the arms and legs of the baby will remain bent with the feet held off the ground. As this flexed posture relaxes, the baby gains more selective control of their head and will turn their head to follow objects moved across their visual field. In these first few weeks the neck is not strong enough to hold the head when pulled to sitting from supine. This lagging of the head (head drops back from the trunk) gradually disappears, usually by 4 months, as head control is achieved. This test is sometimes used as a gross, early measure of motor development.

Object Manipulation (Hand Skills)

Holding and exploring objects with the hands is clearly an important developmental process; exploring the physical environment is important for physical and cognitive development. In the first few months, control of the arm and hand is very basic and still dominated by the primitive reflexes (Table 10.2). Movements are gross and stereotypical, and not really under the baby's control. There may be some early success in getting the hand to the mouth, but this is usually brief, although the sensory reward for this success no doubt provides a lot of motivation to keep trying.

The grasp reflex persists through this period so that any object placed in the hand will be held reflexively. By 3 months there may be purposeful arm movements to try and hit objects placed nearby. This will be easier in the supine position without the need to lift the body, so toys such as cot mobiles serve a key role in this stage, as does a parent's face or hand. The ability to reach for an object and actually grasp it won't fully develop until 7 or 8 months. The reach to grasp movement is actually a very skilled movement, requiring constant fine-tuning to smoothly reach and then grasp a target that could be any shape and weight. Consequently, the mature movement won't be established until around 10 years of age (Schneiberg et al., 2002).

Side lying can be a useful position to encourage hand development as it brings both hands together without too much effort, offering the opportunity for bimanual activities as well as just exploring the other hand. However, these lying positions are limited in that you are stuck in one position. It's hard to find new things to feel and play with, and if you drop anything its hard work to retrieve. Real progress in hand (upper limb) skill comes when the infant can finally sit without falling (careful positioning of cushions advised) at around 6 months. This is a good moment for the infant; suddenly both hands are free to hold and fully experience objects and they have a larger space to explore by moving their trunk. In the early stages of sitting there is a high risk of falling as they struggle to keep their centre of mass within their base of support, especially if there are

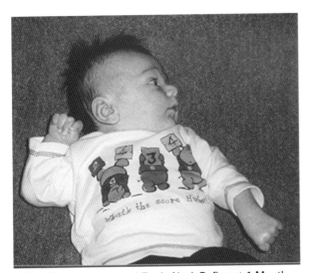

Fig. 10.1 Asymmetrical Tonic Neck Reflex at 1 Month.

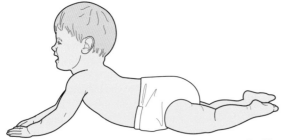

Fig. 10.2 Baby Developing Head Control in the Prone Position.

TABLE 10.2 Overview of Key Physical Milestones.

Age	Physical Milestone
4 weeks	Begins to hold head steady in sitting (head in neutral). This may take up to 3 months to fully develop.
2 months	Can turn from side to back when placed on side. This may take up to 4 months.
2–3 months	Can sit with support with hands-on support to lower trunk. Independent sitting will take 6 months to achieve.
4–5 months	Can roll from back to side.
5 months	Can sit independently for short periods.
6 months	Can roll from back to front.
6–7 months	Can sit independently and use hands to manipulate objects without falling. This may take 8–9 months to master.
7–8 months	Will be able to make crude steps when supported.
8 months	Will begin pulling to standing and maintain standing for brief moments.
9 months	May be able to walk with assistance (and is usually very keen to do so).
10 months	Can crawl (although some babies never crawl).
11 months	Can stand alone (although this may take up to 15 months to acquire).
12–13 months	Can walk alone, with regular falls. This may take 18 months to master.

interesting distractions. To overcome this lack of stability they will, very cleverly, lean forward, and place one hand on the ground to increase their base of support and to ensure their centre of mass is well within its perimeter. One-handed reaching is therefore preferred in the early stages of mastering this precarious skill (Rochat, 1992) (Fig. 10.3). In this position hand control develops rapidly, driven by enormous sensory rewards (e.g. touch, feeding, rattling toys) and new interactions with parents (clapping, pointing and waving). This is an exciting time with new experiences every day.

An odd thing can sometimes happen while the baby is developing these advanced motor skills; they can often regress, albeit briefly, in their established skills. It is not unusual for a baby to lose their sitting ability, for example, as they try to make progress with their hand skills. Movement control requires a lot of attention; even things considered routine, such as sitting, haven't yet become automatic, so lapses in ability are bound to occur as attention is diverted to developing a new skill.

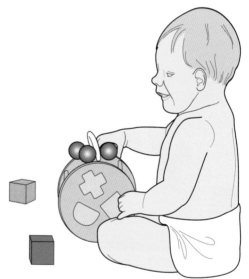

Fig. 10.3 Sitting allows manipulation of objects to begin enabling the child to explore more of their environment.

Primitive Grasp

As we have said, the newborn has a crude grasp ability, but this reflex action disappears over the first 6 months to be replaced with something more useful. One of the problems with this primitive grasp is that it is not functional. The thumb (which is needed for the fun stuff) is usually tucked under the fingers and the grasp is not easily released. Functional grasping techniques (i.e. ones under the infant's control) appear around 5 months. A crude **fist grasp** that does not include independent movement of the thumb allows the baby to grab an object and bring it to their mouth. The grasp is basic and will often fail but it is a good start and brings the reward of the object to the baby to inspire future attempts.

Independent movement of the thumb and fingers is part of the **raking grasp**, which is observed a few months later.

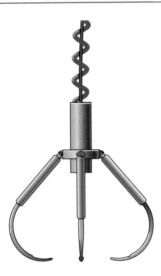

Fig. 10.4 Claw Crane Grabber.

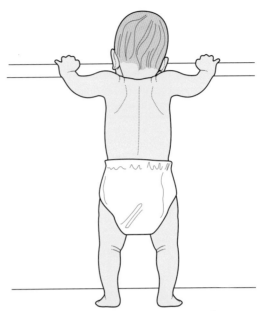

Fig. 10.5 Using Furniture to Stand.

This grasp is very much like the grasp from a claw crane used in arcade games (Fig. 10.4). As we all know from bitter experience, this is not a very effective grasp. The raking grasp is the forerunner of the **pincer and chuck grips**, which will allow the object to be manipulated and held securely even if it has an unusual shape, like a spoon. These refined grasps will take a couple more years to get right, culminating in the ability to hold and manipulate a crayon.

Standing and Walking

We will consider development of standing and walking together; after all, you can't walk without gaining the ability to stand. The stimulus to try and stand may be deeply ingrained but, like so many steps in motor development, it is driven by the need to explore the environment, which often means getting higher, to a table, sofa or bed.

Pulling up to stand will probably start happening around 5 months but can't really be maintained until 7 to 8 months. Achieving a standing posture is the ultimate fight against gravity. Initially this can't be done by the baby alone; they need help, and this may be from a parent, or the strategic use of furniture, chairs, tables etc. (Fig. 10.5). Early attempts will inevitably end in failure due to a lack of strength and balance, so expect to see an infant slowly sink to the ground during this period (as their muscles fail to match the external gravitational moments) or, less gracefully, collapse onto their bottom. The balance system is not yet ready to deal with the demands of controlling the centre of mass, which is now high above the base of support, which is an inherently unstable position (see Chapter 8 for more information on balance). A wide stance is a good strategy and, of course,

this is what the infant does, as well as holding on, very tightly, to anything stable. Once up and steady(ish), many infants will engage in a bouncing action. It seems this rhythmic action is designed to train all the systems involved in standing balance (primarily the visual, vestibular and motor systems). The infant is basically creating their own balance training programme. Rhythmic movements may appear earlier in the developmental process (e.g. in four-point kneeling as a precursor to crawling), and are the inspiration for therapeutic interventions such as hippotherapy, rhythmic stabilisations and rebound therapy, which aim to improve movement and posture in children (and adults) with impaired movement. Rhythm is also considered to be a key element in the development of speech. However, persistent rhythmic movements, such as rocking back and forward in the cot or head banging, are sometimes observed in children deprived of sensory input (e.g. in institutional care) (Smyke et al., 2007). This kind of behaviour may be a sign of neglect, with the infant's movements an attempt at self-soothing (Activity Box 10.1).

Ultimately the goal in standing is to get around more of the environment but it will take a month or two after the first pull to stand before experimentation with the standing position begins. Releasing a hand to touch a toy or lifting a leg will require substantial postural stability; consequently this behaviour might not be observed until 9/10 months. Developing this dynamic standing balance is the first step towards walking.

ACTIVITY BOX 10.1   Baby Bouncers

Baby walkers are a popular toy for children aged 6–12 months.

Have a think about why these baby bouncers are often criticised by physiotherapists working with children. In what way could they interfere with normal development?

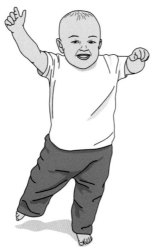

Fig. 10.6 First Steps.

It's interesting that a failure in standing (i.e. a fall) rarely leads to a diminished desire from the baby to stand up, unlike adults. Provided they are not hurt, the baby will want to, probably immediately, get up again (perhaps after a wee cuddle). What do you think are the motivational differences between an adult and a child when it comes to standing up again after a fall?

Moving From Standing to Walking

At first this is achieved by furniture cruising, which might start at around 10 months. Side-stepping along a sofa is a good start. With increasing confidence this will progress to holding a stable moving object such as a parent's hand or a toy with wheels. Making the move to walking on their own will quickly follow (Fig. 10.6) with short distances attempted (with frequent fails) between stable objects. Independent walking will generally appear around 12 months (Capute et al., 1985) but 1 to 2 months earlier or later is absolutely normal. A mature walking pattern, that is, one that accommodates balance disturbances and is sufficiently automated to allow the child to do other tasks, such as talking or balancing an object (egg and spoon), might not be established until around 7 years (Jeng et al., 1997).

Gait Initiation in Standing

Moving from standing to walking is basically learning to avoid a forward fall. When standing, the centre of pressure (see Chapter 8 for reminder) is located in front of the ankle joints (this is the same for adults and infants). This means that we are tipping forwards all the time when we are standing, and are held up by only by the activity of our calf muscles. Think about the video clips of exhausted soldiers or grooms who fall forwards after standing for too long. This is the first step in the gait initiation process from standing. You basically relax your calf muscles, which has the effect of rotating your body forwards (fall forwards like a dehydrated soldier on parade). The trick is to avoid a fall, so within a few milliseconds of relaxing the calf muscles a stepping action must be initiated. This starts the walking sequence. The reemergence of the stepping reflex (see Table 10.1) during this period helps the infant achieve this, but, of course, there are many failed attempts and these first few steps are characterised by the arms already positioned for a fall (see Fig. 10.6).

Over the last few pages we have described the typical development of key motor skills: head control, reaching and grasping, standing and walking. These were examples intended to highlight the motivation (exploration and reward) for movement as well as the general stages and use of rhythmic movements, such as rocking in a crawling position and bouncing in standing. As we stated at the beginning, movement development is a process tied closely to cognitive development. Therefore the next part will consider how a child acquires knowledge and understanding. However, before we move on, it might be worth having a look again a Table 10.2; committing a few of the key stages to memory will serve you well.

Cognitive Development

Maturation of movement and postural control are only part of a child's development; cognitive and social development, of course, takes place concurrently, and they interact with each other. Delayed or limited physical development will, by consequence of imposing a restricted experience of the physical environment, effect cognitive and social development.

Understanding the way a child learns will not only provide insight on the child's problem beyond their physical impairment but also will be invaluable in constructing a meaningful therapy programme that will have a global impact on their physical, cognitive and social development.

This next section will consider cognitive development. It is beyond the scope of this chapter to give an in-depth account of all the theories of cognitive development. Instead we will introduce some of the more popular theories and spend a little more time on Piaget's stages of cognitive development, which, although they have been around for a while, are still regarded as valid and are routinely taught in child psychology courses.

Theories on How a Child Learns

Many people have tried to explain how a child learns. Some early theories postulate that the child is a blank page, ready to be written on when they are born. The early experiences of the child are perceived to be a bit of a muddle; the baby's brain is not mature enough to discriminate between all the different inputs (a bit like semester one in the first year at university). Slowly the child begins to unravel these experiences and starts to make sense of them, sort them out and learn from them. This theory was called **empiricism**.

The scientific (systematic analysis through direct observation) approach to understanding learning in general, and child development specifically, really took off in the early 20th century. Ivan Pavlov was perhaps most famous for his experiments with dogs, but the principles were also applied to the way a child learns. Pavlov measured the volume of saliva produced by his dogs. If a bell was rung there would be no difference in the amount of saliva produced. However, if food was introduced just after the bell was rung, the dogs (after a few times) produced more saliva when the bell was rung on its own. This is not too different from the feeling I get when I hear an ice-cream van—but hopefully with less saliva! This method of behavioural learning was called **classical conditioning** (Activity Box 10.2).

This theory of learning fell out of favour in the 1920s as it was considered too simplistic, and new ideas were proposed. The **law of reinforcement** was the basis for Skinner's theories on learning. This, essentially, is the idea that actions associated with rewards are the ones that are most readily repeated and adopted into everyday behaviour; actions unrewarded are the ones quickly dropped. The inclusion of a reward helps to reinforce behaviour. Can you think of examples from your own life where reward might explain your behaviour? Perhaps you got a comic for tidying your room? Or maybe you gave yourself a reward for studying so hard on a Friday night (e.g. a small glass of shandy).

In modern times, Professor Bandura expanded on reward as the motivation for learning, but placed greater value on intrinsic reward; feelings of pride and satisfaction from an achievement is probably the best way to describe this. These intrinsic rewards then set up the process for gaining a perception of self (self-concept) and how you judge yourself (self-worth), although this is also based on other people's perception. Bandura also thought that imitation played a large part in motor learning, particularly in children. He termed this **observational learning** or **social cognitive theory**. In essence, this is based on the idea that a child can learn simply from watching others. Actually doing it is not a prerequisite for understanding it; this has also been called **vicarious learning**. In support of this theory, a newborn has the ability to copy their parent's behaviour. Endearingly they can copy a mother or father sticking their tongue out. If you get the chance you should try this yourself.

Piaget's Stages of Learning

Jean Piaget is the most quoted psychologist in history, mainly for his descriptions and analysis of the stages in a child's cognitive development, which are still widely taught. There are several ideas underpinning the stages: that a baby is born with innate patterns of movement behaviours called schemas or strategies, which are employed to understand the physical environment and to develop increasingly sophisticated schemas.

The child's process for learning is inherently different from that of an adult but the following processes gradually lead to an adult style of learning.

Assimilation: The child receives information and compares it against what they already know from experience. An early example of this is when the child begins sucking their thumb/finger. This learnt behaviour stems from early feeding experiences.

Accommodation: This is a higher stage of thinking where the child alters their understanding. New experiences, when compared with existing knowledge, will induce a change in their behaviour. For example, the baby finds the thumb more satisfying to suck due to its shape, so deliberately selects this digit.

Equilibration: This is where the child develops new schemas (understandings) as the previous ones just didn't explain everything. One example might be a child who thinks all animals are called 'animal' but learns that this is not true and will develop a new understanding. Of course, this takes time and opportunity to learn (lots of picture books!).

These three processes, suggests Piaget, explain how a child learns about their environment and how to behave within it. The key thing throughout is experiencing the environment; whether that is through touch, sound, movement or social

---

ACTIVITY BOX 10.2 Classic Conditioning

With a partner (not a dog) elicit a stretch reflex on their quads with a patellar tendon tap. Do this a few times (try 10) and note the response. Wait a few minutes (try 10) and elicit the same reflex, only this time blow in their face at the same time (which should cause them to close their eyes. Repeat this a few times. Now try the tendon tap. What happens? Do they close their eyes?

interaction, learning events have to occur for the brain to develop understanding.

Piaget's Stages of Development

According to Piaget there are four stages of development between birth and adulthood, which are broadly categorised as infancy, early childhood, middle childhood and adolescence.

The driving force behind learning at each stage is the child deliberately manipulating the environment to see what happens, much as a scientist would manipulate an experiment to test a hypothesis. These manipulations are termed operations. You can imagine the restricted operations a child with sensory or mobility impairment might have, or even a child deprived of toys or social interactions.

1. **Sensorimotor (birth to 18 months).** A great deal goes on during this period.
   - Birth to 2 months: the child connects with their environment, driven mainly by their primitive reflexes. The child receives a lot of sensory input using just these reflexes, with the focus of the stimulation being the mouth.
   - Two to 4 months: the baby gets pleasure from repeating actions. This may have nothing to do with survival (e.g. kicking legs in the air or sucking a rubbery toy). The actions are essentially their primitive reflexes, except that they are learning how to control them for pleasure (reward).
   - Four to 8 months: the baby pays more attention to external objects, not merely as extensions of themselves but things that have the capacity to amuse them, so they start to directly control their environment. Perhaps they start shaking a rattle to get that nice reaction from people or use that particular cry that brings mummy running back.
   - Eight to 12 months: the baby begins to show coordinated effort. There is evidence of planning. Movement is organised with a goal in mind. In advanced cases this might mean bringing a stool to stand up to reach an object, or simply lifting up one toy to gain access to another. This is early problem solving.
   - Twelve to 18 months: during this period the child experiments a lot with the environment, trying new ways of achieving their goals. For example, they may discover that shuffling with their bottom is the fastest way to get upstairs; bottom, knees, all fours. There is a lot of experimentation; for example, throwing balls at different angles and putting blocks together.
   - Eighteen to 24 months: the child can represent actions/ objects with symbols. They are able to think about objects and people without them being there. They

also use words and perhaps pictures to represent their thinking. A child who looks for their favourite toy in all the usual places is displaying this ability. This way of thinking about an object is sometimes called object permanence. The ability of a child to understand that an object exists even if they can't see it is a key plank of Piaget's theories. The child develops the ability to think beyond its current environment around 6 months. At this age the child will become better at hide and seek; they know the missing object exists, it's just a matter of finding it.

2. **Preoperational (2 to 7 years).** Children are very egocentric, that is, they only perceive the world from their own point of view. They have an understanding of the world so that they begin to represent ideas/situations in the abstract (e.g. pictures to represent home). Children at this age see things very much in black and white and will generalise their understanding of one thing to others, so all grannies wear glasses or all girls like pink, etc. Rules absolutely dominate during this stage.

3. **Concrete operational (7 to 11 years).** Children will become less egocentric and begin to use logic. They begin to understand relationships, such as the amount of ingredients to make a cake of a certain size. They are less able to think of ideas without some experience of them. It's called 'concrete' because they need some definite experience for understanding.

4. **Formal operational (11 to 15 years).** Children in this age group can now think about things that have never happened to them or even been observed by them. They are able to think in a rational, systematic manner. They are also able to grasp abstract concepts of economy, politics and justice. They are also able to separate concrete reality from imagination.

Piaget's theories of cognitive development and stages of learning are obviously more complex than this basic overview. However, some people have criticised the staged approach, but it is a useful starting point for understanding the way a child learns to think. I would encourage you to read more in depth on this subject. It will inform your communication and treatment of children, and you will probably also find it interesting (Activity Box 10.3).

ACTIVITY BOX 10.3   Play Therapy

Human children, and many other young mammals, play instinctively.

What purpose does it fulfil?

What could a child lose if they are unable to play, in terms of cognitive, social and motor skills?

Activity Boxes 10.4 and 10.5 are designed to help you consolidate understanding of child development, putting together motor, social and cognitive development.

PART TWO: DECLINE OF MOVEMENT

Introduction

In the second half of this chapter we will consider the loss of movement capacity through ageing. Being able to live independently in later life will depend on your ability to carry out activities of daily living (ADL), such as washing yourself and preparing food. The physiological changes associated with ageing impinge on these abilities. However, the supportive role of physical activity, rehabilitation and assistive technologies can help individuals maintain their functional capacity for as long as possible. Like child development, age-related decline is complex and multifactorial with interactions between pathological, physiological and psychological processes. Consequently, people do not age at the same rate; however, there are similarities in the sequence

---

ACTIVITY BOX 10.4

Evidence that sudden infant death syndrome, also known as cot death, might be linked to babies sleeping on their front, led to the recommendation that babies should be placed on their back to sleep. Of course this led to some people avoiding the prone position entirely for their baby.*

How could avoiding a prone position alter movement development?

Could there by an impact on social, cognitive pattern?

*There is no suggestion that children with less experience of prone lying do not reach the same physical, social and cognitive milestones but may get there in different ways.

ACTIVITY BOX 10.5

Damage to the brain, at, before or just after birth will result in a condition called cerebral palsy which is a nonprogressive (doesn't get worse) disability characterised by abnormal movement and posture. Depending on which part of the brain has been affected there may also be associated problems with behaviour, learning, vision, hearing and speech.

As a result of this condition the child may be unable to hold or manipulate objects on their own.

What do you think will be the effect of this on social and cognitive development as the child grows?

Consider things like feeding, playing or even using a computer or mobile phone.

---

that we lose functional movements, which generally starts with losing the ability to cut your toenails and ends with the inability to feed yourself (Kingston et al., 2012).

Ageing

The world population of adults aged 60 years and over is growing faster than any other age group. In 2017 there were 962 million people aged 60 or over worldwide (13% of the world's population); this is estimated to increase at a rate of 3% per year (United Nations, Department of Economic and Social Affairs, Population Division, 2017). This increased life expectancy has been accompanied by an increase in the incidence and prevalence of the noncommunicable diseases associated with ageing (World Health Organisation [WHO], 2011a). One example of this is the prevalence (percentage of people within a defined population that have a specific condition) of dementia, which has increased dramatically in recent decades from 2% to 3% for those aged 70 to 75 years, to 20% to 25% for those aged 85 years and older (Rizzi et al., 2014). General levels of disability are also increasing with an ageing population, with a global disability prevalence of 38% among people aged 60 years and over (WHO, 2011b). The shift towards an aged population increases the economic burden on society in terms of increased health care and pension costs (Slottje and Rogers, 2016), which are all to be paid for by a smaller proportion of the population who are of working age.

The age-related physiological changes in body structures and functions, described in Table 10.3, can have a great impact on the quality of life of older adults. Changes in the cardiovascular and respiratory system can lead to fatigue, decreased exercise capacity and, if severe, to diseases such as heart failure (Gupta et al., 2015; Fleg and Strait, 2012; Strait and Lakatta, 2012; Zeleznik, 2003). Changes in the musculoskeletal system can cause muscle weakness, osteoporosis and increased risk of injury from falls (Frontera, 2017; Gomes et al., 2017). Neurological, vestibular and proprioceptive changes can contribute to an increased risk of falls, reduced dual task ability and other balance problems (Allen et al., 2016; Seidler et al., 2010; Goble et al., 2009). Sensory changes in vision and hearing can have a tremendous effect on quality of life in addition to directly affecting mobility (Aqmon et al., 2017; Chader and Taylor, 2013).

Age-Related Changes in Cognition and Psychology

Cognitive Function and Ageing

As with child development, motor skills and cognition are inextricably linked. In addition to the above mentioned age-related structural changes in the brain (e.g. loss of grey matter), cognitive decline is well documented in domains such as memory, fluid intelligence, executive function

TABLE 10.3   Age Related-Changes in Body Structure and Function

Body System	Structural Changes	Functional Changes
Cardiovascular system (Gupta et al., 2015; Strait and Lakatta, 2012)	↑ myocardial thickness ↑ left ventricular wall thickness ↓ in pacemaker cells ↓ myocardial contractility ↑ vascular stiffness ↑ arterial diameter ↑ arterial stiffness	↓ early diastolic filling rate Increased arrhythmias ↑ systolic blood pressure
Respiratory system (Skloot, 2017; Zeleznik, 2003)	Alveolar dilation ↓ alveolar surface area ↓ pulmonary blood volume ↑ elastin to collagen ratio ↓ expiratory airway diameter Calcification of the rib articulations Distal airway enlargement (emphysema) ↓ respiratory muscle mass	↓ ability to transfer oxygen across alveolar capillary membrane ↓ elastic lung recoil ↓ respiratory muscle strength ↓ vital capacity ↓ forced expiratory volume in 1 s ↑ forced residual capacity and residual volume
Neurologic system (Liu et al., 2016; Seidler et al., 2010)	↓ grey matter volume ↓ white matter volume ↓ production of acetylcholine ↓ concentration of serotonin ↓ norepinephrine levels ↓ dopamine transmission	↓ memory and learning Motor dysfunction ↓ motor learning ability
Musculoskeletal system (Frontera, 2017; Gomes et al., 2017)	↓ muscle mass ↓ in type II muscle fibres ↓ number of motor units ↓ tendon elasticity ↓ ligament strength ↓ bone mineral density ↓ chondrocytes	↓ muscle strength ↓ motor control ↑ risk of tendon, cartilage and ligament injury ↑ risk of osteoporosis
Vision (Chader and Taylor, 2013; Gipson, 2013; Petrash, 2013)	↑ lens density ↓ ability of the lens to change in shape (presbyopia) Increased intra-ocular pressure ↓ hydration of the vitreous body ↓ receptors in the retina and macula ↓ tear production	↑ risk for cataract ↓ accommodation to changes in light ↓ visual acuity Floating bodies Dry eyes
Auditory (Chislom et al., 2003)	↑ stiffness of the tympanic membrane ↓ neurons in the cochlea and auditory centre in the brain	Age-related hearing loss
Vestibular (Allen et al., 2016)	↓ hair cells in the semicircular canals Degeneration of vestibular ganglion and nerve ↓ neurons in the vestibular nuclei Decreased cerebellar volume	↑ incidence of benign paroxysmal positional vertigo and dizziness
Proprioception (Goble et al., 2009)	↓ cutaneous and joint receptors Change in the sensitivity of the receptors ↓ central processing of proprioceptive information	↓ joint position sense ↓ kinaesthesia ↓ dynamic position sense

(Activity Box 10.6), attention and processing speed. However, some other cognitive functions seem to be immune to ageing, such as crystallised intelligence (ability to use the knowledge gained through experience, *wisdom*), language and visual recognition (Harada et al., 2013; Activity Box 10.7).

Age-Related Anxiety and Depression

Depression is one of the most common affective disorders in older adults, with a prevalence of 17.1% for depressive and 7.2% for major depression disorders (Luppa et al., 2012). However, there is also contradictory evidence that anxiety and depression may be less prevalent in older adults than in young adults (Jorm, 2000). This has been explained by reduced responsiveness to negative emotions and greater control of emotion among older adults (Jorm, 2000).

Older adults with limitations in mobility or sedentary lifestyle are at a higher risk of developing depression (Lampinen and Heikkinen, 2003). Why do you think this might be the case? Depression is also associated with an increased risk of frailty in older age (Vaughan et al., 2015). So, perhaps it is not the ageing itself but the loss of movement and independence that leads to depression and anxiety.

Age-Related Changes in Motivation and Self-Regulation

Self-regulation is the ability to control your feelings, to cheer yourself up when you are feeling down or to keep yourself calm when you get upset.

ACTIVITY BOX 10.6 Age-Related Changes in Posture

Age-related changes in the musculoskeletal system can affect the posture of older adults.

Think of four postural changes that can be seen in older adults and how these might impact on daily function.

1.
2.
3.
4.

ACTIVITY BOX 10.7 Cognition in Everyday Activities

Ageing can negatively impact on cognitive functions. How can these changes in cognition affect an older adult's everyday life? Think about all the things you do between getting up in the morning to going to sleep at night that requires some thought.

There is conflicting evidence on the changes in self-regulation with ageing. Some findings suggest that older adults have better self-regulation than young adults due to greater emotional stability, while other research has shown that older adults have poorer self-regulation due to a deterioration in their executive function (National Research Council, 2006), which is the decision-making part of your brain.

The relationship between age and health behaviour changes (e.g. becoming more physically active to reduce morbidity) has been described as a U-shaped curve where young adults and young-old adults (60 to 70 years old) are more likely to change their health behaviour, whereas middle-aged and old-old adults show poor health behaviour change (Zanjani et al., 2006). Why do you think middle-aged adults are less able to modify their health-related behaviours, such as alcohol consumption, smoking and sedentary living?

The Impact of Ageing on Mobility

Fatigue

The prevalence of fatigue increases with age (Zengarini et al., 2015). A prevalence as high as 68% has been reported in the population aged 85 years and over (Moreh et al., 2010) and up to 98% in frail older adults living in nursing homes (Liao and Ferrell, 2000). Fatigue is linked to dependency and disability in ADL and to low levels of physical activity (Moreh et al., 2010). Fatigue is a symptom that emerges from a combination of the physiological changes in ageing, for example, decreased muscle mass, reduced exercise tolerance (cardiovascular and respiratory changes) and psychological factors such as depression and anxiety. Poorer sleep patterns are also a likely factor. It is worth noting that the muscles themselves become less efficient with ageing; that is, they need more energy to create a contraction. Even activities such as bed making show higher energy expenditure when compared to values recorded by healthy young/middle-aged adults (Christie et al., 2014).

Activities of Daily Living

In general terms, ADL performance declines with age (Hortobágyi et al., 2003). However, this is not consistent across the population with factors such as health and social support (Femia et al., 1997) affecting people differently. Medical conditions associated with ageing (e.g. diabetes, coronary heart disease, hypertension, osteoporosis and cognitive impairment) are associated with poorer ADL performance in older adults (Wang et al., 2002). Hospital admission also negatively affects ADL performance in older adults, with 35% of them having poorer performance on discharge than when they were admitted (Covinsky et al., 2003; Activity Box 10.8).

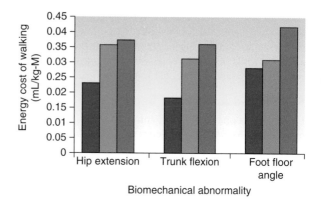

Fig. 10.7 Energy Cost of Walking With Different Grades of Biomechanical Abnormalities (Reprinted with permission from VanSwearingen, J.M., Studenski, S.A., 2014. Aging, motor skill, and the energy cost of walking: implications for the prevention and treatment of mobility decline in older persons. J. Gerontol. A Biol. Sci. Med. Sci. 69 [11], 1429–1436.)

Longitudinal data suggest that the capacity to perform basic ADL deteriorates with age in a predictable manner; the sequence is loss of ability to: (1) walk, (2) bathe, (3) transfer, (4) dress, (5) toilet and then (6) feed (Kingston et al., 2012). Becoming dependent in three or more ADL suggests general frailty and has been found to be a strong predictor for nursing home admission (Gaugler et al., 2007). These are useful things to know as they can help individual therapists and the whole health service develop targeted interventions to stop an older adult moving from being unable to walk to being unable to bathe, or at least to slow this process down through assistive technologies and rehabilitation.

Gait

The age-related changes, outlined above, can lead to observable postural and movement abnormalities during gait (e.g. increased trunk flexion, decreased foot-to-floor angle and decreased hip extension), creating a slower, more energy inefficient walking pattern, that is, it takes more energy to take each step (VanSwearingen and Studneski, 2014) (Fig. 10.7). So, not only is it mechanically more difficult to walk but the muscles required to propel the body forward need more energy. Therefore walking endurance is, unsurprisingly, reduced in older adults.

Differences in temporo-spatial gait characteristics (step/stride length, plus gait speed and cadence) have been consistently reported between young and older adults, such as decreased gait speed, increased step time variability, shorter step length and increased double support time in the older population (McKay et al., 2017; Menz et al., 2003).

One of the clearest predictors of decline in function and mortality in older adults is gait speed (Studenski et al., 2011; Abellan Van Kan et al., 2009). Older adults walking faster than 0.82 m/s (about 3 km/h) are less likely to die in the following 5 years than those who walk slower than 0.82 m/s (Stanaway et al., 2011). This intriguing statistic, quoted as being the speed that death walks, reinforces the importance of maintaining a good walking speed to keep ahead of death! The relationship between gait speed and falls risk in older adults has been described as a U-shaped relationship where both fast and slow gait speeds are associated with a greater risk of falls (Quach et al., 2011) than a normal gait speed (1 to 1.3 m/s) (Fig. 10.8).

Age-Related Changes in Other Functional Movements
Stair Negotiation

Stair negotiation is considered to be one of the most difficult activities to perform by older adults (Verghese et al., 2008). Based on peak knee joint moments, this activity requires near maximal force production in older adults compared to young adults (Hortobágyi et al., 2003). Of deaths from falls, 10% occur on stairs (Startzell et al., 2000). The variety in stair structure and environment, the physiological changes associated with ageing and the burden of disease contribute to the difficulty of this activity in this population (Startzell et al., 2000).

Reduced foot clearance during stair negotiation is considered to be a major contributor to these stair falls (Hamel et al., 2005) and has been the subject of several research studies (Muhaidat et al., 2011). Reduced foot clearance may be caused by a number of age-related changes, such as reduced muscle strength, fatigue, loss of joint flexibility, impaired sensory perception (proprioception) and reduced motor control (Chiu et al., 2015).

Sit-to-Stand

Older adults perform an average of 71 sit-to-stand transitions per day (Grant et al, 2011). Sit-to-stand performance has

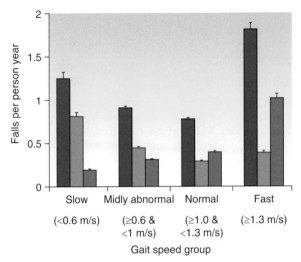

Fig. 10.8 U-Shaped Relationship Between Gait Speed and Falls. (Reprinted with permission from Quach, L., Galica, A.M., Jones, R.N., Procter-Gray, E., Manor, B., Hannan, M.T., Lipsitz, L.A. 2011. The non-linear relationship between gait speed and falls: The MOBILIZ Boston Study. J. Am. Geriatr. Soc. 59 (6), 1069–1073.)

been associated with factors such as proprioception, lower extremity muscle strength and balance (Lord et al., 2002)—all of which decline with age. A reduced ability to perform this activity is associated with sarcopenia reduction in skeletal muscle mass in older adults unable to perform 10 continuous sit-to-stand movements (Abe et al., 2016) and is a predictor of becoming institutionalised within a year. After all, if you cannot stand up from a chair on your own, then dressing, toileting and feeding will be very difficult. The association between sarcopenia and sit-to-stand performance may simply be due to reduced muscle activation. If you are not doing many sit-to-stand movements you are (probably) not standing up very much. Reduced muscle activation will result in reduced muscle mass.

As a mechanically difficult task (lifting your body weight up against gravity) and at the same time being functionally very important, the sit-to-stand task has been used as a single general physical test in older people. For example, poor performance on the 30-second sit-to-stand test (number of successful repetitions completed in 30s) is associated with a higher risk of falls among institutionalised older adults (Applebaum et al., 2017).

Stooping Down to Pick Up an Object

Bending down to pick up an object from the floor has been identified as a difficult dual task by older females, requiring

substantial strength, balance and coordination (Muhaidat et al., 2010). Stooping, crouching and kneeling have been reported as difficult activities by older adults (Hernandez, Murphy and Alexander, 2008). Factors such as self-reported lower limb impairment, low balance confidence and weak knee muscles have been associated with increased difficulty in this task by older adults (Hernandez et al., 2008).

Upper Extremity Tasks

Upper extremity function is of high importance to maintain independence in later life, especially in ADL (Desrosiers et al., 1995). Upper extremity function is affected by the above-mentioned age-related physiological changes. Performing upper extremity tasks by older adults necessitates the activation of more brain regions compared to younger adults, highlighting the amount of attention required to complete these skilled movements. Moreover, reaction times and joint coordination are poorer in older adults, affecting performance time (they get slower) and accuracy (greater number of errors) (Sebastjan et al., 2017; Coats et al., 2016). These changes in upper extremity task performance become more evident with increasing task difficulty (Coats et al., 2016), as you might imagine.

Slower elbow flexion speed has been associated with frailty in older adults (Toosizadeh et al., 2015) and again this is likely to result from the loss of muscle fibres, predominantly the fast twitch (type 2a and 2b) involved in for high velocity contractions, as well as reduced joint flexibility and coordination/motor control.

Falls in Older Adults

Annually, 30% of adults aged 65 years and older, and 50% of those aged 80 years and older experience falls (Rubenstein and Josephson, 2002). There are over 400 identified multifactorial risk factors for falls (Masud and Morris, 2001). The risk factors can be (1) intrinsic, such as age, female gender, previous history of falls, gait and balance problems, and reduced muscle strength and power, and polypharmacy (≥4 medications); or (2) extrinsic, such as environmental hazards, footwear, and wrongly used assistive devices (Skelton and Todd, 2004).

Most falls do not result in serious injuries. However, 10% to 15% of falls result in fractures (Berry and Miller, 2008), 25% of which occur at the hip with potentially fatal consequences (Nevitt et al., 1989). Falls can also result in the person lying on the floor for a long time, risking dehydration, hypothermia, pneumonia and death (Fleming and Brayne, 2008).

Falls can result in depression, anxiety and fear of falling. This is termed the post-fall syndrome (Skelton and Todd, 2004). These psychological consequences can lead to activity and movement avoidance, which unintentionally increases the risk of falls due to muscle weakness and balance impairments caused by the lack of activity (Rubenstein and Josephson, 2002).

Ageing and Physical Activity

The benefits of physical activity for older adults have been well established in the literature (see chapter 14 for more details). Physical activity can have a positive impact on the physical, psychological and cognitive well-being of older adults. Some of these benefits are highlighted in Fig. 10.9.

Physical activity guidelines devised by the WHO state that older adults should engage in at least 150 minutes of moderate, or 75 minutes of vigorous, intensity aerobic physical activity per week or a combination of both. This should be performed in bouts of 10 minutes. Moreover, they should perform strengthening exercise for the major muscle groups at least twice a week, and if they are at risk of falling, they should perform balance exercise at least three times a week (WHO, 2010). The percentage of adults meeting the guidelines for physical activity declines with age, with almost half of adults aged 80 years and over not meeting recommended levels (Bauman et al., 2016).

Time spent being sedentary (sitting and lying) is being increasingly recognised as a factor for poor health and well-being in adults, young and old. Older adults spend on average 5.3 to 9.4 hours in sedentary behaviour per day (Harvey et al., 2015). Sedentary behaviour has been associated with poor health outcomes (Dogra and Stathokostas, 2012); therefore efforts should be made to break up periods of sedentary behaviour in addition to increasing physical activity in older adults.

Plasticity in Older Adults

These age-related changes in physiology, cognition and general function described above probably come across a little negatively. These are the hard facts, but many of the changes are modifiable through activity and exercise. Muscle mass can be maintained and even increased in older adults (Martins et al., 2015) and the brain retains its plasticity (Calero and Navarro, 2004) (i.e. it can learn [or re-learn] new movements). This has been shown even in older adults with neurological conditions such as Parkinson disease (Petzinger et al., 2013). There is plenty of scope to recover functional abilities among older adults through physical activity and rehabilitation. The next section will take you through a case study aimed to get you thinking about geriatric rehabilitation.

Geriatric Rehabilitation Case Study
History

ML is an 82-year-old female, who has been referred to physiotherapy for management of falls risk due to having five falls in the previous year. ML lives alone in a one-bedroom apartment on the second floor of a high-rise building.

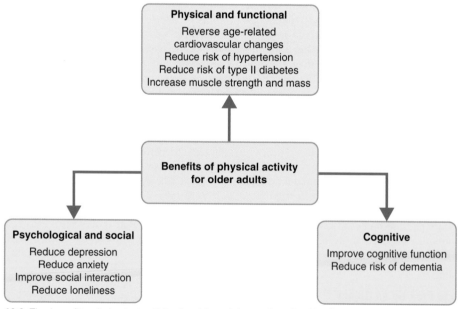

Fig. 10.9 The benefits of physical activity for older adults as described by Bauman et al. (2016) and Taylor et al. (2004).

TABLE 10.4   Performance on Clinical Scores.

Assessment Tool	Score	Interpretation
TUG	20 s	High risk of falling
FES-I	19	High concern about falling
30-s chair stand test	6	Risk of falling
POMA	16	High risk of falls
Osteoporosis Risk Score	10	Moderate risk

FES-I, Falls Efficacy Scale-International; *POMA*, Performance-Oriented Mobility Assessment; *TUG*, Timed Up and Go test.

Her daughter helps her with the house chores and grocery shopping once a week. ML was a very active person and used to enjoy going on walks with her dog and meeting her friends at the sewing club. However, in the last year she has limited her outings and stopped going to the sewing club as she is afraid of falling and injuring herself. Her goal from physiotherapy is to be able to take her dog on walks again.

Physiotherapy Assessment

The physiotherapist assessed ML's functional balance using the Timed Up and Go test, fear of falling using the short form Falls Efficacy Scale—International, lower extremity muscle strength using the 30-second chair stand test, gait using the Performance-Oriented Mobility Assessment test and osteoporosis risk using the Osteoporosis Risk Score. The results of the assessment are in Table 10.4.

Management

ML was referred to a group falls prevention exercise class that consisted of a multicomponent exercise programme (strengthening, balance, flexibility and endurance). This has been shown to be effective in reducing the incidence of falls and in increasing balance confidence in older adults (Kumar et al., 2016; Sherrington and Tiedemann, 2015). ML was advised to perform an individualised home exercise to improve her strength and balance as this also has been shown to help reduce the risk of falls (Hill et al., 2015).

ML agreed to install an automatic fall detection system in her home, which could reduce the chance of a long time

ACTIVITY BOX 10.9   Assistive Devices

Technology can have a great impact on improving the quality of life. Older adults are no exception to this.

Think of two different assistive technologies that might have been used to help ML remain independent in daily living.

Think of two barriers to the use of these technologies by older adults.

lying on the floor and improve her confidence (Hawley-Hague et al., 2014).

She will continue to be reviewed annually by the team and has been referred to the mobility centre to consider the use of assistive devices to keep her independent in the home and the local community for as long as possible (Activity Box 10.9).

The Motivation to Move

The motivation to move has been mentioned throughout this chapter. Early movement was reflexive, but volitional movement required a starting point; for example, the baby's desire to touch the object they are staring at, to find out what it feels like. There are plenty of sensory rewards for the baby: touch, sound, vision, taste. The sensory reward for movement strengthens the pattern and provides the motivation to do it again and again. Repetition is critical if the movement is to become automatic. What motivates an older adult to move (what rewards their efforts) is quite different. The desire to maintain independence and avoid illnesses caused by sedentary living may be important motivators for older adults to move. Ultimately, as Bandura suggests, motivation is an intrinsic thing, and individuals have their own motivations to move. As therapists you have to find that motivation.

This chapter has looked at movement from both ends of the life curve. In the development and decline of movement ability, the physical, cognitive and psychological functions have been considered and the importance of motivation stressed. Before you finish the chapter have a look at the following self-assessment questions and then go back to the learning outcomes and reflect on whether you have achieved them.

SELF-ASSESSMENT QUESTIONS

1. Describe the upper and lower limb response of a newborn baby if their head is turned to the left.
2. By what age (an estimate is fine) would you expect an infant to start pulling themselves up into standing?
3. What happens during observational learning, according to Bandura?
4. What kind of thing motivates an infant/child to move?
5. When does movement begin?
6. What are the physical benefits of physical activity for older adults?
7. What are the age-related changes in the musculoskeletal system?
8. Describe the physical activity guidelines for older adults.
9. Provide three intrinsic and three extrinsic risk factors for falls in older adults.
10. What type of exercise is effective in reducing falls risk in older adults?

REFERENCES

Abe, T., Yaginuma, Y., Fujita, E., Thiebaud, R.S., Kawanishi, M., Akamine, T., 2016. Association of sit-up ability with sarcopenia classification measures in Japanese older women. Int. Med. Appl. Sci. 8 (4), 152–157.

Abellan van Kan, G., Rolland, Y., Andrieu, S., Bauer, J., Beauchet, O., Bonnefoy, M., et al., 2009. Gait speed at usual pace as a predictor of adverse outcomes in community-dwelling older people an international Academy on nutrition and aging (IANA) task force. J. Nutr. Health Aging 13 (10), 881–889.

Allen, D., Rbeiro, L., Arshad, Q., Seemungal, B.M., 2016. Age-related vestibular loss: current understanding and future research directions. Front. Neurol. 19, 7–231. doi:10.3389/fneur.2016.00231.

Applebaum, E.B., Breton, D., Feng, Z.W., Ta, A.T., Walsh, K., Chassé, K., et al., 2017. Modified 30-second sit to stand test predicts falls in a cohort of institutionalized older veterans. PLoS ONE 12 (5), e0176946. doi:10.1371/journal.pone.0176946.

Aqmon, M., Lavie, L., Doumas, M., 2017. The association between hearing loss, postural control, and mobility in older adults: a systematic review. J. Am. Acad. Audiol. 28 (6), 575–588.

Bauman, A., Merom, D., Bull, F.C., Buchner, D.M., Fiatarone Singh, M.A., 2016. Updating the evidence for physical activity: summative reviews of the epidemiological evidence, prevalence, and interventions to promote "active Aging". Gerontologist 56 (S2), S268–S280.

Berry, S.D., Miller, R.R., 2008. Falls, Epidemiology, pathophysiology and relationship to fracture. Curr. Osteoporos. Rep. 6 (4), 149–154.

Calero, M.D., Navarro, E., 2004. Relationship between plasticity, mild cognitive impairment and cognitive decline. Arch. Clin. Neuropsychol. 19 (5), 653–660.

Capute, A.J., Shapiro, B.K., Palmer, F.B., Ross, A., Wachtel, R.C., 1985. Normal gross motor development: the influences of race, sex and socioeconomic status. Dev. Med. Child Neurol. 27 (5), 635–643.

Chader, G.J., Taylor, A., 2013. The aging eye: normal changes, age-related diseases, and sight-saving approaches. Invest. Ophthalmol. Vis. Sci. 54 (14), ORSF1–ORSF4. doi:10.1167/iovs.13-12993.

Christie, A.D., Tonson, A., Larsen, R.G., DeBlois, J.P., Kent, J.A., 2014. Human skeletal muscle metabolic economy in vivo: effects of contraction intensity, age, and mobility impairment. Am. J. Physiol. Regul. Integr. Comp. Physiol. 307 (9), R1124–R1135.

Chislom, T.H., Willot, J.F., Lister, J.L., 2003. The aging auditory system: anatomic and physiologic changes and implications for rehabilitation. Int. J. Audiol. 42 (Suppl. 2), 2S3–2S10.

Chiu, S.L., Chang, C.C., Dennerlein, J.T., Xu, X., 2015. Age-related differences in inter-joint coordination during stair walking transitions. Gait Posture 42 (2), 152–157.

Coats, R.O., Fath, A.J., Astill, S.L., Wann, J.P., 2016. Eye and hand movement strategies in older adults during a complex reaching task. Exp. Brain Res. 234 (2), 533–547.

Covinsky, K.E., Palmer, R.M., Fortinsky, R.H., Counsell, S.R., Stewart, A.L., Kresevic, D., et al., 2003. Loss of independence in activities of daily living in older adults hospitalized with medical illness: increased vulnerability with age. J. Am. Geriatr. Soc. 51, 451–458.

de Vries, J.I.P., Fong, B.F., 2006. Normal fetal motility: an overview. Ultrasound Obstet. Gynecol. 27, 701–711.

Desrosiers, J., Hébert, R., Bravo, G., Dutil, E., 1995. Upper extremity performance test for the elderly (TEMPA): normative data and correlates with sensorimotor parameters. Arch. Phys. Med. Rehabil. 76 (12), 1125–1129.

Dogra, S., Stathokostas, L., 2012. Sedentary behavior and physical activity are independent predictors of successful aging in middle-aged and older adults. J. Aging Res. 190654. [Epub 2012].

Femia, E.E., Zarit, S.H., Johansson, B., 1997. Predicting change in activities of daily living: a longitudinal study of the oldest old in Sweden. J. Gerontol. Psychol. Sci. 52B (6), P294–P302.

Fleg, S.L., Strait, J., 2012. Age-associated changes in cardiovascular structure and function: a fertile milieu for future disease. Heart Fail. Rev. 17 (4–5), 545–554.

Fleming, J., Brayne, C., 2008. Inability to get up after falling, subsequent time on floor, and summoning help: prospective cohort study in people over 90. BMJ 337, a2227. doi:10.1136/bmj.a2227.

Fox, A.T., Palmer, R.D., Davies, P., 2002. Do "shufflebottoms" bottom shuffle? Arch. Dis. Child. 87 (6), 552–554.

Frontera, W.R., 2017. Physiologic changes of the musculoskeletal system with aging: a brief review. Phys. Med. Rehabil. Clin. North Am. 28 (4), 705–711.

Gaugler, J.E., Duval, S., Anderson, K.A., Kane, R.L., 2007. Predicting nursing home admissions in the u.S: a meta-analysis. BMC Geriatr. 7, 13. doi:10.1186/1471-2318-7-13.

Gipson, I.K., 2013. Age-related changes and diseases of the ocular surface and cornea. Invest. Ophthalmol. Vis. Sci. 54 (14), ORSF48–ORSF53. doi:10.1167/iovs.13-12840.

Goble, D.J., Coxon, J.P., Wenderoth, N., Van Impe, A., Swinnen, S.P., 2009. Proprioceptive sensibility in the elderly: degeneration, functional consequences and plastic-adaptive processes. Neurosci. Behav. Rev. 33 (3), 271–278.

Gomes, M.J., Martinez, P.F., Pagan, L.U., Damatto, R.L., Cezar, M.D.M., Lima, A.R.R., et al., 2017. Skeletal muscle aging: influence of oxidative stress and physical exercise. Oncotarget 8 (12), 20428–20440.

Grant, P.M., Dall, P.M., Kerr, A., 2011. Daily and hourly frequency of the sit to stand movement in older adults: a comparison of day hospital, rehabilitation ward and community living groups. Aging Clin. Exp. Res. 23 (5–6), 437–444.

Gupta, D., Verma, S., Pun, S.C., Steingart, R.M., 2015. The changes in cardiac physiology with aging and the implications for the treating oncologist. J. Geriatr. Oncol. 6 (3), 178–184.

Hamel, K.A., Okita, N., Higginson, J.S., Cavanagh, P.R., 2005. Foot clearance during stair descent: effects of age and illumination. Gait Posture 21 (2), 135–140.

Harada, C.N., Natelson Love, M.C., Triebel, K., 2013. Normal cognitive aging. Clin. Geriatr. Med. 29 (4), 737–752.

Harvey, J.A., Chastin, S.F., Skelton, D.A., 2015. How sedentary are older people? A systematic review of the amount of sedentary behavior. J. Aging Phys. Act. 23 (3), 471–487.

Hawley-Hague, H., Boulton, E., Hall, A., Pfeiffer, K., Todd, C., 2014. Older adults' perceptions of technologies aimed at falls prevention, detection or monitoring: a systematic review. Int. J. Med. Inform. 83 (6), 416–426.

Hernandez, M.E., Murphy, S.L., Alexander, N.B., 2008. Characteristics of older adults with Self-Reported stooping, crouching, or kneeling difficulty. J. Gerontol. A Biol. Sci. Med. Sci. 63 (7), 759–763.

Hill, K.D., Hunter, S.W., Batchelor, F.A., Cavalheri, V., Burton, E., 2015. Individualized home-based exercise programs for older people to reduce falls and improve physical performance: a systematic review and meta-analysis. Maturitas 82 (1), 72–84.

Hortobágyi, T., Mizelle, C., Beam, S., DeVita, P., 2003. Old adults perform activities of daily living near their maximal capabilities. J. Gerontol. A Biol. Sci. Med. Sci. 58 (5), M453–M460.

Jeng, S.F., Liao, H.F., Lai, J.S., Hou, J.W., 1997. Optimization of walking in children. Med. Sci. Sports Exerc. 29 (3), 370–376.

Jorm, A.F., 2000. Does old age reduce the risk of anxiety and depression? A review of epidemiological studies across the adult life span. Psychol. Med. 30 (1), 11–22.

Kingston, A., Collerton, J., Davies, K., Bond, J., Robinson, L., Jagger, C., 2012. Losing the ability in activities of daily living in the oldest old: a hierarchic disability scale from the newcastle 85+ study. PLoS ONE 7 (2), e31665.

Kumar, A., Delbaere, K., Zijlstra, G.A.R., Carpenter, H., Iliffe, S., Masud, T., et al., 2016. Exercise for reducing fear of falling in older people living in the community: cochrane systematic review and meta-analysis. Age. Ageing 45 (3), 345–352.

Lampinen, P., Heikkinen, E., 2003. Reduced mobility and physical activity as predictors of depressive symptoms among community-dwelling older adults: an eight-year follow-up study. Aging Clin. Exp. Res. 15 (3), 205–211.

Liao, S., Ferrell, B.A., 2000. Fatigue in an older population. J. Am. Geriatr. Soc. 48 (4), 426–430.

Liu, H., Yang, Y., Xia, Y., Zhu, W., Leak, R.K., Wei, Z., et al., 2016. Aging of cerebral white matter. Ageing Res. Rev. 34, 64–76.

Lord, S.R., Murray, S.M., Chapman, K., Munro, B., Tiedemann, A., 2002. Sit-to-stand performance depends on sensation, speed, balance, and psychological status in addition to strength in older people. J. Gerontol. A Biol. Sci. Med. Sci. 57 (8), M539–M543.

Luppa, M., Sikorski, C., Luck, T., Ehreke, L., Konnopka, A., Wiese, B., et al., 2012. Age and gender specific prevalence of depression in latest life: systematic review and meta-analysis. J. Affect. Disord. 136 (3), 212–221.

Martins, W.R., Safons, M.P., Bottaro, M., Blaszcyk, J.C., Diniz, L.R., Fonseca, R.M.C., et al., 2015. Effects of short term elastic resistance training on muscle mass and strength in untrained older adults: a randomized clinical trial. BMC Geriatr. 15 (1), 99.

Masud, T., Morris, R.O., 2001. Epidemiology of falls. Age Ageing (Suppl 4), 3–7.

McKay, M.J., Baldwin, J.N., Ferreira, P., Simic, M., Vanicek, N., Wojciechowski, E., et al. 1000 Norms Project Consortium, 2017. Spatiotemporal and plantar pressure patterns of 1000 healthy individuals aged 3-101 years. Gait Posture 58, 78–87. doi:10.1016/j.gaitpost.2017.07.004.

Menz, H.B., Lord, S.R., Fitzpatrick, R.C., 2003. Age- related differences in walking stability. Age. Ageing 32 (2), 137–142.

Moreh, E., Jacobs, J.M., Stessman, J., 2010. Fatigue, function, and mortality in older adults. J. Gerontol. A Biol. Sci. Med. Sci. 65 (8), 887–895.

Muhaidat, J., Kerr, A., Rafferty, D., Skelton, D.A., Evans, J.J., 2011. Measuring foot placement and clearance during stair descent. Gait Posture 33 (3), 504–506.

Muhaidat, J., Skelton, D.A., Kerr, A., Evans, J.J., Ballinger, C., 2010. Older adults' experiences and perceptions of dual tasking. Br. J. Occup. Ther. 73 (9), 405–412.

National Research Council, 2006. When I'm 64. Committee on aging frontiers in social psychology, Personality, and adult developmental psychology. In: Carstensen, L.L., Hartel, C.R. (Eds.), Board on Behavioral, Cognitive, and Sensory

Sciences, Division of Behavioral and Social Sciences and Education. The National Academies Press, Washington, DC.

Nevitt, M.C., Cummings, S.R., Kidd, S., Black, D., 1989. Risk factors for recurrent nonsyncopal falls: a prospective study. JAMA 261 (18), 2663–2668.

Petrash, J.M., 2013. Aging and age-related diseases of the ocular lens and vitreous body. Invest. Ophthalmol. Vis. Sci. 54 (14), ORSF54–ORSF59. doi:10.1167/iovs.13-12940.

Petzinger, J.M., Fisher, B.E., McEwen, S., Beeler, J.A., Walsh, J.P., Jakowec, M.W., 2013. Exercise-enhanced neuroplasticity targeting motor and cognitive circuitry in Parkinson's disease. Lancet Neurol. 12 (7), 716–726.

Quach, L., Galica, A.M., Jones, R.N., Procter-Gray, E., Manor, B., Hannan, M.T., et al., 2011. The non-linear relationship between gait speed and falls: the MOBILIZ Boston study. J. Am. Geriatr. Soc. 59 (6), 1069–1073.

Rizzi, L., Rossit, I., Roriz-Cruz, M., 2014. Global epidemiology of dementia: Alzheimer's and vascular types. Biomed Res. Int. doi:10.1155/2014/908915.

Robson, P., 1984. Prewalking locomotor movements and their use in predicting standing and walking. Child Care Health Dev. 10 (5), 317–330.

Rochat, P., 1992. Self-sitting and reaching in 5- to 8-month-old infants: the impact of posture and its development on early eye–hand coordination. J. Motor Behav. 24, 210–220.

Rubenstein, L.Z., Josephson, K.R., 2002. The epidemiology of falls and syncope. Clin. Geriatr. Med. 18 (2), 141–158.

Schneiberg, S., Sveistrup, H., McFadyen, B., McKinley, P., Levin, M.F., 2002. The development of coordination for reach-to-grasp movements in children. Exp. Brain Res. 146 (2), 142–154.

Sebastjan, A., Skrzek, A., Ignasiak, Z., Sławińska, T., 2017. Age-related changes in hand dominance and functional asymmetry in older adults. PLoS ONE 12 (5), e0177845. doi:10.1371/journal.pone.0177845.

Seidler, R.D., Bernard, J.A., Burutolu, T.B., Bling, B.W., Gordon, M.T., Gwin, J.T., et al., 2010. Motor control and aging: links to age-related brain structural, functional, and biochemical effects. Neurosci. Behav. Rev. 34 (5), 721–733.

Shea, C.A., Rolfe, R.A., Murphy, P., 2015. The importance of foetal movement for co-ordinated cartilage and bone development in utero. Bone Joint Res. 4 (7), 105–116.

Sherrington, C., Tiedemann, A., 2015. Physiotherapy in the prevention of falls in older people. J. Physiother. 61 (2), 54–60.

Sibley, B.A., Etnier, J.L., 2003. The relationship between physical activity and cognition in children: a meta-analysis. Pediatr. Exerc. Sci. 15 (3), 243–256.

Skelton, D.A., Todd, C., 2004. What Are the Main Risk Factors for Falls Among Older People and What Are the Most Effective Interventions to Prevent These Falls? WHO Regional Office for Europe, Copenhagen. http://www.euro.who.int/document/E82552.pdf. (Accessed 7 December 2017.) (Health Evidence Network report [online].)

Skloot, G.S., 2017. The effect of aging on lung structure and function. Clin. Geriatr. Med. 33 (4), 447–457.

Slottje, D., Rogers, B., 2016. Some thoughts on the economics of ageing, geriatrics and end-of-life. J. Health Med. Econ. 2 (1), 1–7.

Smyke, A.T., Koga, S.F., Johnson, D.E., Fox, N.A., Marshall, P.J., Nelson, C.A., et al. The BEIP Core Group, 2007. The caregiving context in institution-reared and family-reared infants and toddlers in Romania. J. Child Psychol. Psychiatry 48, 210–218.

Stanaway, F.F., Gnjidic, D., Blyth, F.M., Le Couteur, D.G., Naganathan, V., Waite, L., et al., 2011. How fast does the grim reaper walk? Receiver operating characteristics curve analysis in healthy men aged 70 and over. BMJ 343, d7679.

Startzell, J.K., Owens, D.A., Mulfinger, L.M., Cavanagh, P.R., 2000. Stair negotiation in older people: a review. J. Am. Geriatr. Soc. 48 (5), 567–580.

Strait, J.B., Lakatta, E.G., 2012. Aging-associated cardiovascular changes and their relationship to heart failure. Heart Fail. Clin. 8 (1), 143–164.

Studenski, S., Perera, S., Patel, K., Rosano, C., Faulkner, K., Inzitari, M., et al., 2011. Gait speed and survival in older adults. JAMA 305 (1), 50–58.

Taylor, A.H., Cable, N.T., Faulkner, G., Hillsdon, M., Narici, M., Van Der Bij, A.K., 2004. Physical activity and older adults: a review of health benefits and the effectiveness of interventions. J. Sports Sci. 22 (8), 703–725.

Toosizadeh, N., Mohler, J., Najafi, B., 2015. Assessing upper extremity motion: an innovative method to identify frailty. J. Am. Geriatr. Soc. 63 (6), 1181–1186.

United Nations, Department of Economic and Social Affairs, Population Division, 2017. World Population Prospects: The 2017 Revision, Key Findings and Advance Tables. Working Paper No. ESA/P/WP/248.

VanSwearingen, J.M., Studenski, S.A., 2014. Aging, motor skill, and the energy cost of walking: implications for the prevention and treatment of mobility decline in older persons. J. Gerontol. A Biol. Sci. Med. Sci. 69 (11), 1429–1436.

Vaughan, L., Corbin, A.L., Goveas, J.S., 2015. Depression and frailty in later life: a systematic review. Clin. Interv. Aging 10, 1947–1958. doi:10.2147/CIA.S69632.

Verghese, J., Wang, C., Xue, X., Holtzer, R., 2008. Self-reported difficulty in climbing up or down stairs in nondisabled elderly. Arch. Phys. Med. Rehabil. 89 (1), 100–104.

Von Hofsten, C., Rosander, K., 1997. Development of smooth pursuit tracking in young infants. Vis. Res. 37 (13), 1799–1810.

Wang, L., van Belle, G., Kukull, W.B., Larson, E.B., 2002. Predictors of functional change: a longitudinal study of nondemented people aged 65 and older. J. Am. Geriatr. Soc. 50, 1525–1534.

World Health Organization, 2010. Global recommendations on physical activity for health. Available at: http://apps.who.int/iris/bitstream/10665/44399/1/9789241599979_eng.pdf. (Accessed December 7, 2017.)

World Health Organization, 2011a. Global health and aging. Available at: http://www.who.int/ageing/publications/global_health.pdf?ua=1. (Accessed December 7, 2017.)

World Health Organization, 2011b. World report on disability. Available at: http://www.who.int/disabilities/world_report/2011/report.pdf. (Accessed December 7, 2017.)

Zanjani, F.A.K., Schaie, W.K., Willis, S.L., 2006. Age group and health status effects on health behavior change. Behav. Med. 32 (2), 36–46.

Zeleznik, J., 2003. Normative aging of the respiratory system. Clin. Geriatr. Med. 19 (1), 1–18.

Zengarini, E., Ruggiero, C., Pérez-Zepeda, M.U., Hoogendijk, E.O., Vellas, B., Mecocci, P., et al., 2015. Fatigue: relevance and implications in the aging population. Exp. Gerontol. 70, 78–83.

Measurement of Movement

11

Nine Key Things That Define Physical Movement

Philip Rowe

LEARNING OUTCOMES

After reading this chapter, you will be able to:
1. List and define the nine things (parameters) that are generally used to quantify movement.
2. Understand linear and angular definitions of movement and how they mirror each other.
3. Explain how movement parameters are related to each other.
4. Understand how Newton's laws and concepts can be used to understand movement and how it is generated.
5. Understand how combining our understanding of the relationships between the nine parameters used to define movement and Newton's laws allows us to look at the causes of movement in three different but complimentary ways.

INTRODUCTION

When looking at biomechanical and movement studies published in the literature it can seem like there are an endless number of possible movement measures requiring a whole plethora of equipment. In addition, considerable variation is apparent in the processing, analysis and reporting of data and in the selection of variables used to combine or summarise the data. A couple of hours spent browsing the movement analysis literature will illustrate this apparent diversity.

When first accessing the movement analysis literature, it is not immediately apparent that, while techniques of measurement and reporting vary, the vast majority of these studies record one or more of nine key mechanical variables associated with motion, which are:

1. Time
2. Linear displacement
3. Linear velocity
4. Linear acceleration
5. Angular displacement
6. Angular velocity
7. Angular acceleration
8. Force
9. Moment of force.

This chapter seeks to explore these nine basic measures, their definitions, meanings and interrelationships, and how they may be combined and transformed to produce derived variables of value in the study of human motion.

WHAT IS MOTION AND HOW DO WE DESCRIBE IT?

Motion analysis often involves comparison of the subject(s) under examination with a group of their peers. For this comparison to be valid we require a consistent definition of motion to be employed in all tests; hence our discussion of the description of motion should begin with a definition of motion itself.

Although we understand the concept of motion and can recognise it when we see it, defining motion actually proves quite a difficult task. Probably the best definition of motion is given by the following:

> *Motion is the act or process of changing place or position with respect to some reference point or object.*
>
> ### Oxford English Dictionary

This definition contains three important concepts regarding motion.

Motion is an 'act or process'. This implies that motion, and the movement it produces, take place over a period of time. The movement of matter takes time and has a maximum rate of travel set by the speed of light (3×10^8 m/s). According to Einstein's theory of relativity movement velocities in excess of this value are impossible; hence movement will always take time. Therefore time is an important element of movement studies and one of the nine key mechanical variables.

Motion involves 'changing place or position'. In order to 'change place' we are required to change location within the universe. Our position within the universe can be fully described using three parameters; this is the concept of three-dimensional (3D) space. In most motion analysis situations, the distances (translations) along three axes at right angles to each other (orthogonal) are used to define a point in space. These axes are often labelled X, Y and Z, but conventions vary as to which axis is defined as the X, Y or Z axis. This method is known as the Cartesian system and gives 3D Cartesian coordinates. However, other coordinate systems (polar, helical etc.) do exist and are sometimes employed in motion studies.

Changing 'position' can be thought of as involving a change in the orientation of the object (a rotation) rather than a change in the location of the object (a translation). In other words, the object stays where it is but is spinning and hence changing orientation. An example is given by an ice skater executing a spin at one point on the ice. Again in 3D space, three parameters are required to fully define the rotational movement of an object. In human motion analysis studies, it is normal to define these rotations relative to the three orthogonal axes already defined, that is, rotations around the X, Y and Z axes.

Thus the assertion that motion involves 'changing place or position' leads us to the realisation that movement can be fully described by reporting the translation of the centre of the object (in 3D space) and the rotation of the object around its centre (in 3D space). Thus, motion in 3D space has 6 degrees of freedom, three translations and three rotations.

The description of motion using these concepts is known as 'kinematics'. Kinematics is concerned with the geometry of motion. It seeks to describe motion rather than to explain why it occurs, and for this reason it is considered an observational rather than an analytical discipline. The description of translatory motion is known as 'linear kinematics'. Linear kinematics use three mechanical variables to describe linear motion, namely linear displacement, linear velocity and linear acceleration (often abbreviated to displacement, velocity and acceleration). The description of rotary motion is known as 'angular kinematics'. Angular kinematics can be described using a similar set of three mechanical variables, namely angular displacement, angular velocity and angular acceleration. The general motion of an object can therefore be fully described by considering the linear and angular kinematics of the object in 3D space. The description of linear and angular kinematics therefore introduces six more of the key mechanical variables used to investigate human movement.

The third and final point of interest in this definition of motion is that motion takes place 'with respect to some reference point or object'. The reference point or object can be any point in the universe and is very influential in determining what we 'see'. As an example, consider passengers on a train passing a station. They will 'see' the station pass by through the windows while their fellow travellers on the train remain in the same position. They will interpret this as the train moving through the station and leaving it behind. However, it could be that the train is not moving and the station is! The passengers would receive the same visual information as before and would be likely to interpret it as before. It is not very often that you see stations on the move, so in this case the chances of being wrong are small.

However, if you take two objects that we know move around then it is not always so clear which is moving and which is stationary. Imagine sitting in a train in a station when the train at an adjoining platform starts to move. Initially we may think that our train has begun to move and the other train is stationary. It is only when we fail to 'feel' the motion of our train or we observe that other objects, such as the station, have not changed location that we interpret the situation as the other train moving while we are stationary.

Luckily for motion analysis, mechanics recognises no difference in any of these situations except that the reference point or object from which motion is measured is changing. We would say that if the passengers on the train interpret what they see as the train moving and the station staying still, they have chosen the station as the reference point or object for measuring motion. If they choose to see themselves and the train as stationary and the station passing by the window as moving, they have chosen to name the train as the reference point or object from which to measure motion. All motion must be described relative to some other point or object and hence the statement that 'all motion is relative'.

Therefore, when describing motion, we must define the origin of motion against which we will measure movement. The choice of reference point or object will affect the data obtained in human motion studies. For example, consider measuring the angle of inclination of the upper body during gait. Some studies have reported the angle of inclination relative to the vertical, while others have reported it relative to the pelvis. Each method gives a characteristic trace for inclination angle against time. However, the shapes of the curves and the magnitudes of the angles are not the same, and it is not possible to convert from one form to the other because the angle of the pelvis to the vertical is not known. The definition of an appropriate reference point or origin is therefore an important aspect of the protocol of any motion analysis study.

While the definition of motion we have used highlights three key points regarding motion, it is deficient in one aspect. It does not indicate the cause of motion. In our discussion of relative motion above, we often relied on 'feel' to determine whether we were moving or not. Mechanical receptors in the body 'feel' the pushes and pulls applied to the body by gravity, inertia and other objects in contact with the skin. These pushes and pulls are known as forces and it is the interactions of these forces with the body that determine the motion of the body.

By pushing or pulling, forces attempt to change the motion of objects. Forces can stop objects, make them move faster or slower or in different directions; that is, they affect the linear kinematics of the object. In addition, forces applied with a line of action, which does not pass through the centre of mass of an object, produce an effect that causes the object to spin. This effect is known as a moment of force and effects the angular kinematics of the object. Forces and moments control the changes in motion of the object. An analysis of the forces and moments acting on an object can be used to predict its subsequent motion. Therefore forces and moments explain the causes of motion rather than simply describing the motion occurring. This branch of

mechanics is called 'kinetics', which seeks to explain the causes of motion. Kinetics is therefore considered an analytical rather than a purely observational discipline.

This discussion of the causes of motion has introduced the last two of our nine key mechanical variables, namely: 'force' and 'moment of force'. Forces can be defined as 'that which acts to change (or to try to change) the motion of an object'. If the forces acting on an object are not balanced then there will be a net force on the object and the object will begin to move in the direction of the net force, thereby altering the linear kinematics of the object. If the moments of the forces applied to an object do not balance there will be a net moment on the object and the object will begin to spin in the direction of the net moment, thereby altering the angular kinematics of the object. The way in which these interactions effect motion is governed in all circumstances relevant to human movement by Newton's laws of motion, which will be covered later in this chapter. Forces and moments have an important role in changing the motion of objects; hence they are commonly recorded in human movement studies.

By recording all of these nine mechanical variables, we are able to describe motion and analyse the causes of motion. By recording one or more we can use the data to evaluate human movement. The subsequent sections of this chapter will introduce each variable, plus its definition and points of note relevant to human movement studies. We will also explore the interrelationships between these nine variables and how they can be combined or transformed to produce other measures of use in movement studies. Let's begin this process by considering time.

TIME

Time is a vital element of motion. Without a change in time we can have no motion. Conversely, motion must take place over time. This relationship between time and motion is often illustrated in popular fiction using statement such as 'time stood still' and 'frozen in time'. It is only in science fiction that we find motion occurring in the absence of time.

The recording of time is therefore an important element of motion analysis. Some studies record the time required to conduct a task, for example, the time taken to walk 10 m, the time taken to rise from a chair or the time taken to reach and grasp an object. Timings are also used to investigate subcomponents of a task, for example, the stance and swing phase timings in gait and the timing of specific key actions in a task (e.g. back off the seat, thighs off the seat and upright stance during rising to stand from a chair).

While much can be gained from these simple and global measures of performance, the data do not indicate how or why the motion occurred to produce these changes over time. We have little information on the nature or quality of the movement that occurred to produce these overall effects. If we wish to examine the movement more closely, we must record one of the other eight variables and it is here that we encounter the other important issue related to time in motion analysis.

As we have seen, time and motion occur simultaneously. It is usual (though not compulsory) to use time as the independent variable (the variable under our control) and one of the other eight variables as the dependent variable. Put more simply, it is common to record changes in, for example, force against time rather than vice versa. Time has a unique property in that it always advances; hence no ambiguity can occur when recording variables relative to time. It is usual to use time as the independent variable against which other variables are recorded.

Having decided to use time as the control variable for recording, we encounter a second issue that requires resolution. Time is a continuum. The progression of time occurs in infinitesimally small amounts of time. Time is therefore a continuous variable otherwise known as an analogue signal. Most transducers designed to record linear or angular kinematics or kinetics produce a continuous output. In days gone by, such signals were fed into analogue recording devices, such as chart recorders or oscilloscopes, which also gave out a continuous recording. It was up to the investigator to sample this output and to measure data at key points or regular intervals using, for example, a ruler. This process turns the continuous analogue signal into a series of discrete measures usually at regular intervals, which is known as a digital signal. The decisions about when and where to sample the data stream can be left until the results are available. However, this process of sampling the data by hand, after the event, is inaccurate and extremely tedious for the investigator.

The advent of high-speed personal computers has transformed the data collection process. The analogue signal produced by the transducer is often fed directly to an 'analogue to digital converter' device. This device—as its name implies—converts the continuous analogue signal into a series of digital samples (numbers) at regular intervals. The sampling interval can be controlled and can often be made to vary from as much as 20,000 samples per second to as little as one sample per hour.

The use of computers for data recording and analysis has greatly expanded the possibilities for, and the potential of, human motion analysis. However, in order to exploit these gains, the researcher must select a frequency for sampling the incoming signal prior to data recording.

At first sight it might appear a good strategy to 'sample as fast as possible in order to approximate a continuous signal and delay the choice of ultimate sampling frequency until after the data has been recorded'. However, computers have a limited capacity to store data in their memory and at fast sampling speeds they do not have time to store the data to disc. Hence the storage capacity of the computer is limited at high sampling speeds. While the memory capacity of computers has massively expanded, this strategy leads to very large data files, which can be difficult to store, handle and analyse. Alternatively, we might choose to sample slowly to minimise the size of the data files; however, if the sampling rate is too slow, we will miss important events or misrepresent the shape of the curve recorded. This is known as aliasing. Therefore the question is how slowly should we sample in order to properly record the signal and yet store as little data as possible? This is a difficult question to answer. Sampling theory suggests that sampling should occur in excess of twice the highest frequency of interest in the signal you are recording. However, in many motion analysis studies, the frequency distribution of the signal is unknown. Even if the frequency distribution is known, the significance of different frequency components of the signal is often unknown. Hence it is difficult to decide upon a sampling frequency from theory alone.

A more direct and practical approach is to insure the sampling speed is sufficient to record the signal but does not produce an excess of data points. To do this, data representing the activity of interest are recorded at the fastest available sampling speed. Graphs are then drawn of the data including every data point (i.e. at the maximum available sampling frequency), then with every second data point included (i.e. at half the chosen sampling frequency), then with every fourth data point include (i.e. at a quarter of the chosen sampling frequency) etc. The graphs are compared to see at what point the shape of the graph begins to change and the previous sampling frequency (i.e. the last one not to show change) is then selected.

This is a pragmatic method to solve the sampling frequency. As we will see later, we might also be calculating one variable from another; for example, linear velocity is given by the change in linear displacement divided by the time taken for the change to occur. It may be that a particular sampling frequency is sufficient to record linear displacement without aliasing but because linear velocity is based on the rate of change of linear displacement with respect to time, a higher sampling frequency of linear displacement is required to calculate the linear velocity. When deciding on a sampling frequency it is important to make sure all variables recorded and all derived variables calculated from those variables are unaliased. In general, the higher the sampling frequency the more likely it is to reflect the true analogue signal.

In some fields sufficient work has been undertaken to establish typical sampling frequencies. In gait analysis a sampling frequency of 50 to 60 Hz is common, and for running, frequencies between 100 and 200 Hz have been used. However, these frequencies, while they faithfully represent linear displacements of the body during walking, have been shown to be deficient when calculating linear velocity and particularly linear acceleration during gait. Ideally, we would wish to sample faster if linear velocity and linear acceleration were the focus of our attention, but many optical motion capture systems are limited to these frame rates. This is because the 'gold standard' sampling frequency of 50 Hz used in many gait studies (60 Hz in the USA) can be attributed to the use of television and video cameras, which operate from the electrical mains and hence produce pictures (frames) at the same frequency as the oscillations in the alternating current of the mains; that is, 50 Hz in the UK and 60 Hz in the USA.

In conclusion, for most movement studies, time is used as the controlling variable for data collection. The influence of time may subsequently be eliminated either partially as in gait, where it is common to report measurements relative to the percentage of the gait cycle or completely as, for example, when plotting angle versus angle diagrams for a reaching task of the upper limb. However, in order to use modern data recording and sampling methods, a consideration of the time-dependent properties of the variables to be measured is often a vital component of the planning and piloting of a movement measurement study.

LINEAR KINEMATICS

The linear motion of an object over a period of time can be fully described using three mechanical variables, namely: 'linear displacement', 'linear velocity' and 'linear acceleration'. This section of text will define each variable and then explore the relationships between them.

As we have seen, one aspect of movement is the ability to undergo translation. If an object undergoes translation alone it will move from one location in space to another while maintaining the original orientation of the object, that is, without rotating. The mechanical variable that describes the location of an object in space is called 'linear displacement', which (as a definition)

indicates the present position of an object relative to a reference point or origin

and is measured in metres.

As we discussed earlier, the object is free to translate in three dimensions (X, Y and Z axes, or left/right, forwards/backwards and up/down). Therefore the linear displacement of an object can be described using three coordinates that indicate the displacement of the object parallel to the three orthogonal axes. The combination of these three coordinates

indicates how far away the object is from the origin and in what direction. In order to describe the linear displacement of an object we must therefore define both an origin for measurement and a set of three orthogonal axes centred on that origin. We are free to choose any combination of origin and axes orientation provided we then use this definition throughout the analysis. However, it is usual to pick axes set with either a geographical significance (vertical, forwards and sideways) or with an anatomical significance (cranial, anterior and lateral).

Linear motion in which the object translates in only one dimension (i.e. a change in only one of the three coordinates) will produce movement in a straight line. This type of motion is known as 'rectilinear motion'. If translation occurs in two dimensions, then the object will move within a plane. This is known as two-dimensional 'curvilinear motion'. Finally, if the objects exhibit motion relative to all three axes, the motion will occur in a 3D volume; this is known as '3D curvilinear motion'.

It is interesting to note that if none of the three coordinates of the linear displacement change then the location of the object remains the same; that is, the object is stationary. Conversely, if any of the three coordinates change then the object will change location. This change in location will take time, and this leads us on to the second linear kinematic descriptor: 'linear velocity', which is defined as

the rate of change of linear displacement with respect to time

and measured in metres per second.

It can be quantified by considering the change in linear displacement in a given unit of time; that is, as

$$\text{Linear velocity} = \frac{\text{The change in linear displacement}}{\text{The time taken for the change to occur}}.$$

The linear velocity of an object therefore describes how rapidly the object is moving and in what direction the movement is occurring. The linear velocity of an object can again be described using three components of velocity parallel to the three orthogonal axes of the axes set chosen.

Again, it is interesting to note that if all three velocity components are zero the object is stationary, and that if none of the three components of the object's velocity change the object will continue to travel in the same direction at the same speed ad infinitum. In this case the motion of the object would appear the same at any point in time even though its location will have changed. The object would be undergoing straight line motion at constant speed.

Conversely, if any of the three components of the object's velocity change then the motion of the object will change, and this leads us to our third and final linear kinematic descriptor; 'linear acceleration', defined as

the rate of change of linear velocity with respect to time

and measured in metres per second per second or, in other words, metres per second squared.

It can be quantified by considering the change in linear velocity in a given unit of time, that is, as

$$\text{Linear acceleration} = \frac{\text{The change in linear velocity}}{\substack{\text{The time taken for} \\ \text{the change to occur}}}.$$

The linear acceleration of an object therefore describes how rapidly the velocity of an object is changing and in what direction the change is occurring. The linear acceleration of an object can again be described using three components of acceleration parallel to the three orthogonal axes of the axes set chosen.

From these definitions it is apparent that linear displacement, linear velocity and linear acceleration are interrelated. Linear acceleration is the rate of change of linear velocity with respect to time and linear velocity is itself the rate of change of linear displacement with respect to time.

Changes in linear displacement can therefore be used to calculate linear velocity, and changes in linear velocity can be used to calculate linear accelerations. Likewise, linear accelerations can be used to predict changes in linear velocity, and linear velocities can be used to predict changes in linear displacement. These interrelations can be described using a series of kinematic equations for linear motion, which will now be derived.

Consider an object undergoing linear motion from the origin of measurement to some other location in space with constant acceleration.

Let's define

u	as the linear velocity of the object at the original position of the object
v	as the linear velocity of the object at the final position of the object
s_1	as the original linear displacement of the object
s_2	as the final linear displacement of the object
a	as the constant linear acceleration of the object, between one point and the other, and finally
t	as the time taken for the change in location to occur.

Then from the definition of acceleration:

$$\text{Linear acceleration} = \frac{\text{Change in linear velocity}}{\text{Time taken for change}} \quad \text{or}$$

$$a = \frac{v - u}{t}$$

hence

$$a \bullet t = v - u$$

or

$$v = u + a \bullet t.$$

In addition, from the definition of linear velocity:

$$\text{The average linear velocity} = \frac{\substack{\text{Change in linear} \\ \text{displacement}}}{\text{Time taken for change}}$$

$$\text{or} \quad v = \frac{s_2 - s_1}{t}$$

or

$$s_2 = s_1 + v \bullet t.$$

Consider a graph of linear displacement against time. The definition of linear velocity is a change in linear displacement (on the vertical axis) by a change in time (on the horizontal axis). Linear velocity is therefore indicated by the slope (or gradient) of the curve at any point. We can calculate the slope between two points on the curve by taking the change in their linear displacement and dividing it by the time taken for the change to occur. This will give us the average linear velocity occurring between the two points in time. The faster we sample the smaller will be the change in time; hence the better we will calculate and represent the linear velocity. The slope of the linear displacement time curve therefore indicates the linear velocity of the object. The process of calculating slopes (i.e. the rate of change) is known as differentiation; hence linear velocity is also defined as the first differential of linear displacement.

The use of high-speed computer-controlled sampling and data processing has meant that this process can now be implemented relatively easily. However, two important restrictions are that the sampling frequency must be sufficiently fast to characterise the signal; and that the signal must be sufficiently smooth to allow sensible estimation of the slopes.

Turning our attention now to linear acceleration, it is apparent that similar rules apply. Linear acceleration is defined as the rate of change of linear velocity with respect to time. The linear acceleration is therefore indicated by the slope of the linear velocity time curve. Linear acceleration is the first differential of linear velocity and therefore the second differential of linear displacement. We can use the same numerical process to estimate linear accelerations from linear velocities that we used to estimate linear velocities from linear displacement. Again, care must be taken to sample at a sufficiently high frequency and to ensure that the signal is sufficiently smooth for valid estimation of the accelerations.

From this discussion, it is possible to see that by measuring linear displacement it is possible to estimate linear velocities and linear accelerations. These three variables are 'chained together'. Also, it may be apparent that the process can be operated in the opposite direction, that is, using linear accelerations to predict linear velocities, and linear velocities to predict linear displacements. In our discussion of linear kinematics above, we saw that from the definition of linear acceleration:

$$v = u + a \bullet t.$$

Inspection of this equation indicates that the final linear velocity of an object is dependent on its initial linear velocity and the product of linear acceleration and time. If you have a graph of linear acceleration versus time it can be seen that between two points in time the product of linear acceleration and time is given by the area under the linear acceleration versus time curve between the two time-points. If this area is positive, then the object will accelerate and its linear velocity will increase. If the area is negative, then the object will decelerate (a negative linear acceleration) and its linear velocity will decrease.

The linear velocity of the object can therefore be determined by calculating the area under the curve from the beginning of the movement, provided we know the initial linear velocity of the subject on commencement of activity. This can be estimated by multiplying the linear acceleration for each period of time by the time between samples and then summing these values over the entire activity. This process of area calculation is called 'integration' and therefore linear velocity is the first integral of acceleration.

This process of integration assumes that the linear acceleration can be considered constant for the short periods of time between samples without producing significant error. In effect, the area under the linear acceleration time curve is calculated using a series of rectangular strips (a histogram). This process will only be valid if the linear acceleration is near constant for each strip and hence the area can be estimated appropriately using this approximation. The sampling frequency is key in this respect and we must ensure that the samples are sufficiently frequent that little change in acceleration occurs between samples.

Finally, as we have seen, a similar relationship is evident between linear velocity and linear displacement as that illustrated between linear acceleration and linear velocity.

The final linear displacement of an object is therefore directly related to its initial linear displacement and the product of its linear velocity and the time this linear velocity acts. Again, provided we know the initial linear displacement of the object (usually we define this point as the origin) we can estimate the linear displacement of the object at any point in time after that by calculating the cumulative area under the linear velocity versus time curve. Positive areas will cause the linear displacement to increase and negative areas will cause the linear displacement to decrease. Linear displacement is therefore the first integral of linear velocity and the second integral of linear acceleration.

These interrelationships between the kinematic variables aid our understanding of motion and can be used by the movement scientist to predict variables that are not directly measurable with the available instrumentation. It is therefore possible for optical movement analysis systems to measure displacements but to infer velocity and acceleration data. Likewise, it is possible to use acceleration data from an accelerometer to predict the velocities and displacements of a subject.

ANGULAR KINEMATICS

The angular motion of an object over a period of time also can be fully described using three mechanical variables, namely 'angular displacement', 'angular velocity' and 'angular acceleration'. This section of text will define each variable and then explore the relationships between them.

If an object undergoes angular motion (rotation) alone it will change orientation with respect to one or more of the three axes used to define motion. However, its centre will remain at the same location. The mechanical variable that describes the orientation of an object in space is called 'angular displacement' and (by definition) it:

indicates the present orientation of an object relative to a reference point or origin and a line,

and is measured in radians (or degrees).

As we discussed earlier, the object is free to rotate around any of the three axes (X, Y and Z axes, or left/right, forwards/backwards and up/down). The angular displacement of an object can therefore be described using three angles that indicate the orientation of the object relative to each orthogonal axis. The combination of these three angles indicates the orientation of the object.

It is interesting to note that if none of the three angles of the angular displacement change then the orientation of the object remains the same; that is, the object is stationary. Conversely, if any of the three angles change then the object will change orientation. This change in orientation will take time, and this leads us on to the second angular kinematic descriptor: 'angular velocity', which is defined as:

the rate of change of angular displacement with respect to time

and measured in radians per second or degrees per second.

It can be quantified by considering the change in angular displacement in a given unit of time, that is, as:

$$\text{Angular velocity} = \frac{\text{The change in angular displacement}}{\text{The time taken for the change to occur}}.$$

The angular velocity of an object therefore describes how rapidly the object is spinning and in what direction the movement is occurring. The angular velocity of an object can again be described using three components of angular velocity related to the three orthogonal axes of the axes set chosen.

It is interesting to note that if all three components are zero the object is stationary, and that if none of the three components of the object's angular velocity change the object will continue to spin in the same direction at the same rate ad infinitum. In this case, the motion of the object would appear the same at any point in time.

Conversely if any of the three components of the object's angular velocity change then the motion of the object will change, and this leads us to our third and final angular kinematic descriptor: 'angular acceleration', which is defined as:

the rate of change of angular velocity with respect to time

and measured in radians per second squared (or degrees per second squared).

It can be quantified by considering the change in angular velocity in a given unit of time; that is, as:

$$\text{Angular acceleration} = \frac{\text{The change in angular velocity}}{\text{The time taken for the change to occur}}.$$

The angular acceleration of an object therefore describes how rapidly the angular velocity of the object is changing and in what direction the change is occurring. The angular acceleration of an object can again be described using three components of angular acceleration related to the three orthogonal axes of the axes set chosen.

From these definitions it is apparent that angular displacement, angular velocity and angular acceleration are of a similar form and are interrelated in a similar manner as their linear equivalents. Angular acceleration is the rate of change of angular velocity with respect to time, and angular velocity is itself the rate of change of angular displacement with respect to time. Changes in angular displacement can therefore be used to calculate angular velocity, and changes in angular velocity can be used to calculate angular accelerations. Likewise, angular accelerations can be used to predict changes in angular velocity, and angular velocities can be used to predict changes in angular displacement. These interrelations can again be described using a series of kinematic equations for angular motion, which are a direct parallel to those for linear motion.

Consider an object undergoing angular motion from the origin of measurement to some other orientation in space with constant angular acceleration.

Let's define

ω_i	as the initial angular velocity of the object
ω_f	as the final angular velocity of the object
Ω_i	as the initial angular displacement of the object
Ω_f	as the final angular displacement of the object
α	as the constant angular acceleration of the object, and finally
t	as the time taken for the change in orientation to occur.

Then from the definition of angular acceleration:

$$\text{Angular acceleration} = \frac{\text{Change in angular velocity}}{\text{Time taken for change}}$$

$$\text{or} \quad \alpha = \frac{\omega_f - \omega_i}{t}$$

hence

$$\alpha \bullet t = \omega_f - \omega_i$$

or

$$\omega_f = \omega_i + \alpha \bullet t.$$

In addition, from the definition of angular velocity:

$$\text{The average angular velocity}$$
$$= \frac{\text{Change in angular displacement}}{\text{Time taken for change}} = \frac{\Omega_f - \Omega_i}{t}$$

or

$$\Omega_f = \Omega_i + \omega \bullet t.$$

As we have seen, the situation for angular kinematics is a direct parallel of that for linear kinematics. We can therefore use the same numerical methods for differentiation and integration in angular motion as those we developed for linear motion earlier in this chapter. In addition, the interrelationships between the variables are parallel; hence we can conclude that angular velocity is the first differential of angular displacement, and angular acceleration is the second differential of angular displacement. Likewise, angular velocity is the first integral of angular acceleration, and angular displacement is the second integral of angular acceleration. We have the same 'chain' between the variables as was apparent for the linear kinematic variables.

The linear and angular kinematic variables and their interrelationships provide much of interest to the motion scientist. They can be used to describe normal, pathological and excellent performance. They can be used to compare and contrast subjects and groups of subjects and may indicate in what aspect the motion is abnormal, allowing the clinician to focus in on problem areas.

However, a more careful consideration of this issue will indicate that even if we can fully describe the accelerations of the object, and hence predict its subsequent motion, we have no knowledge of the cause of the motion. A cyclist coming down a hill may have a given acceleration due to the effects of gravity alone, the effects of gravity and propulsion from the legs, the effects of gravity and resistance from the brakes, or—if very undecided, from gravity—propulsion from the legs and resistance from the brakes.

Similarly, during the later stages of swing phase in gait the lower leg may descend and straighten due to the effects of gravity alone, the effects of gravity and propulsion from the quadriceps group of muscles, the effects of gravity and the resistance of the hamstrings muscle group, or—most likely—the effects of gravity and the quadriceps and hamstrings muscle groups.

Therefore, if we wish to analyse the causes of motion, we need to consider the forces acting on the object. It is the combined effect of these forces that determines the acceleration of the object, and hence the subsequent motion of the object. If we remove these forces from the object (e.g. in space), then the motion of the object will remain unaltered for infinity.

FORCES AND MOMENTS

Much of the credit for our current understanding of mechanics and, in particular, the relationship between forces and motion can be ascribed to Sir Isaac Newton (1672–1727). His book *Principia* (or 'Principles') revolutionised the study of mechanics and was one of the outstanding scientific contributions of the age. Newton, who was self-educated, can be said to have to have established the field of mechanics

by setting out the rules that govern the relationship between forces and motion.

Newton carried out many meticulous observations of experimental situations and reduced what he saw to three basic principles or 'laws' as they are often called. Initially these were regarded as absolute laws governing all motion in the universe. However, towards the turn of the 20th century, the 'laws' were brought into question when physicists tried to apply them to motion at very high speeds (near the speed of light, 3×10^8 m/s). Einstein showed that at these very high velocities, Newton's 'laws' needed correction. However, for human motion the correction factors are minute and can be ignored without any loss of accuracy. Newton's laws are now regarded as 'rules of thumb' for all movements except those at very high speeds.

Newton observed the motion of objects on the Earth in a highly meticulous way. If he did (as legend would have it) think up his laws sitting under an apple tree with a bruise on his head, then his thoughts were clearly affected by long hours of experimentation in his laboratory. These are the three principles he proposed.

Newton's First Law of Motion

A body which is at rest will remain at rest unless some external force is applied to it, and a body which is moving at a constant speed in a straight line (a constant velocity) will continue to do so unless some external force is applied to it.

Newton's first law implies that matter has a built-in reluctance to change its state of motion. If it is stationary it will stay stationary, or if it's moving at a certain speed in a certain direction it will continue to do so unless a force is applied to it from outside. We are all quite familiar with this finding. We know it is often difficult to make things move. We also know it is often difficult and sometimes painful to make things stop. The property that objects have by which they resist changing their motion is known as 'inertia'.

Inertia is possessed by all objects to some degree or another. Inertia can occur in two forms; (1) a reluctance to undergo linear motion, which is known as 'mass'; and (2) a reluctance to undergo angular motion, which is called 'moment of inertia'. Because the first law is associated with the property of inertia it is sometimes referred to as the law of inertia.

During his experiments, Newton also observed that the rate of change of velocity with respect to time (or the acceleration) of an object was:
1. directly proportional to the force applied, and
2. inversely proportional to the inertia (mass) of the object.

And from this he proposed his second law.

Newton's Second Law of Motion

When an unbalanced force acts on a body it produces an acceleration which is proportional to the force and inversely proportional to the inertia of the body, and is in the direction of the force.

This is often simplified to:

$$Force = Mass \bullet Acceleration$$

or

$$F = m \bullet a$$

(where the force and acceleration are in the same direction).

Finally, Newton observed the interactions between objects and developed a third law.

Newton's Third Law of Motion

If a body exerts a force on a second body then the second body will exert an equal and opposite force on the first body, or for every action there is an equal and opposite reaction.

For obvious reasons this is sometimes referred to as the law of reaction.

The crux of the relationship between force and linear acceleration is given in the numerical summary of Newton's second law (i.e. F = m•a). This equation indicates that the acceleration produced by a force will be in the direction of the force, and will be directly proportional to the size of the force and indirectly proportional to the mass of the object. Larger forces will cause larger accelerations and subsequent changes from straight line motion at constant speed (i.e. changes in velocity). The greater the mass of the object the less it will accelerate under the influence of a given force. If multiple forces act on an object then it is the net or resultant force produced when all the forces have been added together which will determine the movement of the object.

If we are able to measure the force(s) on an object and we know the mass of the object, we can determine the acceleration that this force or group of forces will produce; hence we will be able to predict the subsequent velocities and displacements of the object over time. Therefore our chain of mechanical variables should really begin with force, which can be related to linear acceleration and thence to linear velocity and linear displacement. Force is the cause of linear motion; hence it is common in movement studies to record the forces used in an activity.

Exploiting the chain in the opposite direction (i.e. using accelerations to predict forces) is more problematic. We can use Newton's second law to predict the net force required

to produce this acceleration. However, the human body can often produce this net force in a variety of ways using the musculature of the body. For example, there are 22 muscles that cross the hip joint. Many of these muscles have similar actions, so considerable redundancy exists in the system. We may predict that a certain net force is required to produce the desired linear acceleration, but this can be achieved by one muscle alone, a group of muscles with similar actions working in combination, an agonist and antagonist pair, or even a combination of an agonist group and an antagonist group. If we then add the influence of pathology and possible spasticity, the problem becomes a complex one with many solutions, and we require some method to predict the actual behaviour of the body.

Electromyography (EMG) studies of certain key muscles are often used to determine which muscles are active at which point in the movement, and hence to determine the solution the body has selected. It is also usual to assume that the body will pick a solution that minimises the amount of force produced or the energy consumed in contraction.

Turning to angular motion, the factor that determines changes in the angular kinematics is not the magnitude of the force but the moment it produces about the centre of mass of the object. Large moments will cause the object to have a large angular acceleration. In addition, objects that have a lot of mass distributed away from the centre of the object (i.e. a large moment of inertia) will be difficult to spin (i.e. a large inertia to angular motion). These observations for angular motion parallel those for linear motion, and can be expressed using a version of Newton's second law for angular motion, that is:

$$T = I \bullet \alpha$$

where T is the moment (or torque) applied to the object, I is the moment of inertia of the object around the axis of rotation and α is the angular acceleration of the object.

Larger moments will produce greater angular accelerations, and objects with large moments of inertia will be reluctant to move and hence produce low angular acceleration. Moment (or torque) is therefore the causal factor for angular motion. If we can measure the moments applied to an object and we know its moment of inertia relative to the centre of mass, then we can calculate its angular acceleration and hence predict the angular velocities and angular displacements it will undergo. Likewise, if we can determine the angular acceleration of an object, we can predict the net moment required to produce that movement. Again, this moment can be produced in a variety of ways by the body and EMG can be used to help determine the solution chosen by the body. Moment, then, is a key factor in determining angular motion and it is therefore also commonly recorded in movement studies.

DERIVED VARIABLES

In our discussion we have covered the nine key mechanical variables used to record movement. However, mechanics makes use of certain combinations of these to produce derived variables that can provide a different viewpoint for analysis. Of particular interest to the movement scientist are impulse, momentum, work and energy. What is not often understood is that these variables are simply re-expressions of Newton's second law using the interrelationships between kinematic variables. To illustrate this, we can transform Newton's second law using the kinematic equations we developed earlier in the chapter, and we will arrive at the definitions of impulse and momentum.

$$f = m \bullet a.$$

But

$$v = u + a \bullet t \quad \text{or} \quad a = \frac{(v-u)}{t}$$

hence

$$f = m \bullet \frac{(v-u)}{t}$$

or

$$f \bullet t = m \bullet v - m \bullet u.$$

In this equation the variable on the left-hand side (i.e. the product of the force and time) is called the 'impulse' of the force. The variables on the right-hand side consist of a mass multiplied by a velocity and this is the 'momentum' of the object. So, on the right-hand side we have the final momentum minus the initial momentum, which is the change in momentum. This equation therefore indicates that the impulse of the force is equal to the change in momentum of the object. This redefinition of Newton's second law is useful in that the momentum before and after an event can be calculated, and provided the time between the two points is known we can predict the average force generated. The impulse/momentum equation can be used to give a slightly different perspective on the cause of motion.

An angular version of the impulse/momentum equation can be derived in a similar fashion:

$$T = I \bullet \alpha.$$

But

$$\omega_f = \omega_i + \alpha \bullet t \quad \text{or} \quad \alpha = \frac{(\omega_f - \omega_i)}{t}$$

hence

$$T = I \bullet \frac{(\omega_f - \omega_i)}{t}$$

or

$$T \bullet t = I \bullet \omega_f - I \bullet \omega_i.$$

The variable on the left-hand side of the equation, which is the product of the moment and time, is known as 'the angular impulse' of the force. On the right-hand side we have two variables, which combine the moment of inertia of the object with its angular velocity; this variable is known as the 'angular momentum' of the object. Hence the equation indicates that the angular impulse is equal to the change in angular momentum of the object.

Similarly, we can redefine Newton's second law as:

$$f = m \bullet a.$$

But

$$v^2 = u^2 + 2 \bullet a \bullet s \quad \text{or} \quad a = \frac{(v^2 - u^2)}{2 \bullet s}$$

hence

$$f = m \bullet \frac{(v^2 - u^2)}{2 \bullet s}$$

or

$$f \bullet s = \tfrac{1}{2} m \bullet v^2 - \tfrac{1}{2} m \bullet u^2.$$

In this equation, the variable on the left-hand side (the product of the force times the displacement in the direction of the force) is known as the 'work done' by the force. On the right-hand side we have variables of the form: half the mass times the velocity of the object squared. This is known as the 'kinetic energy' of the object, so the right-hand side of the equation represents the change in kinetic energy. The work/energy equation therefore indicates that the work done by a force is equal to the change in energy of the object (in this case a change in kinetic energy). Many forms of energy exist, but from a mechanical point of view only three are important: the kinetic energy due to the object's linear velocity, the potential energy due to the object position in a gravitational field (which gives it the potential to move and hence do work) and finally the rotational kinetic energy of the object due to its angular velocity.

The potential energy of an object is given by the formula m•g•h, where m is the mass of the object, g is the gravitational constant at that point in space and h is the height above a chosen datum (sea level, floor level etc.).

The rotary kinetic energy is given by $\tfrac{1}{2} I \omega^2$, where I is the moment of inertia of the object and ω is the angular velocity of the object.

The work/energy equation therefore indicates that the work done on the object is equal to the change in the total mechanical energy (the sum of the kinetic, potential and rotary kinetic energies) of the object. By recording the linear and angular kinematics of a body segment and using a knowledge of the mass and moment of inertia of that segment, it is possible to calculate the fluctuations in kinetic, potential, rotary kinetic and total mechanical energy of the segment, and hence to make an inference about the work done on that segment by the muscles that cross its boundaries. This technique has been used in complex pathologies, such as cerebral palsy, to shed light on which muscles are being used to provide energy to various segments of the body. Also, attempts have been made to model the effects of surgery on specific muscles or muscle groups, and hence predict the likely effect of this type of surgery on the subject's subsequent function. These studies are sometimes supplemented by respiratory gas analysis during movement, which can be used to assess the rate of energy consumption for the body as a whole.

Impulse, momentum, work and energy are derived variables that aid our understanding and discussion of human movement. Like Newton's original laws they help to explain the causes of motion, and are therefore grouped alongside forces and moments as kinetic variables.

SUMMARY

In conclusion, a full mechanical analysis of motion can be achieved by describing nine key variables related to motion. These variables can be recorded directly using a variety of equipment or, in some circumstances, they can be inferred from one another. In addition, these variables can be combined in a variety of ways to provide further insight into the mechanics of motion. Finally, these variables can be presented and processed using a variety of different methods. These methods are often specific to the human functional movement which is being evaluated.

This chapter has attempted to report the basic mechanical variables used in motion analysis, their definitions, interactions and combinations. All the equipment systems and functional studies reported in this book have one thing in common: the data they present will be based solely on the recording of one or more of these nine key mechanical variables. Therefore, in planning a movement study, the researcher should think primarily about the aspect or aspects of movement that reflect the desired outcome of the study. Subsequently, consideration can be given to the best method of recording, processing and presenting the data, and to the most appropriate equipment with which to record the required data. In this way we can develop 'outcome-specific' rather than 'equipment-driven' research projects and hence produce research work of greater relevance to the patient, health professional, scientific community and general public.

SELF-ASSESSMENT QUESTIONS

1. How many parameters does it take to typically describe the movement of an object in three dimensional space and what are those parameters?
2. Why is the linear concept of mass invariant while the angular equivalent moment of inertia is able to change?
3. How do we use changes in moment of inertia to our advantage in human movement?
4. Why do objects spin?
5. During walking, does your lower leg translate, rotate or do both?
6. How does velocity relate to displacement?
7. How does velocity relate to acceleration?
8. Can you accelerate while maintaining a constant speed?
9. Can momentum be made and lost?
10. Can energy be made and lost?

Biomechanical Measurements Including Three-Dimensional Motion Analysis Systems

Philip Rowe

LEARNING OUTCOMES

At the end of this chapter, you should be able to:

1. Explain the basic process underpinning the capture of three-dimensional motion data using a camera system.
2. Appreciate the historical landmarks behind modern systems.
3. Provide an overview of common biomechanical movement variables and the instruments used to measure them.
4. Discuss the possibilities for incorporating modern motion analysis techniques into everyday clinical rehabilitation.

INTRODUCTION

Having established how we define movement using nine key variables in the previous chapter, we will now discuss how we measure these variables in practice. Systems for motion capture can be thought of as either systems that will capture (or predict) all nine parameters of human motion in three dimensions, what I would call 'full three-dimensional biomechanical analysis systems' or those that measure one or more of the variables in one or more dimension, what I would call 'movement assessment systems'. That is not to say one is better than the other. If it is clear what the movement parameter of interest is that defines success or failure for a particular medical technology, then a simple system that measures just that maybe ideal. For example, an accelerometer that measures the acceleration

of a body part can easily be turned into a step-counting device and used by a mass market to encourage activity, or a time piece, such as a stopwatch, can be used to measure the walking speed of a subject. However, if we want to comprehensively measure in three-dimensional space the kinematics and kinetics of the human body in motion then one method comes into its own—optical motion capture—and this will be the initial focus of this chapter.

FULL THREE-DIMENSIONAL MOTION CAPTURE

Following the Second World War there was a need to help rehabilitate the disabled and a growth in life expectancy such that people's joints began to wear out. Both these factors gave a boost to the subject of biomechanics and motion

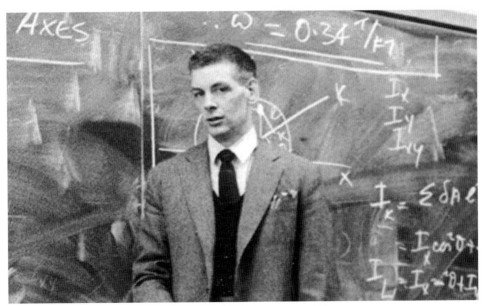

Fig. 12.1 Prof. J.P. Paul, circa 1965.

capture. We needed to know the loading on joints if we were to develop successful implants to replace them, and we needed to know the mechanics of human locomotion if we were to enable amputees and other war disabled to function independently. During the late 1940s and 1950s, pioneering work was undertaken to report biomechanical movement, and much of it was based on serial photographs or interrupted light photography. In the 1960s cine cameras became more widely available and were used to record moving images. By combining multiple cine cameras synchronised together it became possible to record motion from more than one point of view, which lead to the field of stereo-photogrammetry and biomechanical motion capture.

In the UK these developments were led by J.P. Paul (Fig. 12.1) and co-workers at the University of Strathclyde. Paul, then a mechanical engineer, was approached by the local Professor of Surgery as to why the hip implants they were using to repair damaged and worn out human hips kept failing. In a seminal work for his PhD thesis, Paul used two synchronised cine cameras to record the movement of a subject wearing body markers while walking across his laboratory and treading on a plate that measured force in three dimensions. He then projected the film on to the wall of the laboratory and hand-digitised the locations of the markers in each frame of movement. Using the data from the two cameras and knowing their locations he was able to use triangulation to work out where in space each marker must be (Fig. 12.2) and to join these together to give a linked model of human walking in three dimensions.

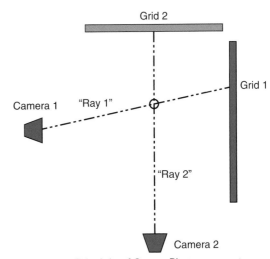

Fig. 12.2 Principle of Stereo Photogrammetry.

He then combined this information with data from the force plate in the floor and worked out the forces and moments being generated at the ankle, knee and hip of both limbs. Using the moment information and a model of the locations and lines of actions of the muscles of the lower limb he was able to determine which muscles must be active in order to counter these moments at the joints, and to estimate the forces in the muscles of the leg. Finally, he was able to combine the force information to give the direct loading of the limb caused by both the ground reaction force and the forces generated by the muscles crossing a joint to calculate the total load on the joint.

You might think that when you stand on one leg you would get one body weight acting across your hip and, indeed, you would if your body weight was directly above your hip. However, in normal human movement your centre of mass (the point through which your body weight can be thought to act) is medial to your hip. In other words, your body weight presses down in the middle of your pelvis but your hip is to the side of the pelvis with the femur pushing up. If nothing were to happen, the pelvis would rotate downwards around the head of the femur; it would list. This is problematic as the swinging leg would be more likely to hit the ground, and at transfer between one leg and the other the pelvis would need to list rapidly the other way giving rise to rapid movements of the pelvis and the centre of mass, and a very jerky gait.

To prevent this, we must provide a counter moment to that generated by our mass about the hip. This counter moment is generated by the hip adductors, which connect the pelvis to the lateral thigh, and when they contract they pull the pelvis back up by generating a counter moment. These muscles are close to the hip while the centre of mass is some distance away medial to the hip. The muscles are therefore at a mechanical disadvantage (approximately three to one) and have to produce a force much greater than body weight (approximately three times body weight). Both this force and the ground reaction force cross the hip and compress it; hence the actual force on the joint is more like four times body weight. This effect is clearly shown in Paul's original data (Fig. 12.3).

This remarkable piece of work was conducted by Paul using paper, pen and slide rule only, and by hand calculation of all the data. The data revolutionised orthopaedic surgery and implant design. For the first time it was clear why implants failed and what forces they would need to withstand if they were to survive during walking. An understanding of the loadings at other joints and during other activities followed. This process of analysis has become known as inverse dynamics. In dynamics, as we saw in the previous chapter, forces and moments can be used alongside Newton's second law to predict accelerations, velocities and displacement. Hence in dynamics we measure forces and moments directly and predict movement. This can be done in engineering as it is possible to apply force and moment sensors to the moving parts. However, in human motion this is not so easily done and therefore we rely on the reverse process of inverse dynamics in which we record the movement and predict the forces and moments. Inverse dynamics is the mainstay of biomechanical analysis of movement.

In the 1970s and 1980s Paul and his co-workers, particularly Mike Jarett and Brian Andrews, converted the cine

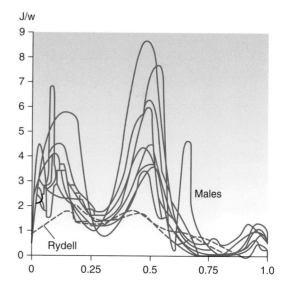

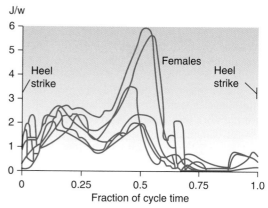

Fig. 12.3 Paul's Original Diagrams of Hip Joint Loading in Males and Females. Courtesy of Professor John P. Paul. From http://theses.gla.ac.uk/3913/1/1967PaulPhD.pdf

camera method to use the newly emerging technologies of television cameras (Fig. 12.4) and mainframe computers. They also turned from using visible light to capture sequential pictures to invisible infrared light. This had the benefit that retro reflective markers would show up as bright dots, while clothes and flesh did not reflect infrared light strongly and so appeared black. The infrared light source was flashed (strobed) to give 50 pictures (frames) per second.

Using three of these camera and strobe combinations synchronised together and a computer, it was possible to reconstruct the position of a limited number of markers on the body in real time at a frame rate of 50 Hz (Fig. 12.5).

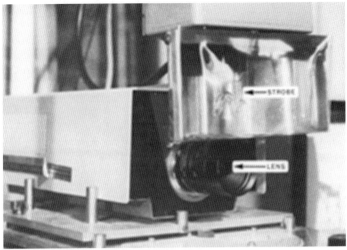

Fig. 12.4 An Early Motion Capture TV Camera With Infrared Strobe Light.

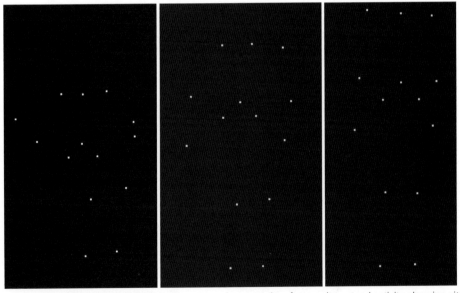

Fig. 12.5 Three typical reconstructed motion capture images taken from a sit-to-stand activity showing sitting prior to leaving the seat, rising to stand prior to hands leaving the arm rests and upright standing, circa 1980.

The image above shows three typical reconstructed images from a sequence of images of someone rising to stand from a sitting position while using arm rests. There are 14 individual markers in use to describe the body motion. In this case the markers are placed at the joints, but in reality this was often difficult due to skin movement and folding at the joints. Also, while these markers can be joined together to form a stick-man figure the analysis is incomplete. In the figure above consider the body segment linking the ankle to the knee (the shank). If this body segment was to rotate about a line joining the knee marker to the ankle marker then neither of these markers would appear to change place in three-dimensional space. The markers would simply spin about themselves. This would change how the bones in the knee articulate, but would not be captured by our motion capture protocol; hence we could not do full three-dimensional motion capture and reconstruction.

In order to capture the full three-dimensional movement of a body segment we need at least three markers on the segment, and those markers must not be collinear (or near collinear) but must form a triangle. If the triangle translates in three dimensions or if the triangle rotates around any of three axes then at least one marker will change position in space and we will be able to reconstruct the movement in the full 6 degrees of freedom required.

In the mid-1980s the technology began to be exploited and developed commercially. In the UK, Vicon Ltd was founded in 1984 as part of the Oxford Metrics Group of companies.

Vicon launched their own marker system called 'plug-in gait' to work with this system for full body capture (Fig. 12.6).

Since the 1980s there has been a revolution in the availability of computing power and in the availability of high-speed, high-definition video imagery. As a result, the world of motion capture and biomechanics has expanded significantly. Modern Mocap systems have been combined with computer technology and video projectors to produce real-time visualisation of the human body in motion. A leading example of this is the Computer-Assisted Rehabilitation ENvironment (CAREN) System from Motek Medical of Amsterdam (part of the DIH group). The CAREN system uses a comprehensive set of single markers (Fig. 12.7) called human body model (HBM) attached to key anatomical

locations of the body to recreate the three-dimensional pose of the whole body

It also uses force plates and subject anatomical data to recreate a full three-dimensional model of the human muscular skeletal system and to solve this model in real time to predict the forces in individual muscles in the body. Fig. 12.8 shows this musculoskeletal model being projected in real time while the subject is standing in the field of view.

The calf muscles are active while in quiet standing as the centre of mass of the body is in front of the ankle, which creates a moment tipping the body forward and, when left unopposed, would lead to the subject falling flat on their face, as happens when you faint. To prevent this, a counter moment is required from the muscles at the back of the ankle joint, primarily the gastrocnemius muscle. This is predicted by Motek's HBM model, which displays these muscles 'in different colours to signify the muscle being on or off'. The system allows the operator to provide feedback to the subject in various forms. In Fig. 12.8 two spheres are being projected on either side of the subject. The diameter of these spheres represents the size of the force in the right (dark orange) and left (orange) gastrocnemius, respectively, as predicted by the HBM model. You can see that the subject

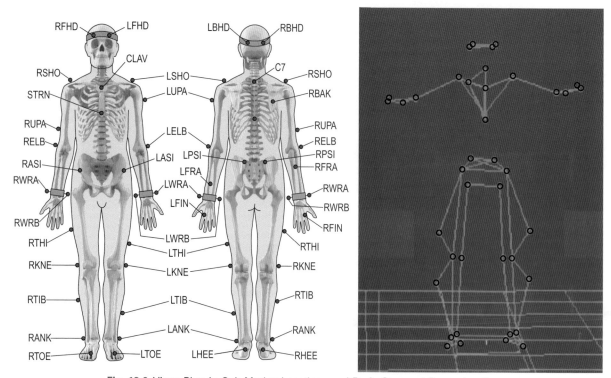

Fig. 12.6 Vicon Plug-in Gait Marker Locations and Body Segment Reconstructions.

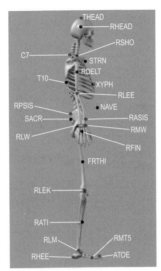
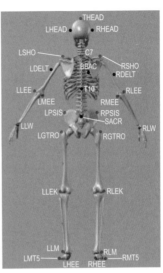
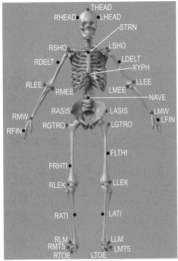

Fig. 12.7 The Motek Human Body Model Marker Model.

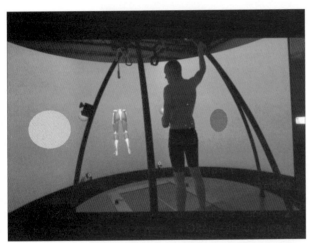

Fig. 12.8 Motek's Computer-Assisted Rehabilitation ENvironment System and Human Body Model in Action.

is standing asymmetrically and is using their right arm to support them. As a result, the predicted force in the right gastrocnemius (the size of the dark orange sphere) is less than that predicted in the left gastrocnemius (the size of the orange sphere). Finally, due to the visualisation capabilities of the system, it is possible to project virtual environments for the subject to explore as shown in Fig. 12.9 where they are 'walking through the woods' to provide simultaneous visual feedback and to make this part of a purposeful game, and hence make rehabilitation more engaging and motivating for the subject.

In the animation industry (Fig. 12.10) multiple actors can interact over a large volume and the animated characters can be recreated and visualised in real time. This level of sophistication has so far not been deployed in rehabilitation, although in the future one could imagine its use in group classes or in competitive purposeful gaming for rehabilitation.

One limitation of the single-marker approach is that either the individual markers have to be stuck to the skin using double-sided tape, which is a slow process requiring near total undressing of the subject (see Fig. 12.8), or they need to wear a special suit to which the markers are attached (see Fig. 12.10), which takes time to put on, must be cleaned between users and does not usually accommodate the body shapes of patients rather than actors.

Therefore a number of biomechanical research groups including ourselves at Strathclyde University have adopted the 'cluster method'. In this approach a series of rigid plates with typically four individual markers permanently fixed to each plate are used. One plate is strapped to each body segment to be recorded (Fig. 12.11). The location of a key anatomical point on the body can be recorded relative to the clusters using a pointer (a stick with markers on it) prior to visualisation. The clusters are tracked by the camera system and by knowing the location of the key anatomical locations of the body relative to these clusters it is possible to reconstruct the body as a three-dimensional avatar (Fig. 12.12).

When dealing with patients with chronic disabilities, such as children with cerebral palsy or muscular dystrophy, full biomechanical analysis provides a powerful technique for the scientific assessment of the functional and neurological

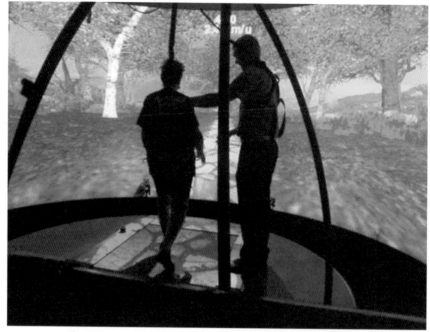

Fig. 12.9 Motek's 'Walking Through the Woods' Application.

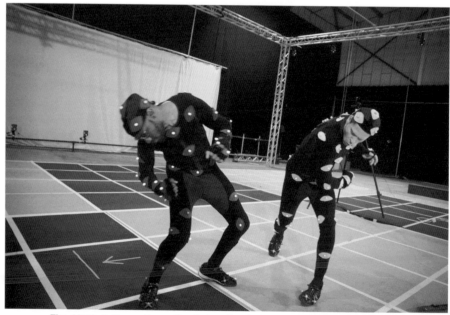

Fig. 12.10 A Scene From the Animation Industry From Vicon's Website.

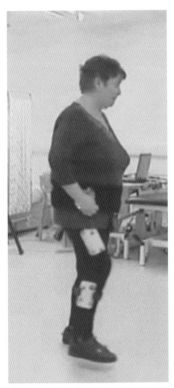

Fig. 12.11 A Cluster Marker System in Action.

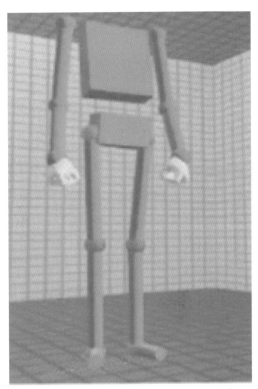

Fig. 12.12 A Typical Reconstructed Avatar of Someone Standing.

impairment of the patient, and hence can be used to determine the success of a treatment regime. In addition, full biomechanical analysis of normal and pathological function is vital in order to determine the loads on joints, and therefore influence the design and strength of joint replacements. Full biomechanical analysis is considered essential to provide a fundamental understanding of human movement, and to provide normative data for comparison, and in the clinical assessment of patients with complex disabilities or those undergoing complex operations. There is a growing area of rehabilitation concerned with providing knowledge of performance and knowledge of the results of physical task performance in order to enhance motor relearning and rehabilitation. This process has been used to great effect in sports biomechanics for the improvement of athletic activity. There is hope that if such methods can be made low cost and ubiquitous, they may find widespread use in rehabilitation. Leading manufacturers of motion analysis systems include Vicon, Motion Analysis Corporation, BTS, Coda Motion, Qualys and Northern Digital.

However, full biomechanical analysis has some limitations. The initial capital costs incurred in setting up a motion

analysis system are considerable, and may include expenditure on buildings, decor, testing equipment and computer systems. Running costs, such as staff wages, staff education, consumables, equipment maintenance and patient transport, may be considerable. A fully equipped biomechanical analysis laboratory therefore represents a large monetary investment that few clinical departments—apart from specialist centres—can afford. In the next decade we are likely to see the cost and complexity fall by an order of 10 and I would predict that multiple camera systems will be portable and available for less than £10,000.

The testing procedure can be long and arduous for the patient, particularly if pain is present. Few systems are currently capable of providing immediate results and data processing times may lead to considerable delays before the results can be studied. With more advanced recognition and labelling techniques, and the use of clusters, one would hope that real-time results also will be achievable in the next few years. The data themselves are complex and a considerable amount of education and training is required before they can be interpreted. Visual feedback methods may help in this regard. The use of force plates places spatial restrictions on the testing procedure and may make testing difficult. A growing use of self-paced instrumented treadmills may overcome this limitation in the future. In order to improve accuracy, the fields of view of the optoelectronic sensing devices are often concentrated on a small volume, making it difficult to follow the action during a number of steps, for example. Again, the use of advanced treadmill technology may overcome this restriction in the future.

Despite these limitations, full biomechanical analysis systems remain a powerful and impressive analysis tool with which to study issues in human movement and clinical rehabilitation. The capital costs, running costs and complexity of these systems currently limit their use to the more complex analytical situations in which the initial outlay is offset by the analytical insight gained from the data they produce. In other circumstances, the evaluation needs of clinical practice can often be met in simpler, less expensive and more direct ways.

MOVEMENT ASSESSMENT SYSTEMS

Visual Movement Evaluation

Perhaps the most common and complex evaluation of human movement is made by the unaided human eye. Our ability to detect abnormal patterns of movement is remarkable. The brain's ability to process the data from our binocular vision system is highly tuned, complex and versatile. Despite this ability to recognise abnormality, visual movement evaluation has some serious limitations. It is dependent on the 'skill' of the individual observer. Even with considerable training and formalised methods of recording the movement (Brunnstrom, 1964; Olney et al., 1979; Tracy et al., 1979; Koerner, 1984), it is often difficult to get agreement between observers. Krebs et al. (1985) found visual gait analysis to be 'only moderately reliable', while Saleh and Murdoch (1985) indicated that visual gait analysis missed many gait abnormalities, which could be detected by full biomechanical analysis systems.

Visual movement analysis is a 'real-time', one-off activity. It is not possible to repeat the observation or to provide a permanent record of the activity. In addition, many human functions and activities take place at relatively high speed, which cannot be observed in detail by the human eye. As an example, it is often difficult to observe heel strike in gait. This leads to problems when evaluating children with cerebral palsy where it may appear that they produce an acceptable heel strike, but on subsequent analysis it can often be shown that they strike the ground with the metatarsals alone. Finally, visual observation only allows estimates of linear and angular displacement to be made. Velocities may sometimes be construed, but accelerations, forces and moments cannot be observed; hence the causes of motion remain unrecorded.

In order to overcome these limitations, the clinical researcher has attempted to produce scientifically objective measures of aspects of movement.

Timing

Arguably the most basic objective measure available is the time taken to perform some or all of a task. Timing can be achieved using clocks, wrist watches, stopwatches and switches connected to computers. Considerable clinical information can be obtained from such simple measures. Simply recording the time taken to rise from a chair, walk 10 m or reach for a cup can provide objective information regarding the extent of functional impairment in a patient group. Their performance can be compared to matched normal subjects and be used to chart their recovery or deterioration. Additionally, it is often possible to break down functional tasks into separate phases of activity and to time these phases individually. For example, a gait cycle can be split into stance and swing, and stance itself can be split into double support and single support phases (Perry et al., 1979). Climbing stairs also can be split into periods of stance and swing, while rising from a chair can be split into a phase of leaning forward, a phase of ascent and a phase of establishing stability in standing.

In many situations, the timing of activities and phases of activities can be greatly facilitated by the use of a video camera and recorder. The video allows repeated observation of the function. Therefore it is possible to time different phases or activities on different showings of the video. Repeated estimates can be made, allowing both inter- and intra-observer variability to be measured, and the video provides a permanent record of the activity for future reference and further analysis. Video recorders with slow-motion playback are built into most mobile phones and tablets, and are particularly valuable as they allow the phases to be timed at a reduced speed. Therefore events take longer to occur and this allows transitory events, such as double support in gait, to be measured. The resulting values can then be converted to real-time values, provided the playback speed of the recorder is known or can be calculated.

Wall and Crosbie (1997) produced a quick and sophisticated gait analysis system using a camcorder mounted on a tripod, a video and a multi-memory stopwatch. A video recording is made of the subject walking. The operator attempts to focus in on the feet while keeping both feet in the field of view of the camera. This can easily be done by panning the camera to follow the subject across the floor. The video is played back in slow motion and the time between successive heel strikes and toe offs is recorded using the multi-memory stopwatch. In this way it is possible to record all the temporal parameters of gait, quickly and efficiently, for a number of consecutive gait cycles. This technique lends itself to the analysis of other functional activities and can be computerised as an app.

Timing also can be facilitated using beams placed across the path of the movement. As the body, or a body part, passes through the beam, the continuity of the beam is interrupted. Using two such beams it is possible to time the passage of the body part from one location to the other. Timing can also be facilitated by switches attached to anatomical landmarks (e.g. footswitches during gait, running or stair climbing) or attached to objects which the body contacts (e.g. the back rest and seat of a chair during rising to stand). Arrays of switches built into a flat surface, such as those seen in walk mats or pressure distribution plates, can be used to identify the timing and pattern of contact between them and various parts of the body. Leading pressure plate and walk mat manufacturers include Novel, Tekscan, RSScan, Gaitmat II, Gaitrite, Pressure Profile Systems and Phoenix.

Linear Displacement

Linear displacement in one-, two- or three-dimensional space is probably the next most commonly reported kinematic variable. Most of the systems used to measure linear displacement have been developed for applications in gait analysis. More recently, these techniques have been adapted to record other functional activities. Since humans first left footprints in the primeval mud, the effect of human weight-bearing on the Earth's surface has been used to study the spatial patterns of gait. By coating a subject's feet with water-soluble paint or talcum powder, it is possible to produce a record of the footfalls used during gait. However, the technique is rather messy and quite laborious to analyse. Recognising this, Boenig (1977) used markers soaked in coloured ink attached to the soles of the shoes to record the spatial positioning of the feet during locomotion along a half-metre-wide strip of white paper. The position of the resultant ink marks was then measured by hand using a ruler. A similar system using felt-tip marker pens was reported by Cerny (1983). This testing method, although simple and quick to conduct, had three main disadvantages. The results were analysed manually requiring 20 minutes data processing time per traverse of the paper; considerable quantities of paper were used; and the system gave no information on the temporal asymmetries of gait.

Wall and Crosbie (1997) developed a similar but more efficient technique for recording the spatial parameters of gait. The subject walks along a 10 m walkway, which is marked with a regular grid. A video recording is made of the subject simultaneously from the side and from behind, using two camcorders mounted on tripods. Each camera is panned to follow the subject by an operator. By playing back the video and freezing it at points where the foot is flat on the floor, it is possible to measure, from the grid, the forward and mediolateral displacement of the feet, and hence calculate step and stride length and step width. In addition, the video can be used to calculate the temporal parameters of gait, which leads to a comprehensive analysis of the footfalls during gait.

Various authors have attempted to automate this type of analysis using a walk mat capable of measuring the contact between the feet and the floor. Wall et al. (1976) used an instrumented walkway, which consisted of two sets of parallel conducting rods set into groves in a corrugated walking surface at right angles to the direction of forward progression. The rods were connected by a series of electrical resistances to a power supply. Conductive strips placed on the soles of the subject's shoes linked two adjacent rods, which completed the electrical circuit. The current flowing through the circuit could be used to calculate the position of the foot relative to the beginning of the mat. The system gave the temporal parameters of gait as well as step and stride length, and has been used to investigate normal subjects, total hip replacement patients and subjects with neurological problems (Wall et al., 1978; Wall et al., 1981). Similar systems have been reported using pressure-sensitive rod switches (Gabel et al., 1979), photochemically etched boards (Gifford and Hutton, 1980; Durie and Farley, 1980) and longitudinal resistive wires (Arenson et al., 1983). Two-dimensional walk mats capable of measuring step width and foot angle, as well as step and stride length, have been developed by Gabell and Nayak (1984) and Hirokawa and Matsumara (1987). Al-Mijalli et al. (1993) reported the design of a portable, two-dimensional walk mat suitable for use in the clinical environment. Currently, a number of manufacturers produce these types of systems including Tekscan, Gaitrite, Emsphysio and Podotech.

Walk mats, while providing information on the contact between the feet and the floor, are essentially intermittent devices. Nothing is known about the displacement of the foot while in the air. Various authors have attempted to develop systems that can give a continuous recording of one-, two- or three-dimensional linear displacement. A simple, continuous displacement recording system was reported by Mukherjee and Ganguli (1977). In this system a tachogenerator (a wheel that gives an electrical signal as it is turned) and continuous loop string were used to record the forward progression of the pelvis during gait. Law (1987) used two tapes and two recorders to monitor the forward progression of the left and right feet during gait. This system allowed the temporal and spacial patterns of the feet to be recorded and gave information regarding the velocity of the feet during swing (Law and Minns, 1989). Crosbie and Eisenhuth (1993) have reported a similar device that uses an optical encoder attached to a wheel to record movement of a weighted string wrapped round the wheel. The encoder is made up of a small, lightweight disc with 500 slots cut in it. The slots pass between the source and sensor of a light emitting diode as the disc rotates. Each slot causes the output of the device to produce a pulse of electricity; by counting these pulses and the direction of spin of the disc it is possible to record the movement of the encoder and hence the string. Crosbie et al. (1996) have used this device to record upper and lower trunk translations associated with stepping. The device has since been modified by Rowe et al. (1999) to allow direct connection to a computer. By using two of these devices attached to the same anatomical landmark it is possible to record planar motion. By using three devices it is possible to record three-dimensional displacements in a hemispherical volume. Rowe and co-workers have used this device to measure a range of functional activities including gait, sitting, rising to stand, standing, sitting down, reaching and pointing (Baer et al., 1995; Rowe et al., 1999). While this technique is in its infancy it is simple to use and is inexpensive, costing a few hundred pounds. The data produced are accurate and three dimensional. As such this system has much to commend it as an alternative to camera systems when undertaking a three-dimensional analysis of motion in a limited volume of space and where information is required on only one or two anatomical landmarks. However, it has not found widespread clinical use and no manufacturers of this type of technology exist.

Angular Displacement

Angular displacement is also of considerable interest to the researcher and clinician. Mobility in the human is produced by a series of angular displacements at adjacent joints, and it is often the function of these joints that is the focus of rehabilitation. Therefore it is not surprising that a number of attempts have been made to directly record angular displacement. Perhaps the simplest and most common clinical measurement made in a rehabilitation setting is that of joint range using a manual goniometer. While of interest, these passive measures of joint motion do little to reveal the function of a joint during dynamic activities. Fluid-filled and gravity goniometers attached to the subject can be used to record the range of motion of the subject during quasi-static movements and this may be assisted by video recordings. However, these devices have poor dynamic characteristics as they take time to 'settle' before a reading can be taken. This makes them impractical for functional analysis. Therefore researchers have looked for devices that respond more rapidly to angular displacement changes.

Electric goniometers or electrogoniometers that record angular displacement as a changing electrical voltage have been widely reported in the literature. Finley and Karpovich (1964) reported an electrogoniometer that consisted of a rotary

potentiometer wired to a battery as a variable resistor (or potential divider) and which was attached to the subject using two lever arms. They used this device to investigate normal and pathological gaits. Finley and Karpovich's device was unidimensional in that it used one potentiometer placed on the lateral side of the joint at the level of the joint centre to measure the flexion–extension angle of the joint. Electrogoniometers were developed for both the knee and ankle. They were held in position using a metal chassis strapped to the limb, and the output was recorded using a chart recorder. A similar method was reported by Trnkoczy and Badj (1975).

However, human joints are complex structures and often allow motion (both rotational and translational) in more than one plane. The centre of rotation often alters during the joint range, giving rise to a polycentric joint. The use of this type of unidimensional electrogoniometers with a single fixed axis of rotation to measure polycentric joints inevitably leads to restriction in the motion of the joint under observation, or to unwanted movement of the instrument relative to the joint. Tala et al. (1978) attempted to provide a polycentric unidimensional electrogoniometer using a three-bar linkage with a potentiometer at each of the two hinges. The joint angle was determined using a trigonometric combination of the outputs of the two potentiometers. However, this device was essentially planar and did not allow abduction, adduction or rotation of the joint.

Lamoreux (1971) introduced a 'self-aligning' electrogoniometer, which used an exoskeleton of metal bars and straps attached to the leg. The various sections of the device were connected using parallelogram linkages, which allowed abduction, adduction and translation but not rotation. Johnson and Smidt (1969) developed a three-dimensional potentiometer goniometer with linkage bars and this has been used Wadsworth et al. (1972) and Stauffer et al. (1974) and Kettlekamp et al. (1979) to study gait. Similar devices have been developed and extensively used to study motion by Townsend et al. (1977), Gore et al. (1979), Chao (1980) and Perry (1981). Potentiometer goniometers are commercially available from Biokinetics, Chattex and MIE Medical Research. These potentiometer devices with their single fixed axis of motion have found widespread use. However, they remain limited due to the restrictions of the exoskeleton needed to allow for the polycentric and the three-dimensional nature of joints.

Nicol (1988) developed a new form of 'flexible' electrogoniometer, which used a long strain gauged shim as the measuring device, and which could accommodate the polycentric and three-dimensional nature of joints. Rowe et al. (1987, 1989) adapted these devices for clinical use and recorded flexion/extension of the hip and knee of both legs during gait, rising from and sitting to a chair, and ascending and descending stairs in a group of normal subjects and a group of patients undergoing total hip replacement (Paul and Hamblen, 1986; Rowe, 1990). Using the same device Macmillan (1989) investigated elbow function in rheumatoid arthritis and elbow replacement. The device was made commercially available by Biometrics Ltd and comes in one- and two-dimensional versions. Hazelwood et al. (1994) has used these devices to investigate the effect of electrical stimulation on the function of children with cerebral palsy, and Myles et al. (1995) have used the devices to study hip, knee and ankle movement during stair climbing in the elderly and subjects following a fractured neck of femur. These flexible electrogoniometers have found widespread applications in human movement analysis. When care is taken to look after them and mount them on the body in an appropriate manner, they can provide accurate, valid and reliable results. Recently, a number of alternative flexible electrogoniometers have been introduced including the Greenleaf Wristsystem from Greenleaf Medical Systems and the Bioback system from Proteo Service. This system remains available from Biometrics, and other manufacturers have copied the design.

An alternative to electrogoniometry was introduced by An et al. (1988). They used a magnetic tracking device called a 3-Space Isotrak system from Polhemus Navigation Sciences Division, McDonald Douglas Electronics Company. The Isotrak consists of a source that develops a three-dimensional electromagnetic field and a small sensor able to record its position and orientation relative to the source. By attaching the source and sensor to the proximal and distal limb segments of a joint, the experimenter is able to record linear and angular displacement of the joint in all three dimensions. Therefore the 6 degrees of freedom of the joint can be examined simultaneously without a direct physical connection across the joint. The system has been used by Pearcy and Hindle (1989) and Hindle et al. (1990), among others, to measure the range of motion of the lower back, and by Rowe and White (1996) to measure the three-dimensional kinematics of the lumbar spine during gait in patients with back pain. Subsequent versions of this technology are available from Polhemus and Xsens.

Accelerometers and Inertial Measurement Units

As was mentioned in the previous chapter, if the displacement of an object is recorded carefully and rapidly, it is possible to process the data to estimate the velocity and acceleration of the body. Acceleration is particularly useful as it is directly related to motive force by Newton's second law of motion ($F = ma$). Accelerations, in some circumstances, can be measured directly using accelerometers (Vivoda, 1986). These devices contain a small mass connected to a spring or flexing beam, and an electronic device that can measure the deflection of the mass when the device is accelerated. This deflection is proportional to the acceleration experienced by the small mass. Accelerometers have been used to measure accelerations directly and, theoretically, can be used to predict velocity and displacement. However, this procedure is more problematic than when using displacement to predict velocity and acceleration, as it is severely affected by any form of drift or system inaccuracy. These errors are integrated and therefore continue to affect the data even when the noise and drift have abated. As a result, accelerometers have not found widespread use in motion analysis on their own. However, when a three-dimensional accelerometer is combined with a three-dimensional gyroscope (which gives angular velocity) and a three-dimensional magnetometer (a three-dimensional compass) the data from the other devices can be used to help correct for the accelerometer drift. This device is known as an inertial measurement unit (IMU) and is manufactured as a small computer chip. It is very cheap as it is used in almost every smart phone on the planet. The fusion of the nine channels of information can provide motion-capture capability; therefore these IMUs are finding application in human body motion capture. They have yet to become widespread and their accuracy and stability overtime have yet to be established, but these devices may offer a cheap form of motion capture in the future. Manufacturers of such systems include Xsens, Pedavatar, Technaid, Jimfit and LpMocap.

Force Transducers

A number of force-measuring devices have been used to evaluate human motion. Most popular has been the force plate, a three-dimensional force-measuring device mounted in a floor or other surface. Force plates have been extensively used to investigate abnormalities and asymmetries in the loading patterns of the lower limbs in various pathologies during gait (Charnley and Pusso, 1968; Jacobs et al., 1972; Andriacchi et al., 1977; Pedotti, 1977; Jansen et al., 1982). The three-dimensional components of the ground reaction force and the moments generated about the three principal axes of the plate were recorded. These systems require that the foot of the limb under investigation be placed wholly upon the upper surface of the plate and that the contralateral limb remain clear of the plate. This and the need to conceal the plate to avoid targeting mean that it is often necessary to conduct a series of walks before a successful recording is made. In patients with pain and severe functional limitation this represents a substantial problem. Despite these issues, force plates are now widespread and commonly form part of a gait analysis system. Commercial force plates are available from Kistler Instruments Ltd, the

Bertec Corporation and Advanced Mechanical Technology Incorporated.

Force plates also have been used to assess balance in both sitting and standing. Sackley and Baguley (1993) used a force plate mounted in the seat of a chair to measure balance in patients with stroke. Durward and Rowe (1995) have developed a system that uses eight force plates: four mounted in the seat of a chair and four mounted under the feet to examine the load distribution during sitting, rising to stand, standing and sitting down in normal and stroke subjects. Various commercial balance assessment systems are available that incorporate one or more force plates, including the Nottingham Balance Platform from Nottingham Rehabilitation Services and the Balance Master from Neurocom International Incorporated. A system for superimposing the output of a force plate, as a force vector, on top of a video image of the subject was reported by Tait and Rose (1979) and subsequently by Cook (1981). This device called a 'Video Vector' is commercially available from MIE Medical Research Limited as the 'Video Vector Generator'. A similar but inexpensive device has been reported by Rowe (1996). Other force transducers have been used to study functional activities. Most notable of these is the use of instrumented force-measuring walking aids to record the supportive forces generated during gait (Bergmann, 1978; Bennett et al., 1979; Opila, 1986, 1988; Rowe, 1990).

Attempts have been made to record the pressure distribution under the feet, which gives rise to the ground reaction force using a matrix array of force transducers. These systems have tended to be less accurate than their force plate counterparts but are useful in that they indicate not only the force being generated but the points of high pressure between the foot and floor. This is of particular benefit for those interested in foot problems, such as bunions, excessive pronation or diabetes. Commercial systems include the Musgrave Footprint from WM Automation, the Computer Dyno Graphy System from Infotronic, the Emed System from Novel GmbH and the Pedobaragraph from Baltimore Therapeutic Equipment. Both Infotronic and Novel also make flexible, in-shoe devices, which can record the pressure distribution between the sole of the foot and the shoe during activity. However, the sole of the foot is a curved surface and when wearing shoes there is little room in normal shoes for a transducer and wiring. For these reasons the sensors are usually clustered at key anatomical points, such as the heel and metatarsals, and do not cover the whole of the sole of the foot.

Moments

Moments generated at the joints by concentric, eccentric and isometric muscle activity can be measured during non-weight-bearing, prescribed activities using 'isokinetic' measuring devices such as the Akron, KinCom and Cybex. The moments exerted by a subject on a number of different manual tools can be measured during a number of work-related activities using the Baltimore Therapeutic Equipment (BTE) Work Simulator produced by the BTE Company. However, no direct measurement system exists to measure joint moments during functional activities.

Other Scientific Measures of Human Movement

Electromyography (EMG), which is the measurement of the electrical activity of muscles caused by contraction of the muscle, has been widely used in studies of human movement. Various methods of detecting the electrical noise produced by muscles are available including surface electrodes, fine wire electrodes and needle electrodes. EMG recordings are very difficult, if not impossible, to equate with the force developed by the muscle. While EMG can be used to indicate the activity of a muscle, morphological differences, muscle-length–tension relationships and fatigue all complicate the relationship between the electrical activity of the muscle and the force generated by the muscle. Even if the force generated by the muscle could be obtained by EMG, the anatomical position of the muscle would also need to be recorded before the data could be used to calculate the muscle moment produced, and hence determine the nature of the motion likely to be produced. EMG is therefore useful as an adjunct to movement studies but cannot be thought to evaluate movement itself. An excellent expose of the issues related to EMG can be obtained from reading Muscles Alive by Basmajan (1974). EMG manufactures include Biometrcis, Delsys, Cranlea, B and L, MIE and Noraxon.

In summary, a number of 'movement assessment systems' are available to the clinical researcher. These systems are able to record one or more kinematic variable for one or more joints or limb segments. However, comprehensive coverage of all nine aspects of movement for a number of joints or body segments would not be practical with such equipment. Therefore these systems are useful to characterise motion and movement deficits but are usually unable to identify the cause of such deficits. To identify the cause of the deficit a full biomechanical assessment is often required. However, these systems can be usefully employed to produce outcome measures for a number of clinical movement measurement purposes. In comparison to full biomechanical analysis, such systems are currently less expensive, are relatively simple to use and are portable; hence they may offer a valuable alternative for clinical measurement of motion.

SUMMARY

At the present time there exists a considerable spectrum of motion measurement systems available to the clinical researcher. In presenting these tools and systems, the author has attempted to indicate that, for a particular research topic, a number of outcome measures are available and that these measures can often be recorded in a number of ways. Therefore, when initiating a clinical research project, the investigator must select an appropriate outcome measure (e.g. angular displacement of the knee during gait in knee replacement surgery) and a system by which this outcome measure can be recorded (cameras, electrogoniometer, IMU).

The measure and the system will be affected by the nature of the research question being asked. For example 'does the patient use their knee replacement normally?' may be more efficiently investigated by kinematic systems, such as electrogoniometers or IMUs, which are simple to use and inexpensive, while the question 'why is the motion of the knee different in patients with knee replacements?' may require a full biomechanical analysis using cameras, force plates, EMG and the calculation of kinetic parameters such as energy transfers between segments and the muscle work done.

While it is not possible to predict the exact nature or cost of motion measurement systems that will be available in the near future, it seems likely that the human movement scientist will continue to need to commission a system that addresses the measurement issues of specific interest to that project. It would be overkill, indeed (but not unheard of), for a £200,000, full biomechanical analysis system to be used to record the walking speed or stance time of a group of subjects when a stopwatch and video could be used to achieve the same ends with considerable saving in time and money.

The author encourages those who read this chapter to plan their investigation based on the nature of the research question posed, the type of data needed, the level of accuracy considered appropriate and the detail required from the results. Having established these requirements the investigator can then seek a method that can determine the required data with the maximum efficiency and minimum expenditure of time and money. In other words, the question should precede the measurement system and not vice versa.

By presenting some of the historical developments in this chapter it is hoped that the reader will be encouraged to create systems and solutions that are appropriate to their situation. Most of the current analysis systems have been developed by medical engineers with an eye to clinical assessment needs. Some have included input from orthopaedic surgeons, sports scientists and physiotherapists. However, the field of human movement analysis remains in a developmental stage. Direct involvement of clinicians in the design, operation and reporting of these measurement systems is vital, if the recording of human movement is to become a regular activity in the clinical environment.

SELF-ASSESSMENT QUESTIONS

1. What nine things can be recorded by a full biomechanical motion analysis system?
2. How does a movement assessment differ from a full biomechanical motion analysis?
3. What is stereo photogrammetry?
4. What type of light do most motion capture systems use?
5. What are the disadvantages of single marker systems?
6. What is a cluster?
7. What is the disadvantage with visual motion analysis?
8. What is an electrogoniometer?
9. How does electromyography help biomechanical motion analysis?
10. What is an IMU?

REFERENCES

Al-Mijalli, M., Solomonides, S., Spence, W., et al., 1993. Design specification of a walkmat system for the measurement of temporal and distance parameters of gait. Gait Posture 1, 119–120.

An, K.N., Jacobsen, M.C., Berglund, L.J., Chao, E.Y.S., 1988. Application of a magnetic tracking device to kinesiologic studies. J. Biomech. 21 (7), 613–620.

Andriacchi, T., Ogle, J., Galante, T., 1977. Walking speed as a basis for normal and abnormal gait measurements. J. Biomech. 10, 261–268.

Arenson, J., Ishai, G., Bar, A., 1983. A system for monitoring the position of feet contact during walking. J. Med. Eng. Technol. 7 (6), 280–284.

Baer, G.D., Rowe, R.J., Crosbie, J., Fowler, V.E., Durward, B.R., 1995. Measurement of body segment displacement during functional activities. Physiotherapy 81 (10), 643.

Basmaijan, J.V., 1974. Muscles Alive: Their Functions Revealed by Electromyography. Williams & Wilkins.

Bennett, L., Murray, P., Murphy, E., Sowell, T., 1979. Locomotion through cane impulse. Bull. Prosthet. Res. 10 (31), 38–47.

Bergmann, G., Kolbel, R., Rohlmann, A., 1978. Walking aids–their effect on forces transmitted at the hip joint and proximal end of the femur. Biomechanics VI (B), 264–269.

Boenig, D., 1977. Evaluation of a clinical method of gait analysis. Phys. Ther. 57 (7), 795–798.

Brunnstrom, S., 1964. Recording gait patterns of adult hemiplegic patients. Phys. Ther. 44, 11.

Cerny, K., 1983. A clinical method of quantitative gait analysis. Phys. Ther. 63 (7), 1125–1126.

Chao, E., 1980. Justification of a triaxial goniometer for the measurement of joint rotation. J. Biomech. 13, 989–1006.

Charnley, J., Pusso, R., 1968. The recording and analysis of gait in relation to surgery of the hip joint. Clin. Orthop. 58, 153–164.

Cook, T., 1981. Vector visualizaion in gait analysis. Bull. Pros. Res. (Conf. Rep.) 10–35 (18/1), 308–309.

Crosbie, J., Eisenhuth, J., 1993. Transducer for the measurement of linear displacement of body segments. Med. Biol. Eng. Comput. 31, 430–432.

Crosbie, J., Durward, B.D., Rowe, P.J., 1996. Upper and lower trunk translations associated with stepping. Gait Posture 4 (1), 26–33.

Durie, N., Farley, R., 1980. An apparatus for step length measurement. J. Biomed. Eng. 2, 38–40.

Durward, B.R., Rowe, P.J., 1995. Measurement of total vertical force and time during rising to stand in normal and hemiplegic subjects. Physiotherapy 81, 640.

Finley, F., Karpovich, P., 1964. Electrogoniometric analysis of normal and pathological gaits. Res. Q. 35 (Suppl.), 379–384.

Gabel, R., Johnston, R., Crowninshield, R., 1979. A gait analyzer/trainer instrumentation system. J. Biomech. 12, 543–549.

Gabell, A., Nayak, U., 1984. The effect of age on variability in gait. J. Gerontol. 39, 662–666.

Gifford, G., Hutton, W., 1980. A microprocessor-controlled system for evaluating treatments for disablilities affectiing the lower limb. J. Biomed. Eng. 2, 46–48.

Gore, T., Flynn, M., Stevens, J., 1979. Measurement and analysis of hip joint movements. Eng. Med. (ImechE) 8, 21–25.

Hazlewood, M.E., Brown, J.K., Rowe, P.J., Salter, P.M., 1994. The use of therapeutic electrical stimulation in the treatment of hemiplegic cerebral palsy. Dev. Med. Child Neurol. 36, 661–673.

Hindle, R.J., Pearcy, M.J., Cross, A.T., Miller, D.H., 1990. Three-dimensional kinematics of the human back. Clin. Biomech. 5, 218–228.

Hirokawa, S., Matsumara, K., 1987. Gait analysis using a measuring walkway for temporal and distance factors. Med. Biol. Eng. Comput. 25, 62–74.

Jacobs, N., Skorecki, J., Charnley, J., 1972. Analysis of the vertical components of force in normal and pathological gait. J. Biomech. 5, 11–34.

Jansen, E., Vittas, D., Hellberg, S., Hansen, J., 1982. Normal gait of young and old men and women. Acta Orthop. Scand. 53, 193–196.

Johnston, R., Smidt, G., 1969. Measurement of hip joint motion during walking, an evaluation of an electrogoniometric method. J. Bone Joint Surg. Am. 51 (A), 1083–1094.

Kettlekamp, D., Johnston, R., Smidt, G., et al., 1979. An electrogoniometric study of knee motion in normal gait. J. Bone Joint Surg. Am. 52 (A), 775–790.

Koerner, I., 1984. Observation of Human Gait (a study guide to accompany videocassettes). Health Sciences Audiovisual Education, University of Alberta.

Krebs, D.E., Edelstein, J.E., Fishman, S., 1985. Reliability of observational kinematic gait analysis. Phys. Ther. 65, 1027–1033.

Lamoreux, L., 1971. Kinematic measurements in the study of human walking. Bull. Prosthet. Res. 10 (15), 3–84.

Law, H.T., 1987. Microcomputer-based, low-cost method for measurement of spatial and temporal parameters of gait. J. Biomed. Eng. 9, 115–120.

Law, H.T., Minns, R.A., 1989. Measurement of spatial and temporal parameters of gait. Physiotherapy 75, 81–84.

Macmillan, F.S., 1989. Performance of the Rheumatoid Elbow following Elbow Arthroplasty. PhD thesis, University of Strathclyde, Glasgow.

Mukherjee, P., Ganguli, S., 1977. Detection of gait abnormality from tachographic data. J. Med. Eng. Technol. 1 (2), 106–107.

Myles, C., Rowe, P.J., Salter, P.M., et al., 1995. An electrogoniometry system used to investigate the ability of the elderly to ascend and descend stairs. Physiotherapy 81, 639.

Nicol, A., 1988. A new flexible electrogoniometer with widespread applications. Biomechanics X, 1029–1033.

Olney, S.J., Elkin, N.D., Lowe, P.J., et al., 1979. An ambulation profile for clinical gait evaluation. Physiother. Can. 31, 31–85.

Opila, K., Nicol, A., Paul, J., 1986. Biomechanical analysis of limb loads in aided gait using elbow crutches. In: Perren, S., Schneider, E. (Eds.), Biomechanics and Current Interdisciplinary Research. Martinus Nijhoff, pp. 567–572.

Opila, K., Nicol, A., Paul, J., 1988. Quantification of the function of walking aids. Biomechanics XA, 147–172.

Paul, J., Hamblen, D., 1986. Clinical and Biomechanical Investigation of the Lower Limb Function in Patients with Polyarthritis following Single Joint Replacement. Report to the Scottish Home and Health Department. Contract Number K/RED/4/C42. University of Strathclyde, Glasgow.

Pearcy, M.J., Hindle, R.J., 1989. New method for the noninvasive three-dimensional measurement of human back movement. Clin. Biomech. 4, 73–79.

Pedotti, A., 1977. Simple equipment used in clinical practice for evaluation of locomotion. IEEE Trans. Biomed. Eng. 24 (5), 456–465.

Perry, J., 1981. The techniques and concepts of gait analysis. Bull. Prosthet. Res. (Conf. Rep.) 18 (1), 279–281.

Perry, J., Bontgranger, E., Antonelli, D., 1979. Footswitch definition of basic gait characteristics. In: Kennedi, Paul, Hughes (Eds.), Disability. Proceedings of a Seminar on Rehabilitation of the Disabled, August 1978. Macmillan.

Rowe, P.J., Crosbie, J., Fowler, V., Durward, B., Baer, G., 1999. A new system for the measurement of displacements of the human body with widespread applications in human movement studies. Med. Eng. Phys. 21, 265–275.

Rowe, P.J., 1990. The Evaluation of the Functional Ability of Total Hip Replacement Patients. Thesis, University of Strathclyde, Glasgow.

Rowe, P.J., White, M., 1996. Three-dimensional lumbar spinal kinematics during gait following mild musculoskeletal low back pain in nurses. Gait Posture 4, 242–251.

Rowe, P.J., Nicol, A., Kelly, I., 1987. A microcomputer based system for the assessment of hip function. In: Proc. Conf. Gait Anal. Med. Photogrammetry, pp. 42–44. Oxford Orthopaedic Engineering Centre.

Rowe, P.J., Nicol, A., Kelly, I., 1989. Flexible goniometer computer system for the assessment of hip function. Clin. Biomech. 4, 68–72.

Sackley, C.M., Baguley, B.I., 1993. Visual feedback after stroke with the balance performance monitor. Clin. Rehabil. 7, 189–195.

Saleh, M., Murdoch, G., 1985. In defence of gait analysis. J. Bone Joint Surg. Am. 67B, 237–241.

Stauffer, R., Smidt, G., Wadsworth, J., 1974. Clinical and biomechanical analysis of gait following Charnley total hip replacement. Clin. Orthop. 99, 70–77.

Tait, J., Rose, G., 1979. The real time video vector display of ground reaction forces during ambulation. J. Med. Eng. Technol. 3 (5), 252–255.

Tala, J., Quanbury, A., Steinke, T., Grahame, R., 1978. A variable axis electrogoniometer for the measurement of single plane movement. J. Biomech. 11, 421–425.

Townsend, M., Izak, M., Jackson, R., 1977. Total motion knee goniometry. J. Biomech. 10, 183–193.

Tracy, K.B., Montague, E.C., Gabriel, R.P., et al., 1979. Computer assisted diagnosis of orthopaedic gait disorders. Phys. Ther. 59, 268.

Trnkoczy, A., Badj, T., 1975. A simple electrogoniometric system and its testing. IEEE Trans. Biomed. Eng. 22 (3), 257–259.

Vivoda, E., Jenkins, S., Stanish, W., Putnam, C., 1986. Gait patterns of accelerometry. Orthop. Trans. (IEEE), 10 (1) (abstract), 93.

Wadsworth, J., Smidt, G., Johnston, R., 1972. Gait characteristics of subjects with hip disease. Phys. Ther. 52 (8), 829–839.

Wall, J.C., Crosbie, J., 1997. Accuracy and reliability of temporal gait measurement. Gait Posture 4, 293–296.

Wall, J., Ashburn, A., Klenerman, L., 1981. Gait analysis in the assessment of functional performance before and after total hip replacement. J. Biomech. Eng. 3, 121–127.

Wall, J., Charteris, J., Hoare, J., 1978. An automated online system for measuring the temporal patterns of foot/floor contact. J. Med. Eng. Technol. 2, 187–190.

Wall, J., Dhanendran, M., Klenerman, L., 1976. A method of measuring the temporal/distance factors of gait. Biomed. Eng. December, 409–412.

Clinical Measures of Mobility Within the International Classification of Functioning, Disability and Health Framework

Andy Kerr

OUTLINE

LEARNING OUTCOMES

After reading this chapter, you will be able to:

1. Distinguish between the International Classification of Functioning, Disability and Health (ICF) categories: body structures/functions, activity and participation.
2. Explain the impact of environmental factors on activity and participation.

3. Understand the need to measure the impact of rehabilitation on mobility across body structure/function, activity and participation.
4. Apply understanding to common clinical problems.

INTRODUCTION

This chapter continues the theme of measurement. It differs from Chapters 11 and 12, which dealt with measurement of the mechanics of movement, joint rotations, forces etc. In this chapter we will consider ways of measuring how a condition or injury might affect movement ability as well as the impact this might have across the life experience; going to school, playing, working, studying, domestic chores, social

activities etc. Voluntary movement is a defining characteristic of humans, and indeed all animals. The Chambers Dictionary defines an animal as 'an organism having life, sensation and voluntary **motion**' (i.e. not a plant). Disease and injury will inevitably have some impact on your ability to move, whether it is a routine daily function, such as brushing your teeth, or a more complex activity, such as playing a musical instrument. In many cases movement will recover as the disease or injury abates; others will need more time and input from rehabilitation experts. The physiotherapist's specialised skills and knowledge mean they are uniquely placed to support this recovery. The Chartered Society of Physiotherapy defines physiotherapy as follows: 'Physiotherapy helps restore movement and function when someone is affected by injury, illness or disability'. It is important that this restorative process considers all aspects of movement, to look beyond the measurement of knee range of motion and see the impact a reduced range might have on activities, such as stair climbing, as well as on a person's ability to participate in their occupations or leisure interests. Of course, physiotherapists are likely to adopt this approach anyway; it makes sense, and is, after all, what the patient wants. What isn't done so well is measuring these different aspects of mobility during clinical practice. Knee range of motion is pretty easy and we have simple, reliable tools for doing this. Measuring the impact of reduced knee motion on daily life is a little trickier, but this wider impact of a movement problem is nevertheless important, which is why research studies often include them. Lord Kelvin said, 'When you can measure what you are speaking about, and can express it in numbers, you know something about it'. In modern health services we could probably add, 'and can put a value on it'; health professionals, like everyone else, have to prove their worth.

In this chapter we will look at some of the many clinical methods for measuring movement with examples from orthopaedics and neurology, and explore how the different aspects of movement inter relate. To do this we will consider mobility within the classification model proposed by the World Health Organisation (WHO); this is called the International Classification of Functioning, Disability and Health (ICF), and is the most widely accepted model for considering human behaviour and health (WHO, 2013), see Activity Box 13.2.

In Chapter 11 the properties of measurement tools (validity, reliability, sensitivity etc.) were explained; we will refer to these properties throughout the chapter, but it is a good idea to remind yourself of the main points; see Activity Box 13.1.

ACTIVITY BOX 13.1 Measurement Properties

Remind yourself what the following terms mean:
- Face validity
- Content validity
- Criterion validity
- Reliability (inter and intra)
- Sensitivity

THE INTERNATIONAL CLASSIFICATION OF FUNCTIONING, DISABILITY AND HEALTH

The International Classification of Diseases (ICD) is a framework used by almost every country in the world to classify disease. It is basically a long and very detailed list of every known disease from arthritis to yellow fever, which are classified into appropriate groups such as 'diseases of the circulatory system' and given a unique code. This is basically a statistical tool to keep track of disease across the globe. It is very useful for governments and health agencies to plan how their resources are distributed in terms of fighting disease. It tells us very little about how a particular disease or condition affects the way an individual lives their life. The impact a disease or condition has on function varies substantially between individuals, with factors as diverse as culture, occupation, local infrastructure and perception all affecting the level of disability. To help us understand how these contexts of the disease or long-term condition alters an individual's disability, the WHO proposed the ICF to complement the ICD. This was endorsed by all 191 members of the WHO in 2001. There is a fully operational online version of this classification system available on the WHO website, so you can check it out yourself: http://apps.who.int/classifications/icfbrowser/.

I will introduce the overall structure of the system and then go through some examples, but first it is worth defining some of the central terms.

Movement and Mobility

I have used these terms interchangeably so far but it is probably worth clarifying what each means. The dictionary definition of mobility is 'the ability to move or be moved freely and easily', so it covers both an individual's voluntary movement and someone/something moving them. You can be mobile with a car, for example. Movement, or to be more specific, voluntary movement, is 'the act of changing body position or orientation'. In practice the terms are used synonymously, so you might mobilise a stiff joint or ask about someone's mobility on the ward following orthopaedic surgery; on the other hand you might practice repetitive arm movements with a stroke patient. Within the ICF model, the term *mobility* is used to describe movement of specific joints (e.g. mobility of the scapula [b7200]). It is also the subject of a whole chapter under Activities and Participation (chapter 4, Mobility) with four main categories of mobility: (1) *changing and maintaining body position*, (2) *walking and moving*, (3) *carrying, moving and handling objects* and (4) *moving around using transportation*. These are illustrated in Fig. 13.1. Think of **mobility** as a general term covering moving yourself and being moved, and **movement** as the

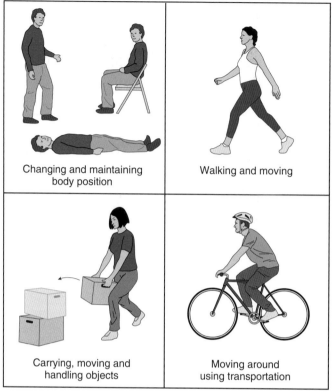

Changing and maintaining body position

Walking and moving

Carrying, moving and handling objects

Moving around using transportation

Fig. 13.1 The Four Categories of Mobility as Defined by the International Classification of Functioning, Disability and Health.

act of moving bits (and all) of your own body. Hopefully that clarifies things.

Body Functions

Denoted With a 'b' in the ICF Coding System

Body functions are the physiological (and psychological) functions of a specific body system. Examples (WHO call them '*chapters*') are: mental functions (chapter 1), voice and speech functions (chapter 3) and neuromusculoskeletal and movement-related functions (chapter 7). These chapters have sub-chapters; for example, chapter 7 has a sub-chapter called 'Functions of the joints and bones' (b710 to b729), which has sub-categories such as 'mobility of joint functions' (b710, i.e. joint movement).

Body Structures

Denoted With an 's' in the ICF Coding System

Body structures are the actual physical systems (again called '*chapters*') contained in a body. Examples include Structures of the Nervous System (chapter 1), The Eye, Ear and Related

Structures (chapter 2), and Structures Related to Movement (chapter 7). Like body functions, structures have sub-chapters; for example, chapter 7 has a sub-chapter called 'Structures of the trunk', which can be further divided into 'muscles of the trunk' (s7601), or 'ligaments and fascia of the trunk' (s7602).

Activities and Participation

Denoted With a 'd' in the ICF Coding System

Activity is the execution of a task or action by an individual. Examples include Learning and Applying Knowledge (chapter 1), Communication (chapter 3) and Mobility (chapter 4). Of course, there are lot of sub-chapters; for example, Mobility has 'Changing and maintaining body position' (codes d410 to d429). D415 in this sub-chapter can be further divided into 'maintaining a kneeling position' (d4152) and 'maintaining a standing position' (dd4154). To highlight how specific the activities are, Walking on Different Surfaces has its own code: d4502.

Participation

Participation, on the other hand, is all about an individual's involvement in life situations. Chapters 7 (Interpersonal Interactions and Relationships), 8 (Major Life Areas) and 9 (Community, Social and Civic Life) are the chapters concerned with participation. Chapter 9, for example, contains the sub-section 'Recreation and leisure' (d920), which includes socialising (d9205) and sports (d9201) among many other codes for participation.

Environmental Factors
Denoted With an 'e' in the ICF Coding System

Finally, we have the environmental factors. These are the physical, social and attitudinal environment in which people live and conduct their lives. They are a major determinant of the limitations placed on how full a life an individual can live. Among these factors we have chapters like Support and Relationships (chapter 3) and Attitudes (chapter 4). Within chapter 4 there are a range of sub-categories such as 'Individual attitudes of people in positions of authority' (e430). Another interesting environmental factor category is Natural Environment (chapter 2, e2), which includes things like Climate (rain, wind, temperature etc.) and Population (e.g. density).

The International Classification of Functioning, Disability and Health Mobility Model

If we consider one of these mobility categories, let's say *carrying, moving and handling objects,* and a simple health related problem that we can all relate to (even if you have to imagine it) we can show how this model works. A 32-year-old female teacher falls and fractures her radius; after 6 weeks of immobilisation she is free to use it, but there is a loss of flexibility at the joints (elbow and wrist) as well as loss of muscle strength (wrist flexors/extensors and finger flexors/extensors).

The **body structures** affected are the muscles (wrist flexors/extensors and finger flexors/extensors) and joints (wrist and elbow).

The **body functions** affected are elbow flexion/extension/supination/pronation (passive and active), wrist flexion/extension (passive and active), digit flexion/extension (passive and active) and all the grips (passive and active).

The **activities** affected by these body structure/function impairments are manifold, including categories such as self-care (toileting/dressing/eating) and recreation/leisure (e.g. sports). If we consider the mobility category alone, affected activities might include lifting, carrying objects in hands, grasping objects, throwing and catching; or she may find it difficult driving her car (d475 within the *moving around with transportation* category). But if she lives in an environment with good public transport this may not be such a big problem (environmental factor).

What about **participation**? You might expect some effect on her ability to fully function at work, although this may be offset by the attitudes of her employers/colleagues; again, this is an environmental factor. Domestic life could be affected; for example, preparing meals may be challenging (d630, within the *domestic life* category), but again this could be mitigated by access to technologies such as microwave ovens and convenience foods; again, access to technology is an environmental factor.

The point here is that a relatively simple health problem can have far-reaching effects on an individual's ability to live their life, which may, or may not, be influenced by their environment (physical, cultural, economic) (Fig. 13.2).

MEASURING MOBILITY ACROSS THE INTERNATIONAL CLASSIFICATION OF FUNCTIONING, DISABILITY AND HEALTH

Now that we have an understanding of body structures/functions, activity and participation we need to figure how to measure them so we can see the full impact of our rehabilitation interventions on mobility, and justify the cost of rehabilitation services!

It would be a bit daft—not to mention dull—to go through all the clinical measurement tools available to measure mobility. So, we will instead tackle two case studies in which I will go through some appropriate ways of measuring mobility across the ICF categories.

Case Study #1: Treadmill Training to Improve Walking Function in Parkinson's Disease
Background

Flora is a 72-year-old woman with mild Parkinson's disease (PD). She has retired after 35 years as a school teacher. She lives at home with her husband. She enjoys playing lawn bowls and is a very sociable person, enjoying trips to restaurants, the cinema and the theatre. The condition is well controlled with her anti-Parkinson drugs; however, she has noticed that her walking has continued to gradually deteriorate, becoming slower with occasional moments of freezing (brief interruptions in forward motion as if her feet are glued to the floor) and difficulty negotiating obstacles, particularly when outside. These problems have started to limit her social outings and has had an impact on her ability to compete at bowls, where she now needs more frequent rests and a bit of understanding from the other bowlers. She sees an advert for treadmill training sessions at her local leisure centre, which are run by physiotherapists, and decides to sign up.

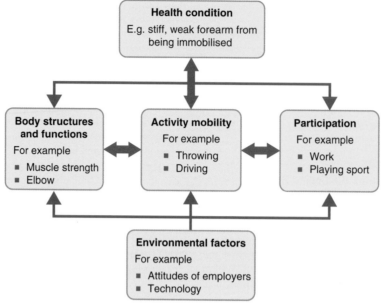

Fig. 13.2 Illustration of the ICF model, adapted from the World Health Organisation

---

ACTIVITY BOX 13.2 Impairment, Disability and Handicap

Before the introduction of the ICF model of body structures/functions, activity and participation, the model used was **impairment** (altered body function; e.g. muscle strength), **disability** (altered ability; e.g. brushing teeth) and **handicap** (limitation in a life role; e.g. occupation)—the latter being strongly influenced by environmental factors.

Why do you think it was changed?

For further information see

World Health Organisation, 1980. International classification of impairments, disabilities and handicaps. WHO, Geneva.

Body Structures and Functions: Parkinson's Disease

PD is a progressive neurological condition, primarily affecting a part of the brain called the basal ganglia due to a lack of dopamine, which is a chemical that helps neurons communicate with each other. The condition affects many aspects of movement; bradykinesia (slow movement), tremor and stiff/rigid muscles are the three main physical symptoms. However, balance problems, flexed posture, depression, insomnia and impaired cognition also can be experienced. The primary body structure involved is therefore the **brain**, which alters the function of the **muscles**. Although muscle strength and endurance are affected, the main problem is **control of voluntary movements** (b760 in the ICF)—specifically, the brain's ability to switch fluently between patterns of muscle activity (Petzinger et al., 2013). For example, to start walking from a standing position you need to first **switch off** the muscles that keep you standing (e.g. soleus) and **switch on** the muscles that start the stepping action (e.g. tibialis anterior and iliopsoas).

Clinical Measurement Options: Body Structure and Function

It is possible to assess the functioning of the basal ganglia using advanced imaging techniques such as radionuclide imaging (Stoessl et al., 2014). However, these techniques are currently outside the capacity of most, if not all, rehabilitation services, so direct measurement of the body structure involved in PD is not possible.

Directly measuring the body functioning problems; for example, motor programme switching (motor control) is possible. Electromyography (EMG) is a technique where electrodes are placed on the surface of a muscle belly to record its electrical activity as it contracts. These systems, once prohibitively expensive, are now commonplace in physiotherapy departments where they are used to provide feedback on muscle activity. We can use this technique to measure the degree of muscle control, or—to be specific—the timing between muscles switching on and others switching off, which is known to be problematic in people with PD (Caliandro et al., 2011).

There was also mention in the background of freezing when walking. This is such a common problem for people with PD that a specific questionnaire has been developed. The Freezing of Gait Questionnaire (FOG-Q) has been validated through comparison with more established, 'gold standard measurements' (Giladi et al., 2009), such as the Unified Parkinson's Disease Rating Scale (UPDRS) (discussed further on); this is called 'criterion validity' (Information Box 13.1). It has also been shown to be reliable when used by patients and carers (Nieuwboer et al., 2009).

While the FOG-Q mainly focuses on the body functioning problem of gait freezing (questions 3 to 6), it also includes a question on activity (question 2) and another on participation (question 1). Like the scores on many rating scales, the numerical result is ordinal. This means that the divisions between the scores are not even. The scale ranges from 0 (i.e. normal, no freezing) to 24 (i.e. severe freezing of gait); however, although a score of 20 is worse than 10 it is not 100% worse. So, we need to apply some caution when interpreting results from these kinds of rating scales, particularly when it comes to using statistical tests. Nevertheless, it is an excellent tool to quantify the degree of gait freezing.

Activity Restrictions: Parkinson's Disease

The activity restrictions mentioned in the background relate to walking (d450), particularly slow walking and avoiding obstacles. In the ICF this would include *walking around obstacles* (d4503) and perhaps *walking on different surfaces* (d4502).

Clinical Measurement Options: Activity

For the past 30 or more years the UPDRS has been the most widely used clinical rating scale for PD, covering body functions and activities but mainly focused on activity. It has recently been clarified, revised and retested for validity/reliability by the Movement Disorder Society (Goetz et al., 2008). It differs from using EMG in that it is a rating scale. The assessor asks the patient and/or carer about various aspects of their life, which they rate on a 5-point scale, 0 (normal) to 4 (severe). This information is then combined with the assessor's rating of the patient's ability to perform tasks such as walking 20 m, turning or standing up from a chair. While it includes all aspects of life, from motor (movement) to mood, it is mainly concerned with movement. For example, there are specific questions on walking (Fig. 13.3) and walking performance is rated by the assessor (Fig. 13.4).

There are 65 questions in the UPDRS, which obviously takes a bit of time to complete although it is acceptable to just do specific sections (e.g. on gait). The scale is used for many purposes, assessing the severity of the condition, identifying the main problem(s) for treatment and evaluating whether a treatment has been effective.

There are other clinical ways of measuring walking function in people with PD, which are used more generally in people with movement disorders such as stroke. I will briefly describe three commonly used ones:

1. *6-Minute walk test:* As the name suggests, this is the distance someone can walk in 6 minutes. It is a test of endurance (Rikli et al., 1998), which is easy to carry out and requires little equipment (or training); it can even be done on a treadmill. Not only is it popular with cardiac and respiratory conditions, but also it is relevant for neurological disorders such as PD. It has good

---

Information BOX 13.1 Freezing of Gait Questionnaire

1. During your worst state—do you walk:
   0 Normally, 1 Almost normally—somewhat slow, 2 Slow but fully independent, 3 Need assistance or walking aid, 4 Unable to walk
2. Are your gait difficulties affecting your daily activities and independence?
   0 Not at all, 1 Mildly, 2 Moderately, 3 Severely, 4 Unable to walk
3. Do you feel that your feet get glued to the floor while walking, making a turn or when trying to initiate walking (freezing)?
   0 Never, 1 Very rarely—about once a month, 2 Rarely—about once a week, 3 Often—about once a day, 4 Always—whenever walking
4. How long is your longest freezing episode?
   0 Never happened, 1 1–2s, 2 3–10s, 3 11–30s, 4 Unable to walk for more than 30s
5. How long is your typical start hesitation episode (freezing when initiating the first step)?
   0 None, 1 Takes longer than 1 s to start walking, 2 Takes longer than 3 s to start walking, 3 Takes longer than 10 s to start walking, 4 Takes longer than 30 s to start walking
6. How long is your typical turning hesitation (freezing when turning)?
   0 None, 1 Resume turning in 1–2 s, 2 Resume turning in 3–10 s, 3 Resume turning in 11–30 s, 4 Unable to resume turning for more than 30 s

> **Walking and balance**
>
> Over the past week, have you usually had problems with balance and walking?
>
> 0: Normal   Not at all (no problems).
>
> 1: Slight   I am slightly slow or may drag a leg. I never use a walking aid.
>
> 2: Mild   I occasionally use a walking aide, but I do not need any help from another person.
>
> 3: Moderate   I usually use a walking aid (cane, walker) to walk safely without falling. However, I do not usually need the support of another person.
>
> 4: Severe   I usually use the support of another person(s) to walk safely without falling.

Fig. 13.3 Example of the Unified Parkinson's Disease Rating Scale: patient rating of walking and balance ability.

> **Gait**
>
> Patient observed (from front/back if possible to see both sides) walking a minimum of 10 m, turning and walking another 10 m.
>
> 0: Normal   No problems
>
> 1: Slight   Independent walking with minor gait impairment.
>
> 2: Mild   Independent walking but with substantial gait impairment.*
>
> 3: Moderate   Requires an assistance device for safe walking (walking stick/cane, walker) but not another person.
>
> 4: Severe   Cannot walk at all or only with another person(s) helping.
>
> *Impairments could include step length, speed, foot lift height, turning, reduced arm swing.

Fig. 13.4 Example of the Unified Parkinson's Disease Rating Scale: therapist rating of a patient's ability to perform a task, for example, walking.

criterion validity and reliability when used in a range of conditions such as spinal cord injury (van Hedel et al., 2005).

2. *10-m walk test:* This is the time it takes for someone to walk 10 m (Rossier and Wade, 2001). Over such a short distance the primary focus is walking speed. The test is well used to evaluate the effect of gait reeducation treatments, such as treadmill training, with the idea being **if** you can walk faster, you **do** walk faster.

3. *Timed up and go:* The timed up and go (TUG) test has been around since the 1980s (Mathias et al., 1986). In this test the patient starts by sitting in a standard chair; on the instruction to go they stand up, walk 6 m to another chair, walk around it, and then return to the first chair to sit down again. This is all timed. It is used to test balance and more complex walking skill (turning, slowing down etc.) and is reliable when used with people who have PD (Morris et al., 2001). In terms of our case study, it might be a good choice as the patient reported difficulty getting around obstacles. It is also closer to an individual's everyday life situations compared with walking 10 straight metres. This is called ecological validity.

Participation: Parkinson's Disease

Maintaining (or improving) levels of participation in sport (lawn bowls) and social events (trips to the cinema and the theatre) is the ultimate goal for any treatment with this lady. It is pretty hard to have an impact on a person's quality of life and levels of participation through physical rehabilitation compared to say improving motor control or walking speed. There are many other personal and environmental factors to consider: confidence, depression, relationships, access to public transport, access to technology etc. Improving walking function through treadmill training will not, necessarily, translate to improved bowling or more frequent and enjoyable social events. Nevertheless, this is what matters to the patient, so we need ways of measuring movement at this level.

Clinical Measurement Options: Participation

Self-evidently, assessing quality of life will mean asking the individual lots of questions, but there are standardised tools we can use. In PD there are a few specific ones available. Long-term conditions, such as PD, tend to have their own quality of life assessment tool, but there are general (non-disease-specific) ones available, such as the EuroQoL, which has been widely tested for validity and reliability. Measuring quality of life is becoming more popular as governments and health services recognise the importance of enabling people to live happier lives, not just longer ones.

The Parkinson's Disease Questionnaire (PDQ-39) covers eight dimensions of life (Table 13.1) and this has been used to evaluate the effect of physiotherapy on quality of life (Chapuis et al., 2005). It has been validated across many languages and its construct validity and reliability has been found to be acceptable (Jenkinson et al., 1997). For the sake of convenience, these quality of life assessments are sometimes abbreviated. While this likely saves time (they can be quite long) it is important to consider all aspects of the life experience. After all, improving an individual's walking ability might have an impact on things like bodily discomfort, fatigue, stigma and not just mobility.

To summarise the main points of case study 1, if the physios running the treadmill training sessions need to demonstrate that that what they are doing is having a meaningful effect on the individual, they should consider measuring a combination of things like:

1. Freezing of gait with the FOG-Q: **Body function** category of ICF

TABLE 13.1 Parkinson's Disease Questionnaire. Dimensions and number of questions.

Dimension	Number of Questions
Mobility	10
Activities of daily living	6
Emotional wellbeing	6
Stigma	4
Social support	3
Cognition	4
Communications	3
Bodily discomfort	3

Adapted from Jenkinson, C., Fitzpatrick, R.A.Y., Peto, V.I.V., Greenhall, R., Hyman, N., 1997. The Parkinson's Disease Questionnaire (PDQ-39): development and validation of a Parkinson's disease summary index score. Age Ageing 26 (5), 353–357.

2. Functional mobility using the TUG test: **Activities** level of ICF
3. Quality of life with the PDQ-39. **Participation** level of ICF.

This is illustrated in Fig. 13.5; further information on the rehabilitation for people with PD is available from ParkinsonNet (http://www.parkinsonnet.info/guidelines), which provides European agreed guidelines on physiotherapy, occupational therapy and speech therapy.

Case Study #2: The Effect of Spinal Mobilisation Techniques on Non-Specific Low Back Pain

Background

Stephen is a middle-aged man who works as a manager in a call centre and has been suffering low back pain for the best part of a year. His main symptoms are pain, loss of flexibility, poor sleep and depression. These problems are now having an effect on his ability to sit for any length of time, and this is affecting his ability to drive to work as well as to actually work. His relationships with his family and friends are also being affected. His family doctor refers him for physical therapy.

Low back pain is a very common problem with a global prevalence (number of people within a population who have the problem) around 12% (Hoy et al., 2012). The pain and disability it causes can last for months with a minority (around 10%) becoming chronic sufferers.

Body Structures and Functions: Low Back Pain

Low back pain can be caused by many things like a vertebral fracture, inflammatory disease (e.g. ankylosing spondylitis) or even a tumour, but what most people experience is called nonspecific low back pain (NSLBP), which simply means we don't know exactly what is wrong. Many causes of NSLBP have been suggested; factors such as obesity, smoking and a sedentary lifestyle, are statistically likely to raise the risk of NSLBP (Activity Box 13.3). There are psychosocial consequences, particularly as the problem becomes chronic; however, the actual mechanism and injured structure are unknown. It is treated by a range of things such as education, exercise, postural advice, pain killers, anti-inflammatory drugs and manual therapy (massage and manipulations) (Balague et al., 2012). There are several potential structures responsible for causing the pain in NSLBP: muscle, joint, vertebral disc, nerves. The actual structure might never be known, although the likelihood is that the disc is involved, particularly if the symptoms are severe enough to cause time off school/work/sport. This is called discogenic NSLBP. The primary body **structures** involved are, therefore, the nerves, joints discs and muscles of the lumbar spine. In the ICF these are grouped together as structures of the lumbar vertebral column (s76002).

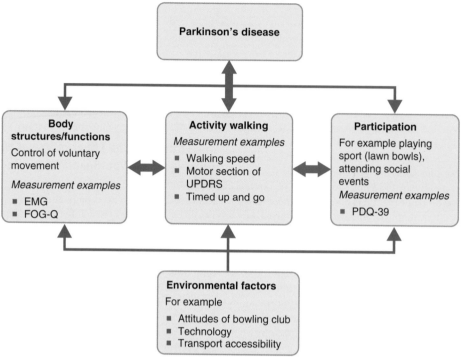

Fig. 13.5 International Classification of Functioning, Disability and Health Mobility Categories With Examples From Parkinson's Disease. *EMG,* Electromyography; *FOG-Q,* Freezing of Gait Questionnaire; *PDQ-39,* Parkinson's Disease Questionnaire; *UPDRS,* Unified Parkinson's Disease Rating Scale.

ACTIVITY BOX 13.3   Risk Factors for Nonspecific Low Back Pain

By definition we don't know what causes NSLBP. However, there are some factors identified as being statistically associated with its incidence. For example, narrowing of the disc space has an odds ratio of 1.9. This means an individual identified with disc narrowing (imaging techniques required) is 1.9 times more likely to get NSLBP. Things like obesity, disc narrowing, even a sedentary lifestyle make intuitive sense, but why do you think cigarette smoking raises the risk by 1.3 times? It is not as much as the other factors, but still.

Is it part of being sedentary?

Is there a physiological mechanism? Tissue weakening?

Is it part of obesity?

Perhaps people just start smoking when they get back pain? Depressed?

For more information try Balagué et al. (2012).

The body **functions** involved mainly relate to mobility, covering all the four categories (see Fig. 13.1). Specifically, it affects muscle power, joint mobility and pain. Pain is also a body function (listed under chapter 2, Sensory Functions and Pain, of the ICF) and back pain has a specific ICF code of b28013 (see Activity Box 13.3).

Clinical Measurement Options: Body Structure and Function

This is an area with an abundance of clinical measurements available to practitioners, probably because it is responsible for 1.3 million annual referrals to physiotherapy in the UK alone (Frost et al., 2004). In terms of structures there are a range of medical imaging techniques available (MR, X-ray, ultrasound), these are mainly used to diagnose a specific problem such as a spinal tumour or fracture. When a diagnosis of NSLBP has been made and the individual is referred for physiotherapy, there are still a number of measurement options open to the physiotherapist; however, they will, by necessity, focus on body function not structure, specifically joint mobility, muscle power/strength and pain. If there are sensory problems (caused by nerve root irritation) there may also be a need to assess sensory functions: touch (b265) and proprioception (b260).

Measuring **joint flexibility** is a little tricky with the lumbar spine compared to a single superficial joint such as the distal interphalangeal joint. Measurements are therefore indirect; for example, the fingertip-to-floor test and Schober's test. Inclinometers have also become a popular way of measuring the slope of the lumbar spine when it is flexed. The digital inclinometers contained in smartphones make this a convenient method (we will talk about the importance of measurement practicality later). When using these methods there is always a problem differentiating between the lumbar spine movement and movement of other parts (e.g. the pelvis). Nevertheless, these techniques give a good indirect measurement of lumbar spine flexibility and have been found to be generally reliable and valid; for example, the inter-rater reliability of the fingertip-to-floor test was found to be excellent (intraclass correlation coefficient = 0.99) (Perret et al., 2001).

Measuring muscle strength/power is clearly important in lower back pain (as well as many other conditions). Despite the development of several technologies, such as handheld dynamometers, isokinetic dynamometers and bioelectrical impedance, we still generally rely on manual testing procedures to measure strength in most muscles, including muscles of the trunk. Of course, this has a lot to do with convenience, but training and tradition may also be factors. The way most practitioners record muscle strength is to use a manual test and grade the muscle's response on a scale. The most widely used scale is the Medical Research Council (MRC) Muscle Scale, which was developed in the 1940s (MRC, 1976), which grades a muscle's maximal performance between 0 (no contraction) and 5 (normal power). See Fig. 13.6 for more details. It has been found to be valid and reliable when used in a range of conditions. There have been various amendments to the original scale (e.g. Paternostro-Sluga et al., 2008), which may be useful to give greater detail to some muscle disorders, such as cerebral palsy, but the original scale has the benefit of simplicity.

The MRC scale fits well into a busy clinical environment, but as a six-point scale it lacks the sensitivity of an instrument that measures the actual force produced by the muscle. A handheld dynamometers is a small device that the therapist holds in their hand when resisting a movement to gauge strength (Fig. 13.7). The device measures the force produced by the muscle using strain gauge technology. They have been shown to be reliable between testing sessions and between raters (Dowman et al., 2016), provided a standard protocol is followed; they also offer an arguably more objective and certainly more sensitive measure of muscle strength.

Power is the rate of generating tension in the muscle, that is, how quickly it can develop the contraction. To

0 = No contraction.
1 = Flicker or trace of contraction.
2 = Active movement, with gravity eliminated.
3 = Active movement against gravity.
4 = Active movement against gravity and resistance.
5 = Normal power.

Fig. 13.6 The Medical Research Council Muscle Scale as Originally Published.

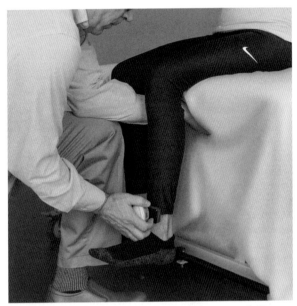

Fig. 13.7 Handheld Dynamometer. (Courtesy of Hoggan Scientific, LLC.)

measure this, we need an idea of time. There are ways of doing this for the upper and lower limbs (e.g. a lower limb power rig; Bassey and Short, 1990), but it is difficult to do with the trunk, so we probably need to rely on functional tests, such as a vertical jump, which indirectly measures power in a number of muscles.

Pain is a multi-dimensional experience involving pain sensation, anxiety, depression, activity restrictions and a number of other psychosocial factors. Consequently, it is very difficult thing to measure, particularly during routine clinical examinations. Visual analogue scales are typically used to assess pain intensity in the clinic and they have been found to be valid, reliable and (importantly) sensitive (Grotle et al., 2004). Essentially, the patient grades their pain intensity on a scale between 1 and 10 (Fig. 13.8). This is clearly the tip of the iceberg when it comes to measuring pain, and there are many more in-depth ways of capturing the whole

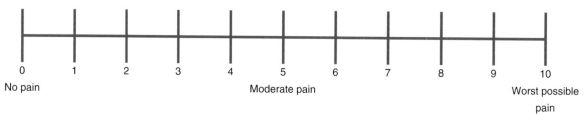

Fig. 13.8 Visual Analogue Scale for Measurement of Pain Intensity.

impact. For more information I refer you to several books written on the subject, such as *Pain: A Textbook for Therapists*, by Strong and Unruh.

I think we have covered a number of possible clinical methods for measuring the body functions involved in NSLBP. Now we will consider Activity.

Clinical Measurement Options: Activity

Again, we will only consider the mobility aspects listed under the ICF. There is a wide impact on activity from NSLBP. If we think of the four mobility categories (see Fig. 13.1) it is highly likely that there will be an effect on each. We already know transportation is a problem (driving car) due mainly to being unable to maintain a sitting position (d4153). Like PD, there are a few condition-specific questionnaires that have been developed. The two most commonly used are the Roland-Morris Disability Questionnaire (RDQ-24) and the Oswestry Disability Index (ODI). They are very similar in what they cover of the body, so we will just consider the RDQ-24.

The RDQ-24 contains 24 questions (surprisingly) dichotomous questions (yes/no) with the score ranging from 0 (no disability) to 24 (maximum disability). The questions cover a range of activities such as walking, sitting, dressing and daily activities. Both the RDQ-24 and the ODI are well used and have good levels of validity and reliability (see Roland and Fairbank, 2000). Change in the overall score can be used to assess whether an intervention has been effective, a decrease in 5 or more points in the RDQ-24 being considered 'clinically important'.

Participation: Low Back Pain

The impact of NSLBP on participation is clear from the background on Stephen (work and relationships). Also, it has been costed in terms of work hours lost (estimated at over 30 million days per year in the United Kingdom alone!). But let's keep our focus on the individual. In many ways the information we are seeking here is similar to the participation section in the PD case study. It differs from the ODI and RDQ-24 in that we are looking at a broad impact on the individual's life. The short form (SF) health survey

---

ACTIVITY BOX 13.4   Utility of Clinical Measurements

Having outcome measures that cover all aspects of movement, from body functions/structures to participation, is very important in understanding the extent of the problem, where the problem lies and to evaluate how effective the interventions and whole rehabilitation service has been. Of course, we need to have confidence in these measures. Knowing that what they measure is true means understanding their measurement properties, particularly validity, reliability and sensitivity. The measurement tools also need to be practical for everyday use in the clinical environment. The tools that have this practicality are the ones that endure to become routinely used in clinical practice; a good example is the MRC muscle scale. Practicality, sometimes called clinical utility, is based on a number of common sense factors:
- The need for equipment.
- Time to complete.
- Need for training.
- Ease of interpretation.
- Need for space or a specialised facility.

From your experience on a clinical site, even if this has been limited to observation, how much time do you think is spent routinely completing outcome measures?

5% of the patient interaction
10% of the patient interaction
20% of the patient interaction
30% of the patient interaction
40% of the patient interaction
50% of the patient interaction

(SF-36) and its smaller version (SF-12) are probably the most widely used in NSLBP for participation levels and quality of life. They have good levels of reliability and validity for people with NSLBP (Luo et al., 2003). An example of a question from the SF-36 is on the next page, so you can see the type of information it gathers.

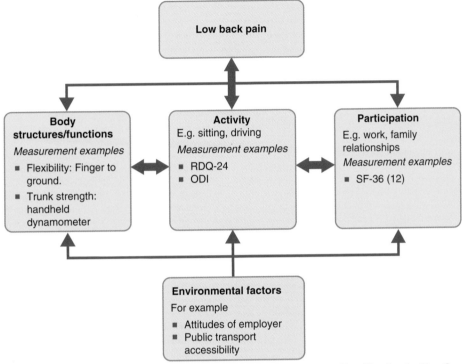

Fig. 13.9 International Classification of Functioning, Disability and Health Classification for Non-Specific Low Back Pain. *ODI*, Oswestry Disability Index; *RDQ-24*, Roland-Morris Disability Questionnaire; *SF*, short form.

SF-36 example question:

During the past 4 weeks, how much of the time has your physical healthy or emotional problems interfered with your social life (visiting friends/relatives etc.)?

(1) All of the time, (2) most of the time, (3) some of the time, (4) a little of the time and (5) none of the time.

To summarise Case Study 2. The physiotherapist treating Stephen needs to bear in mind the chronic nature of the problem and the likelihood that it is having a broad impact on his life. Therefore, they should probably consider measures from the list below:

1. Joint flexibility with fingertip-to-ground. **Body function.**
2. Trunk muscle strength with a handheld dynamometer or MRC muscle scale. **Body function.**
3. Impact on mobility with the RDQ-24. **Activity**
4. Impact on participation with the SF-36 (or SF-12). **Participation.**

This is summarised in Fig. 13.9 with further discussion in Activity Box 13.4.

SELF-ASSESSMENT QUESTIONS

1. Define what is meant by a body function.
2. Is pain a body function or activity?
3. What kind of thing is included in questionnaires designed to consider the participation domain of the ICF?
4. What are the four main classifications of mobility in the activity part of the ICF model?
5. Should walking be considered a body function or an activity?
6. Why is it important for health professionals to measure mobility across the ICF model?
7. If you measured motor control in a stroke would you be measuring in the body structure/function, activity or participation domains of mobility?

8. If you measured sit-to-stand ability (e.g. the five times sit-to-stand test) in someone recovering from a total hip arthroplasty, would you be measuring in the body structure/function, activity or participation domains of mobility?

9. If you measured return to work in someone recovering from cardiac surgery, would you be measuring in the body structure/function, activity or participation domains of mobility?

REFERENCES

Balagué, F., Mannion, A.F., Pellisé, F., Cedraschi, C., 2012. Non-specific low back pain. Lancet 379 (9814), 482–491.

Bassey, E.J., Short, A.H., 1990. A new method for measuring power output in a single leg extension: feasibility, reliability and validity. Eur. J. Appl. Physiol. Occup. Physiol. 60 (5), 385–390.

Caliandro, P., Ferrarin, M., Cioni, M., Bentivoglio, A.R., Minciotti, I., D'urso, P.I., et al., 2011. Levodopa effect on electromyographic activation patterns of tibialis anterior muscle during walking in Parkinson's disease. Gait Posture 33 (3), 436–441.

Chapuis, S., Ouchchane, L., Metz, O., Gerbaud, L., Durif, F., 2005. Impact of the motor complications of Parkinson's disease on the quality of life. Mov. Disord. 20 (2), 224–230.

Dowman, L., McDonald, C.F., Hill, C.J., Lee, A., Barker, K., Boote, C., et al., 2016. Reliability of the hand held dynamometer in measuring muscle strength in people with interstitial lung disease. Physiotherapy 102 (3), 249–255.

Frost, H., Lamb, S.E., Doll, H.A., Carver, P.T., Stewart-Brown, S., 2004. Randomised controlled trial of physiotherapy compared with advice for low back pain. Br. Med. J. 329 (7468), 708.

Giladi, N., Tal, J., Azulay, T., Rascol, O., Brooks, D.J., Melamed, E., et al., 2009. Validation of the freezing of gait questionnaire in patients with Parkinson's disease. Mov. Disord. 24 (5), 655–661.

Goetz, C.G., Tilley, B.C., Shaftman, S.R., Stebbins, G.T., Fahn, S., Martinez-Martin, P., et al., 2008. Movement disorder Society-sponsored revision of the unified Parkinson's disease rating scale (MDS-UPDRS): scale presentation and clinimetric testing results. Mov. Disord. 23 (15), 2129–2170.

Grotle, M., Brox, J.I., Vøllestad, N.K., 2004. Concurrent comparison of responsiveness in pain and functional status measurements used for patients with low back pain. Spine 29 (21), E492–E501.

van Hedel, H.J., Wirz, M., Dietz, V., 2005. Assessing walking ability in subjects with spinal cord injury: validity and reliability of 3 walking tests. Arch. Phys. Med. Rehabil. 86 (2), 190–196.

Hoy, D., Bain, C., Williams, G., March, L., Brooks, P., Blyth, F., et al., 2012. A systematic review of the global prevalence of low back pain. Arthritis Rheumatol. 64 (6), 2028–2037.

Jenkinson, C., Fitzpatrick, R.A.Y., Peto, V.I.V., Greenhall, R., Hyman, N., 1997. The Parkinson's disease questionnaire (PDQ-39): development and validation of a Parkinson's disease summary index score. Age. Ageing 26 (5), 353–357.

Luo, X., George, M.L., Kakouras, I., Edwards, C.L., Pietrobon, R., Richardson, W., et al., 2003. Reliability, validity, and responsiveness of the short form 12-item survey (SF-12) in patients with back pain. Spine 28 (15), 1739–1745.

Mathias, S., Nayak, U.S., Isaacs, B., 1986. Balance in elderly patients: the 'get-up and go' test. Arch. Phys. Med. Rehabil. 67 (6), 387–389.

Medical Research Council, 1976. Aids to Examination of the Peripheral Nervous System. Memorandum No. 45. Her Majesty's Stationary Office, London.

Morris, S., Morris, M.E., Iansek, R., 2001. Reliability of measurements obtained with the timed 'up & go' test in people with parkinson's disease. Phys. Ther. 81 (2), 810–818.

Nieuwboer, A., Rochester, L., Herman, T., Vandenberghe, W., Emil, G.E., Thomaes, T., et al., 2009. Reliability of the new freezing of gait questionnaire: agreement between patients with Parkinson's disease and their carers. Gait Posture 30 (4), 459–463.

Paternostro-Sluga, T., Grim-Stieger, M., Posch, M., Schuhfried, O., Vacariu, G., Mittermaier, C., et al., 2008. Reliability and validity of the Medical Research Council (MRC) scale and a modified scale for testing muscle strength in patients with radial palsy. J. Rehabil. Med. 40 (8), 665–671.

Perret, C., Poiraudeau, S., Fermanian, J., Colau, M.M.L., Benhamou, M.A.M., Revel, M., 2001. Validity, reliability, and responsiveness of the fingertip-to-floor test. Arch. Phys. Med. Rehabil. 82 (11), 1566–1570.

Petzinger, G.M., Fisher, B.E., McEwen, S., Beeler, J.A., Walsh, J.P., Jakowec, M.W., 2013. Exercise-enhanced neuroplasticity targeting motor and cognitive circuitry in Parkinson's disease. Lancet Neurol. 12 (7), 716–726.

Rikli, R.E., Jones, C.J., 1998. The reliability and validity of a 6-minute walk test as a measure of physical endurance in older adults. J. Aging Phys. Activity 6 (4), 363–375.

Roland, M., Fairbank, J., 2000. The Roland–Morris disability questionnaire and the oswestry disability questionnaire. Spine 25 (24), 3115–3124.

Rossier, P., Wade, D.T., 2001. Validity and reliability comparison of 4 mobility measures in patients presenting with neurologic impairment. Arch. Phys. Med. Rehabil. 82 (1), 9–13.

Stoessl, A.J., Lehericy, S., Strafella, A.P., 2014. Imaging insights into basal ganglia function, Parkinson's disease, and dystonia. The Lancet 384 (9942), 532–544.

World Health Organization, 1980. International classification of impairments, disabilities, and handicaps: a manual of classification relating to the consequences of disease, published in accordance with resolution WHA29. 35 of the Twenty-ninth World Health Assembly, May 1976.

WHO, 2013. How to Use the ICF—a Practical Manual for Using the International Classification of Functioning, Disability and Health. WHO, Geneva. Available at: http://www.who.int/classifications/icf/en/. (Accessed 05 December 2018.)

Physical (In)Activity

Daniel Rafferty

LEARNING OUTCOMES

After reading this chapter, you will be able to:
1. Define what we mean by low, moderate and vigorous physical activity.
2. State the current daily recommendations.
3. Understand the strengths and weaknesses of the different ways to measure physical activity.
4. Discuss the relationship between health and being sedentary (physical [in]activity).
5. Appreciate the complexity of changing human behaviour and how it relates to physical activity.

INTRODUCTION

Life has changed over the past 50 years. Labour-intensive work, such as mining, farming and ship building, is being replaced with automation. Many of us now sit in front of phones and computers for long periods. This is the way we now carry out our business; even nurses and physiotherapists will spend some of their time sitting at a personal computer. The way we get to work has also changed, with many studies focusing on the reduction in car use both to combat CO_2 emissions and obesity levels in society (Morency, 2011; Graham-Rowe, 2011).

As has been said before in this book, movement is fundamental to health and well-being. This sedentary life we are increasingly adopting is a major factor in the development of long-term conditions, such as heart disease, stroke and diabetes. In this chapter we will explore what physical activity is, and what we mean by light and moderate to vigorous activity. The idea of sedentary behaviours will also be examined and how these influence our health. We will look at ways of measuring physical activity that are relevant to your practice and take a look at some ways to change physical activity behaviour for your patients (and yourself) so that the daily recommended levels are achieved.

Physical activity is defined as any bodily movement produced by skeletal muscles that requires energy expenditure. Physical inactivity has been identified as the fourth leading risk factor for global mortality causing an estimated 3.2 million deaths globally.

Regular moderate intensity physical activity—such as walking, cycling or participating in sports—has significant benefits for health. For instance, it can reduce the risk of cardiovascular diseases, diabetes, colon and breast cancer and depression. Moreover, adequate levels of physical activity will decrease the risk of a hip or vertebral fracture and help control weight (World Health Organisation [WHO], http://www.who.int/topics/physical_activity/en/) (Activity Box 14.1).

ACTIVITY BOX 14.1   How Physically Active Do You Think You Are?

Being physically active is important for health and well-being. You will have undoubtedly heard that message before, in school for example, but before we get into the details of the chapter have a think about how physically active you are at the moment. Not what you used to do and what you should be doing but actually what you do. Think about the past 7 days using the statements below.

1. I was physically active every day last week.
2. I was physically active on at least 5 days of the week.
3. If you add up my physical activity it would be at least 30 min on every (or most) days.
4. The physical activity I do tends to be:
   a. Light: Does not get you out of breath, e.g. cooking.
   b. Moderate: Gets you a little out of breath, e.g. walking at a reasonable pace or
   c. Vigorous: Gets you breathing rapidly and deeply, e.g. playing squash.

Answering these questions will hopefully get you thinking a bit more about your own physical activity as well as some of the problems measuring it.

ENERGY

Every human action, however small, requires energy. In reading the introduction you make think 'this chapter is going to be interesting'; that required energy for the impulses in the brain to formulate that thought. Even if you adopted the opposite opinion of 'this will be tedious' you still used energy. The very fact of reading and digesting content requires energy. This is low-level energy. Undertaking movement requires a higher level of energy expenditure. So, if your thoughts are now 'I am off to get a biscuit', and you execute this desire, then you will have expended more energy than simply thinking about it. The engagement of our musculoskeletal system requires the activation of thought processes and, through coordination of our central nervous system, the activation and control of the contraction of our muscles is a much more energy-intense requirement than simply thinking about it (see Chapter 6 for more information on muscle contraction).

We get our energy from food. This energy comes in three forms: carbohydrates, fat and protein. It is outside the scope of this chapter to explore the complex relationship as to how to achieve a balanced diet, which is a science in and of itself and is known as nutritional science. Suffice to say that the energy we take in is used in three ways. First, we need energy to keep the basic systems going (resting metabolism), that is, breathing, heartbeat, brain function, all organ functions. Second, we need energy to chew, digest and secrete the food waste. This chapter will focus on the final and largest way we expend energy, through movement. This is often referred to as the energy balance equation. How much energy we take in, in order not to gain weight, must be burned off. We can do very little to affect our resting metabolism. While everyone is different, generally we need similar amounts of energy to keep the systems functioning. The cost of processing food, although somewhat dependant on the type of food consumed, is also similar. The main aspect that we can influence is movement. When we move we use more energy (Fig. 14.1).

PROMOTING PHYSICAL ACTIVITY TO IMPROVE HEALTH

The question then arises: how much and how intense should our physical activity be to accrue health benefits? It is generally accepted, and promoted through a number of recognised nongovernmental as well government agencies (WHO, American College of Sports Medicine, National Health Service UK), that we should do three things:

1. Undertake moderate to vigorous physical activity (MVPA) for 30 minutes/day.
2. Achieve this on at least 5 days/week.

Energy balance equation

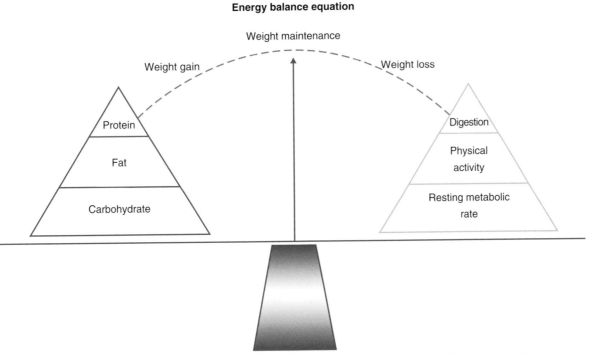

Fig. 14.1 Energy Balance Equation. The types of energy we consume and the activities we undertake.

3. And these bouts of activity should be continuous, lasting for no less than 10 minutes.

Clear and understandable? Number two is straightforward —at least 5 days/week. Numbers 1 and 2 are more open to interpretation.

Let's take number 1. What does MVPA mean? As health professionals you may have a clear understanding of this, but can we assume that the rest of the population are similarly well educated when it comes to understanding physical activity? A recent experience working with schoolteachers, who have a good level of education, provided the answer; no one knew what number 2 meant. Translating this message to the general population is clearly a challenge. As health professionals (future or current), this may be part of your responsibilities; hopefully reading this chapter will fill in some of your knowledge gaps.

What about the final recommendation—achieving physical activity bouts of at least 10 minutes? So, if the bout is interrupted, say 3 minutes, then 7 minutes, does this mean it doesn't count? A colleague power walks to work for a distance of approximately 6 km on most days. Using activity monitors we looked at how they accrued physical activity. Even although on arrival they would be panting and sweaty, at no point did they accrue 10 minutes of continuous physical activity. Why? Well, they walked in an urban environment; therefore they were required to stop, for example waiting for the road to clear to cross it, getting caught behind an annoying student using their smartphone, or going into the shop to buy a newspaper. We know from research by Harvey et al. (2017) that a break in physical activity lasting at least 50 seconds will change the physiological state with a significant reduction in oxygen consumption.

My personal experience, as someone who cycles to work most days, confirms this. It takes me 2 hours/day to cycle to and from work. Using a monitor, only $1\frac{1}{2}$ hours were recorded as activity, and that was without stopping for a newspaper or being held up by students doing impressions of zombies on their mobile phones. As a good cyclist, stopping at traffic lights etc. is a must. It is during these enforced stops that my half hour of activity is lost to inactivity. How we accrue physical activity is a very complex pattern and requires careful measurement and interpretation.

MODERATE TO VIGOROUS PHYSICAL ACTIVITY

So What Is Moderate to Vigorous Physical Activity?

Moderate to vigorous physical activity is considered to be physical activity that has an intensity of been 3 to 6 METs.

Couldn't be clearer, could it? Hold on, what is meant by a MET? A MET is a metabolic equivalent of task, still not making things much clearer, is it? A single MET is considered to be how much oxygen we need to take into our system when sitting at rest to meet our resting metabolic requirements. Or put more simply, the amount of oxygen required to keep the system functioning when sitting at rest. Generally it is considered that we require 3.5 mL/O_2·kg per minute to keep the basic metabolic systems of our body working. That is, for every kilogram of body mass, we consume 3.5 mL of oxygen every minute; this is known as resting metabolic rate. So moderate to vigorous physical activity includes activities that require between three and six times this resting oxygen requirement. The METs for various tasks are listed within the compendium of physical activities (Ainsworth et al., 2011). As examples, walking at a pace of 4.8 km/h (3 mph) is considered to have a MET value of 3.3, or cycling at a pace of less than 16 km/h (10 mph) has a MET value of 4. All MET values in the compendium are only to be considered estimates and will vary between individuals. It has also been demonstrated that the energy requirements of people living with long-term conditions will require additional energy in comparison to healthy controls to undertake everyday activities, such as walking (Paul, 2008; Platts, 2006).

The measurement of oxygen uptake is relatively straightforward. We know the amount of oxygen in air (20.95%); therefore if we measure the amount of oxygen in exhaled air and subtract this from what is present normally in air the difference is the amount of oxygen we require (consume) to perform an activity. Unfortunately, the method for doing this is: (a) relatively expensive, (b) a burden on the participant and (c) requires complex instrumentation. Oxygen uptake can be measured in free living activities; however, the participant could be reluctant to wear the apparatus for long periods of time. The apparatus is known as indirect calorimetry, or is more commonly known as a gas analyser.

WALKING AND METABOLIC ACTIVITIES

For most of us, walking is the most common form of physical activity (McArdle, 1986). The speed of our walking is highly correlated to the oxygen uptake (or METs); the faster we walk the more oxygen we require. The speed of walking is also highly correlated to our cadence. Cadence is the number of steps we take per minute. It is common to consider cadences of 100 steps per minute or more to be MVPA. Is there technology that allows us to measure cadence in free living activities? Yes, most of us will have smartphones. Smartphones have the necessary hardware (accelerometers) and software (applications) that allow us to estimate our cadence in everyday life and therefore enables us to quantify

how much MVPA we actually accrue. There are also a number of more research-orientated devices that improve the accuracy of measuring cadence. We will come on to the technology available to us later in the chapter.

One of the trials that our group undertook was to explore the MVPA of the daily commute. We gathered information using an activPAL activity monitor (PAL Technologies, Glasgow, UK) and synchronised it with a global positioning system (GPS). So, we had the intensity (cadence—activPAL), volume (number of steps taken—activPAL) and context (where the activity was performed—GPS). We discovered that the while the commute, on average, accounted for 32% of daily physical activity, it also accounted for 68% of the MVPA accrued (Rafferty, 2016) (Fig. 14.2).

While less than half of the total number of steps we take is during our commute (32%) it accounts for 68% of over MVPA time. Other activities include: walking at home, in the workplace, going out for lunch, and visiting the supermarket etc.

Think about this in the context of your own activity. How do you get to your place of work or study? What could you do to extend your opportunity to increase your physical activity? (Try Activity Box 14.2.)

Even public transport providers are promoting physical activity as a method for improving public health.

This is not just an attempt by them to be seen to be proactive (and increase their passenger numbers); it is supported by the literature. The Osaka study (Hayashi, 1999) is widely quoted in this area, but more recently Celis-Morales et al. (2017) produced a useful piece of work exploring the relationship between public transport and active travel, and found that small changes can make a difference. Getting off

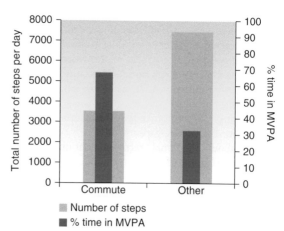

Fig. 14.2 Distribution of Total Steps Taken Per Day and Percentage Time in Moderate to Vigorous Physical Activity *(MVPA)*.

ACTIVITY BOX 14.2 How Do You Get to Work/School/University?

Getting to and from your place of work/study etc. is the most common (and convenient) way of getting your daily fix of physical activity. How do you travel to work?

If you walk or cycle briskly, for at least 30 min (there and back), then you are meeting current physical activity recommendations for health, and there is no need to go to the gym. But, if you don't, then what is stopping you? Have a look at the list below of commonly cited barriers to *active* commuting and see if any apply to you.

1. Time.
2. Distance.
3. Weather.
4. Busy traffic.
5. Too tiring.
6. Don't have the equipment.

ACTIVITY BOX 14.3 How Do You Rate the Intensity of a Physical Activity?

As has been explained in the text, movement requires energy. One way of understanding how much energy an activity takes is to compare it to the resting metabolic rate, i.e. how much energy the body needs, at rest, to keep all the systems going, which is given the value 1MET (see text for further explanation). Have a look at the activities below and put them in order of energy expenditure, i.e. how much energy each activity uses.*

- Watering plants
- Vacuuming
- Spectating at a sports event
- Roller blading
- Sitting on a bus
- Doubles tennis
- Country dancing
- Cycling
- Lying on couch watching TV

*Answers at end of chapter.
Further information:
Ainsworth, B.E., Haskell, W.L., Whitt, M.C., Irwin, M.L., Swartz, A.M., Strath, S.J., et al., 2000. Compendium of physical activities: an update of activity codes and MET intensities. Med. Sci. Sports Exerc. 32 (9; Suppl 1), S498–S504.

---

the bus a stop early, choosing to cycle, not looking for the parking space closest to your office can all play an important role in how we accrue MVPA.

Some Final Thoughts on Moderate to Vigorous Physical Activity

As already stated, MVPA can be a difficult thing to objectively quantify and educate people about, but it is a key part of the physical activity message. We can make reasoned guestimates based on the literature (Activity Box 14.3); however, ultimately, these are guestimates and subject to large differences between people and the context of their activity.

Although appealing, the concept of a MET comes with some uncertainty. The science supporting the value of 1 MET = 3.5 mL/O_2·kg·per minute can be questioned. This value appears to have been derived from a healthy, 40-year-old, 70-kg man, which is not really typical of the general population (Byrne, 2005). Although the underpinning science has some weaknesses, it is still considered, by the scientific community, to be robust.

How MET values translate to people living with long-term conditions is also questionable. The effort of walking is known to be greater in these populations. They require greater energy requirements in order to walk (Paul, 2008; Platts, 2006).

If It Is Not Moderate to Vigorous Physical Activity, Does This Mean It Is Has No Health Benefit?

No, that is not the case!

Any physical activity has health benefit, unless, of course, you are into extreme sports where the risk may outweigh the benefit. Simple tasks, such as doing household chores, can also contribute to health benefits. The important thing is not to be sedentary. We will spend a bit more time on what is meant by sedentary behaviours later in the chapter. Light physical activity (LPA) is considered to be activity that has a MET value of greater than 1.5 and less than 3. These include activities such as typing at your computer and walking slowly (<2.7 km/h). There is a growing body of literature that supports LPA as having health benefit. Again, we come back to the MET value and, as stated previously, this is based on a guestimate of MET.

Vigorous Physical Activity

To round off this discussion on MVAP and LPA it is worth mentioning vigorous physical activity (VPA). VPA is considered to be physical activities that have a MET value of greater than 6. Such activities may include fast cycling (> 20 km/h/12.5 mph), jogging or running. Do you do any VPA on a regular basis? If so, good, and this has been shown to have health benefit.

Banding of Physical Activities

The banding of physical activity outlined above is generally accepted by the scientific community as being an informed and robust manner in which to categorise physical activity. It is not definitive and will vary from individual to individual. In general, it is applicable across a healthy population. As stated, the translation of this banding in people living with long-term conditions is more problematic and should be viewed with caution. For people involved in health care banding provides a useful framework to assess the amount and intensity of physical activity that your patients are undertaking (or not). They also provide useful targets to discuss with your patients.

The bandings also tend to focus on upright activities. Not all activities need be upright to achieve guidelines. For example, a swimmer will normally be operating in the VPA band; however, it is predominately a prone task. Likewise, someone who performs bench presses will undertake this task mainly in a supine position. Again, this would generally be considered VPA. While these bandings provide a reasoned framework they are not exhaustive (no pun intended).

Sedentary Behaviour

When we are not physically active, we consider our behaviour to be sedentary. The current definition of sedentary behaviour is to be in a seated or lying position with a MET value of less than 1.5 (SBR Network, 2012). Again, our old friend the MET raises its head. Sleeping is not going to be discussed in this chapter as it is a science in and of itself (Hirotsu, 2015). Suffice to say, it is not considered a sedentary behaviour but a necessary physiological response.

What would a normal pattern of behaviour look like? The data presented here are data from real people going about their everyday lives. Sleeping time has been estimated using activity diaries (more on these later) but generally it is a fairly consistent pattern and at the same time variable (Fig. 14.3).

If we include sleep then approximately 75% of our day (24 hours) is spent in a seated or lying posture. If we just look at the nonsleep period, then 65% of our active day is still in a seated or lying posture. Remember these are real numbers collected on healthy adults either in various employment types or not currently employed. What does this mean to you? Sedentary behaviour is present in every facet of our everyday lives. Although previously we demonstrated that attending a place of work has an influence on how we accrued MVPA, it is also true in that how we commute to work affects our sedentary time. How many of us stand while commuting on a train/bus? Only if we have to?

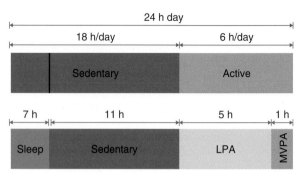

Fig. 14.3 Distribution of Behaviour Throughout a 24-Hour Period. *LPA*, Light physical activity; *MVPA*, moderate to vigorous physical activity.

IS SEDENTARY BEHAVIOUR BAD FOR US?

Too much sedentary behaviour is a threat to health regardless of how much physical activity we undertake. This is known as the active couch potato syndrome (Owen, 2010). We may meet the requirements in terms of physical activity; that is, 5 days/week—MVPA—in bouts of at least 10 minutes. However, if we then spend the majority of our time in a seated or lying position the health risk from this is as high as the health benefits of meeting the physical activity guidelines.

The work by Morris et al. (1953) is considered seminal in exploring sedentary behaviour. They explored the risk of coronary heart disease in London bus drivers, a predominately seated occupation and therefore sedentary, with their counterparts on the bus (the bus conductor). For those of you too young to remember what a bus conductor was, it was someone that moved through the bus taking fares and checking tickets, so it was a predominately upright (nonsedentary) job. Morris et al. found that the incidence of coronary heart disease was elevated in the drivers compared to the conductors.

More contemporary studies also support these findings (Wen, 2011; Lee, 2012). Estimates from observational studies also suggest the majority of our waking day is spent in sedentary behaviours (Matthews, 2008; Hansen, 2012).

A systematic review by Ekelund (2016) perceived that 60 or more minutes of MVPA per day reduced the 'high' risk of death from sedentary behaviour (sitting time). That is more than double the recommended MVPA to garner health benefit. However, it did not eliminate the risk from high levels of television viewing time. Prior to this, Schmid et al. (2014) explored the relationship between sedentary behaviours and television viewing time in relation to cancers. This is now known as 'is sitting the new smoking?'

So far, we have looked at the health benefits of being active and the health detriments from being sedentary. We have also looked at the categories of physical activity and unpicked the current physical activity recommendations. A lot of this information has been gained from direct measurement of physical activity. As discussed in Chapters 11 and 13, we need measurement to understand something. In the next section we will look more carefully at the methods employed to measure physical activity.

HOW DO WE MEASURE THE ENERGY EXPENDITURE OF PHYSICAL ACTIVITY?

In the laboratory there are four recognised methods. Many people consider doubly labelled water as being the criterion measure (the measure against which we should compare all other tests, see Chapter 11). Others debate this and suggest that room calorimetry is a more robust measure. Both can be criticised for being highly specialised and expensive, prohibiting their general use.

Doubly labelled water is a technique where a participant ingests an isotope of hydrogen and oxygen. After a period of time a urine sample is taken from the participant and, dependent on how much of the isotope is still present, this is considered an indication of how much energy the participant has have used over that period of time. During this period of time the participant is free to perform their everyday tasks without restrictions on their function. While completely safe it is a relatively expense method for measuring energy expenditure, requiring considerable laboratory support to analyse the results.

Room calorimetry effectively means we lock the person in a sealed room and measure how much oxygen (oxygen uptake) they consume and how much carbon dioxide they produce. From these measures we can estimate how much energy they have expended. Again, the downside is that such chambers are expensive. Additionally, it means the participants are being confined to a restricted space, raising the question of how reflective this will be of everyday activities.

The next tool in our armoury is indirect calorimetry. In this technique the participant wears a face mask that analyses the expired air. As stated previously, we know the percentage of oxygen in air (20.95%). The output from the mask is fed into a gas analyser to establish the percentage of oxygen in exhaled air. The difference between the two is our old friend, oxygen uptake. This allows us to calculate the energy used during physical activity. While cheaper than doubly labelled water or room calorimetry, these systems still have limitations, as does every method, and still are quite expensive. The participant is free to go about their everyday lives; however, think about how you would feel going about your everyday life with what looks like a gas mask on. First, you would get strange looks from people you interact with. Second, and more importantly, it would not be very comfortable. After a period of about 45 minutes you would be thinking 'take this off!' Obviously eating and other such activities are limited, so again rendering the face validity of using such systems as questionable for measuring free living activity (Fig. 14.4).

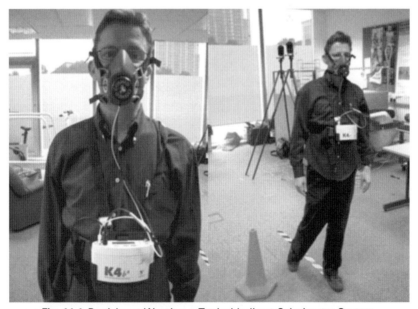

Fig. 14.4 Participant Wearing a Typical Indirect Calorimetry System.

These laboratory-based techniques for measuring the energy requirements of movement present viable, acceptable and potentially very accurate methods; however, they do not readily translate into the free living environment.

We could also focus on mechanical energy. How we go about this would be to use a system that allows us to track the participant's position. These are commonly known as motion analysis systems. If we simultaneously measure the forces that the participant is generating, then by combining the position, velocity, acceleration and forces we can estimate how much energy is being absorbed and expended to undertake physical activity. These systems again are expensive and require considerable technical support. They are also restricted in the volume in which the participant operates, normally about 2 × 3 m. Most of the work in this area concerns the quantification of gait in a very controlled environment and does not readily translate to activities of everyday living. See Chapters 11 and 12 for more details.

What we have explored so far is how to measure energy requirements of undertaking physical activities. All have merits and all add value in understanding the energy requirements of physical activities. However, as already said, they are all very laboratory based, which questions how reflective they are for quantifying real-world physical activity, and how you, as health professionals, can get access to these measures of physical activity to enable you to change someone's behaviour.

PHYSICAL ACTIVITY IN FREE LIVING

This then leads to the question, how do we measure physical activity in free living?

(Why not try Activity Box 14.4?)

Probably, asking the person what they do is the simplest approach. Generally speaking, there are two ways of gathering such information: questionnaire and diaries. The cost of these methods is relatively small, requiring no more than a pen and paper, which makes it a very attractive method when gathering large volumes of data. However, there are, of course, limitations to this approach.

Questionnaires are one of the most common approaches. There are many different types of physical activity questionnaire available to use. Unfortunately, they tend to gather slightly different forms of information, making

---

ACTIVITY BOX 14.4   Measuring Physical Activity

Activity Box 14.1 should have given you a broad idea of how physically active you are and even if you meet recommended levels but it doesn't provide an objective measure which will be useful in changing behaviour or checking whether your advice/rehabilitation programme is working. The text provides a lot of information on measurement systems and guidance on what to use but there is nothing like a practical activity to help you retain some of this information, so your task is to measure the amount of physical activity you do. You can try one of the two choices outlined below:

A. **Physical activity tracking device**: If you have a physical activity monitoring device (e.g. the Moov Now, Fitbit, Apple Watch, Garmin Vivosmart), record the actual minutes you spend in vigorous, moderate and light activity over a three day period AND the amount of time you spend sitting and lying.
  a. Do you believe the numbers?
  b. Do you think your device is overestimating your physical activity or perhaps missing some of the things you are doing?
  c. Do you meet the current guidelines?
  (Note: If you don't have one of these devices you may be able to use an app on your smartphone or you could try option B.)

B. **Physical activity diary**: Get a piece of paper and mark out a table with every hour a column heading for your waking hours, see below for example (but don't stop at 4, go on to your bedtime).

	8–9 a.m.	9–10	10–11	11–12	12–1	1–2	2–3	3–4
Light								
Moderate								
Vigorous								
Sedentary								

In each square insert the amount of time for each hour, each column must equal 60 min. When you have done a whole day, count up the time in light, moderate, vigorous and sedentary activity.

Do you think this is correct? Do you think you might have overestimated your activity or perhaps missed some out?

Do you meet current guidelines?

the integration of such data problematic. They also can use quite confusing language creating a barrier to their use with the layperson. Let's look at an example from the International Physical Activity Questionnaire (IPAQ), shown in Fig. 14.5.

Let's look at how you might answer this question.

As a cyclist I would pick out 'fast cycling' as an example of my regular physical activity, but what is 'fast cycling'? You might consider this to be greater than 20 mph and use a bike computer to define this. If you were not a keen cyclist, you might consider 'fast cycling' to be going at 20 mph down a hill with the wind behind you. The point is that the terms are subjective (open to interpretation).

The next issue is whether you really recall what you did over the last 7 days. Many activities are simply part of the everyday flow of life and quite often will not be committed to memory, making any data based on recall less precise than we would hope. Would we answer honestly? If you are a patient that has been asked by the health professional to increase your physical activity for whatever reason, your response may be influenced by 'trying to please' the health professional to demonstrate you are sticking to the plan (we usually like to please people, or at least avoid disappointing them).

Finally, there is the issue of the fine detail (sometimes called granulation). Can we really recall our lives in segments of '10 minutes at a time'? Maybe this would be possible if you were the suspect in a TV crime drama, but most of us would be pretty useless. This is not an attempt to demonstrate that questionnaires have no worth; THEY DO. Rather, it is meant as a way of exploring their limitations. The IPAQ in particular is a well-recognised questionnaire with established validity and reliability (Hagströmer, 2006).

The other form of physical activity questionnaire is to ask the person to keep an activity diary. How often they record the information varies and is dependent on what information you wish to gather. Some diaries require the participant to complete it every 15 minutes, others every hour, or on a daily basis. All of these are burdensome on the participant. As an active researcher or health professional, the integrity of data is paramount. Having taken part in many studies requiring the completion of diaries, it is not uncommon to forget to do so, or to adopt an approach of stating it was the 'same as yesterday'. Research on variation within physical activity suggests the 'same as yesterday' is actually rarely true. It has also been demonstrated that when comparing a diary or questionnaire to objectively measured physical activity, we tend to overestimate the amount of physical activity recorded in diaries and questionnaires (Slootmaker, 2009). Again, it is worth stating that diaries have their place, providing we understand their limitations.

Where we want to get to is having objective measures of physical activity that accurately reflect both the volume (how much we do) and the intensity (how vigorous the physical activity is). Given the variation within physical activity and inactivity (sedentary behaviour) this is quite a complex task. Is it worth doing? The science supports that increasing physical activity and reducing sedentary behaviour reduces the risks of cardiovascular diseases, diabetes, colon and breast cancer, depression, hip or vertebral fracture and mental illness, and helps to control weight (WHO). Given the huge impact of movement (physical activity) on physical and mental health, it has been recommended that a consultation with your family doctor, or indeed any health professional, should include an assessment of physical activity. Questionnaires and diaries provide a meaningful insight in this situation, provided we acknowledge their limitations, as with all measurement techniques. Both at a macro level (sample of a group) and a micro level (individual patient) measurement of physical activity is important for informing rehabilitation and health improvement strategies.

OBJECTIVELY MEASURING FREE LIVING PHYSICAL ACTIVITY

What is meant by 'objectively measured free living physical activity'? It is the use of technology to eliminate sources of

| 1a. | During the last 7 days, on how many days did you do **vigorous** physical activities like heavy lifting, digging, aerobics or fast bicycling? |
| | Think about *only* those physical activities that you did for at least 10 minutes at a time. |

_____ **days per week** ⇨   1b. How much time in total did you usually spend on one of those days doing vigorous physical activities?

or

☐ **none**   _____ **hours** _____ **minutes**

Fig. 14.5 Example Question From International Physical Activity Questionnaire.

bias present within the collection of physical activity levels when using a questionnaire. The biases present when using questionnaires or diaries are recall bias and interpretation bias (as mentioned above). Objectively measured physical activity removes the participant's subjective input and measures what they have actually done. Does it sound a bit too good to be true? Well on one level it is. It is difficult to quantify all physical activity; however, by using objective measures we can begin to get a better understanding of what people really do. Technology also has limitations. Where do we wear the technology? How much trust do we have in what the technology is telling us? Technology costs much more than a pen and paper. Finally, does it add value to our understanding of how much physical activity and sedentary behaviour we undertake? Let's accept these limitations and explore how we objectively measure physical activity.

As mentioned at the beginning of the chapter, we probably all have smartphones; therefore, we have the technology to measure physical activity. We should be able to download applications that will allow us to quantify our physical activity. Story over, we have solved it! Well not quite. Where do we carry our smartphones? Some of us will have them in our pockets, some in bags, and some in our jacket pockets; these locations all measure very different types of physical activities. Perish the thought that we may, on occasion, venture out into the big bad world without our beloved smartphone. While writing this, my smartphone is plugged in and on charge. In looking for inspiration to inspire you about this chapter, frequently I will get up and pace around, which is not recorded. So, unless it is permanently glued to you, what we are measuring is the physical movement of the smartphone rather than the physical activity of the individual.

Let us explore what an accelerometer signal looks like and what it tells us about activity. These data were collected using a thigh-mounted accelerometer. There are four types of activities represented in Fig. 14.6. The first activity (a) is when the person is in a seated or lying position. Activity (b) is when they are transitioning from seated to lying to an upright posture. Note how the level of the signal changes. The third activity (c) the person is upright and standing still, possibly picking up their smartphone from their desk. The final activity (d) is when they are walking and the thigh is undulating during the gait cycle (see Fig. 14.6).

Obviously, the solution is to get someone to always wear the monitoring technology constantly; that seems simple and solves the problem. Unfortunately, there is still the dilemma of where to wear the technology and how to attach it. Probably the most socially acceptable location of where to wear the technology is the wrist. Most of us wear watches or jewellery on the wrist without drawing attention to it. Commercially available activity monitors, such as the Apple

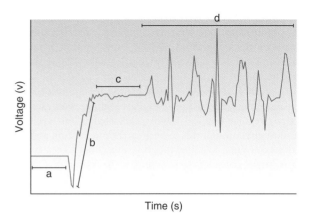

Fig. 14.6 Example of Accelerometer Signal When Worn on the Thigh. a) quiet seated or lying b) transition to upright c) standing upright d) walking.

Watch, Fitbit, Jawbone and others, use this location to quantify physical activity. Think back to our definition of sedentary behaviour, that is, in a seated or lying position. Is the wrist a good indicator for this? Well probably not. When seated or lying we undertake a series of activities that are not really reflective of posture. We will reach to take a drink of tea (or other beverages), brush our hair, click on the mouse as we browse the Internet; the list goes on. The wrist is probably not the best location to determine either postural position or control.

Activity Monitor Placement and Attaching It

There is no ideal location as to where to wear an activity monitor. There are combinations of factors that need to be considered when deciding on which monitor is best suited for your participant: what you are hoping to measure, social acceptability of location, how the monitor is applied and whether location relates to compliance of wear. The list goes on. We will now explore some of the most common body locations.

The lower leg: This has many attractions and is often considered the best site to measure both volume and intensity of activity (total number of steps taken and cadence). However, the lower leg has the same orientation while seated (vertical) and when upright. Therefore, there is a lack of discrimination between seated and upright postures. This makes the identification of sedentary behaviour susceptible to error. From a socially acceptable point of view for those of us that wear shorts or skirts the monitor is also clearly visible, meaning that it may have the appearance of a surveillance monitor to those we interact with. Generally, it can be attached using simple elastic straps that are easy to apply. However, things that are easy to apply are often also easy to remove, raising the issue of reapplication and compliance.

The most common example of such monitors is the Stepwatch. Generally, such devices are considered to be pedometers rather than activity monitors.

The thigh: Consider the orientation of your thigh in everyday life. If your thigh is in a horizontal position then generally you will be in a seated or lying posture. Now, this is beginning to identify sedentary behaviour. If your thigh is vertical, you'll be in one of two activities: standing upright or walking. So, the thigh seems a good indicator of both our posture and activity. Job done; we now know where to locate the monitor. Well true, but how do we attach it? Because of the bulk of the thigh any device is not easily attached by elastic straps; these would prove uncomfortable after a period of wear. So, we need to think of an alternative method to apply the monitor. PAL Technologies are the leading manufacturer for devices worn on the thigh, with the activPAL being their most popular device. The solution suggested by them is to place the device in a neoprene pocket and then attach it using Opsite or a similar type of dressing. This means the device is waterproof to showering and everyday activities, and has been shown to identify seated/lying behaviour, upright posture, and both walking volume and intensity. While the attachment method seems relatively straightforward in practice, it is more problematic. How do you apply the monitor at first? Most participants will have little or no experience of such devices let alone how to make it watertight. What happens when the monitor comes off? While this is rare, it does happen. Allergies to dressings, such as Opsite, are rare but in frail elderly and other populations they do occur. The activPAL provides valid and repeatable measures of posture and physical activity; however, the attachment method is less robust.

The waistband: The leading research monitor for physical activity is probably the ActiGraph. The ActiGraph is predominately worn on the waistband of the participant. It is a well-validated and well-cited monitor in a similar fashion to activPAL. Let's think about how a waistband-worn monitor measures posture. Our waistband, whether we are seated or upright, will largely be in a similar position, that is, vertical. So, this tells us little about the posture we are in. The ActiGraph relies on a measure that is referred to as counts. This is a measure of how often the accelerometer is perturbed and is related to our overall physical activity (movement). There is appeal in wearing a monitor at the waistband. It is covered and unobtrusive in waking hours; however, it is difficult to sleep with a monitor in this location. This means it tends to be removed during sleep, leading to issues surrounding reattachment. Numerous algorithms are available that will compute what is acceptable wear time. All are based around the premise that the device will not always be reapplied and therefore information missing. However, it would be erroneous to dismiss the ActiGraph or other waistband-worn monitors on this basis; instead we should merely recognise this as a limitation in the same fashion as with any monitor.

Other locations: There are other locations that are considered the optimum location for sensor placement. We have already explored—to some extent—location on the wrist. Others include the sternum, the midpoint of the posterior superior iliac spine as this considered to be the best position to reflect the movement of the centre of mass and the upper arm. Consider and critique each of these locations: what do they tell us about the movement of the individual? Are the locations socially acceptable? Can the monitor be worn continuously, or does it need to be removed during sleep? Does it categorise posture?

Activity Monitors Incorporating Physiological Measurement

Some activity monitors will, in addition to monitoring movement, incorporate physiological measures. The accelerometer is good at measuring how much, and the intensity of, movement. However, it is not a measure of physiological response; this can only be inferred from the intensity that the accelerometer is perturbed. It is NOT a measurement of energy expenditure. Monitors that incorporate physiological measures go some way to making this pertinent to measuring energy expenditure. Again, there are still limitations associated with this.

One example of this is the Actiheart. This device is worn at the sternum and also incorporates a heart rate monitor. There is face validity in measuring heart rate as an expression of exertion. However, heart rate is susceptible to other influences, such as caffeine, nicotine, beta-blockers and general fitness. As with other measures of physical activity, there are limitations. These also include social acceptability of wearing the device on the sternum and tolerance to sensor for measuring heart rate.

IMPORTANCE OF WALKING IN PHYSICAL ACTIVITY

We have established the importance of sedentary behaviour and the threats to good health. Let's now consider the banding of physical activity in exploring activity profiles. Walking is the most common form of physical activity we undertake. How do we band this in terms that are meaningful and accessible? Tudor-Locke (2011) developed the classifications listed in Table 14.1.

What is the advantage of understanding behaviour using such bandings? Can we measure it? Well yes, we can measure cadence using activity monitoring or, if not directly, the cadence then the intensity of activity using counts (ActiGraph). It provides a meaningful insight as to how much

TABLE 14.1 Cadence Classifications.	
Descriptor	**Behaviour**
Sedentary behaviour	Seated or lying
Upright	No stepping
Incidental movement	1–19
Sporadic movement	20–39
Purposeful steps	40–49
Slow walking	60–79
Medium walking	80–99
Brisk walking	100–119
Faster locomotion	>120

sedentary time we accrue and the intensity of activity we undertake. We have already suggested that cadences of greater than 100 can be considered MVPA, so this provides a dichotomy between what is and isn't MVPA. However, beneath that there is a series of physical activities that can be further dissected into different bands. Potentially understanding these allows us to influence them and change the activity profiles. It is unlikely that many people living with long-term conditions will be able to achieve cadences of greater than 100 in bouts of no less than 10 minutes. However, quantifying behaviour patterns using these bandings potentially allows the targeting of behaviour change that would be manageable for people living with long-term conditions.

So, what would a day of activity look like? For this example, we are using data collected using activPAL (Fig. 14.7).

The low bars (light orange) indicate periods of sitting or lying; the medium bars (slightly taller dark orange bars) standing upright or stepping with a cadence of less than 20 steps per minute; the higher bars (tallest dark orange bars) walking or running with a cadence of greater than 20 steps per minute. Before we explore in more detail, let us consider the medium bars that represent upright with a cadence of less than 20 steps per minute. All activity monitors have limitations in identifying slow gait. This especially poses a problem in conditions where cadence is limited (e.g. people living with stroke). These data were collected in a healthy individual, so why would their cadence be less than 20 steps per minute? Think about everyday activities. When cooking we will go to the fridge and get vegetables out. We will then move with short steps to the chopping board and stand upright while chopping the vegetables; then we move to the hob and put them in the pan to cook. All such activities require bouts of stepping at a slow cadence. Unfortunately, in people living with long-term conditions this may limit our ability to obtain a clear picture of their physical activity.

Overall, this person spends the hours 12 midnight till slightly before 7:45 a.m., probably in bed. Then there is a period between 7:45 a.m. and before 8:45 a.m. interspersed with sedentary, upright and incidental movement, and purposeful activity probably representing them having breakfast and preparing to go to work. Just before 8:45 a.m. the walking becomes more purposeful, potentially indicating a walk to work. Just before 9.15 a.m., until around 12 noon, their behaviour becomes much more sedentary, indicated by the low bars. What do you think is happening? Yes, they have a desk job and are spending a lot of time seated (sedentary). It is broken with periods of upright activity and sporadic walking. This is common. We all need comfort breaks, or to go to the printer, move to a meeting etc. Try and interpret the rest of the data.

CHANGING PHYSICAL (IN)ACTIVITY BEHAVIOUR

It is all very well understanding how to measure physical activity and knowing the current recommendations for health, but how do you actually change someone's physical activity? Like any behaviour (smoking, eating a poor diet etc.) there are some guidelines based around the individual's readiness to change. People need to have confidence that they can change their behaviour, the social support and perhaps, most importantly, that it will lead to a better and longer life. This may require more than a leaflet; the technique of motivational interviewing might be worth considering (DiClemente, 2002).

Thankfully, the answer does not lie solely in getting people to register for the gym and attend 5 days per week. The answer is much more pragmatic. Get people to do more, within their limits, and to do less sedentary behaviour.

Here are some practical examples of where small changes may help. The scientific rigour behind these is untested and is anecdotal; hopefully they provide an insight as to where small changes in behaviour may have longer-lasting effects.

Scenario 1

Both parents are elderly and infirm. Both are still mobile, although limited, but still able to walk. Entering their home, the usual scenario unfolds:

Parent—'Would you like a cup of tea?'
Offspring—'Yep, that would be nice'.
The parent gets up and makes a cup of tea.
Second offspring comes into the home.
Parent—'Would you like a cup of tea?'
Offspring—'Yes, that would be great. You sit there and I'll make us tea'.

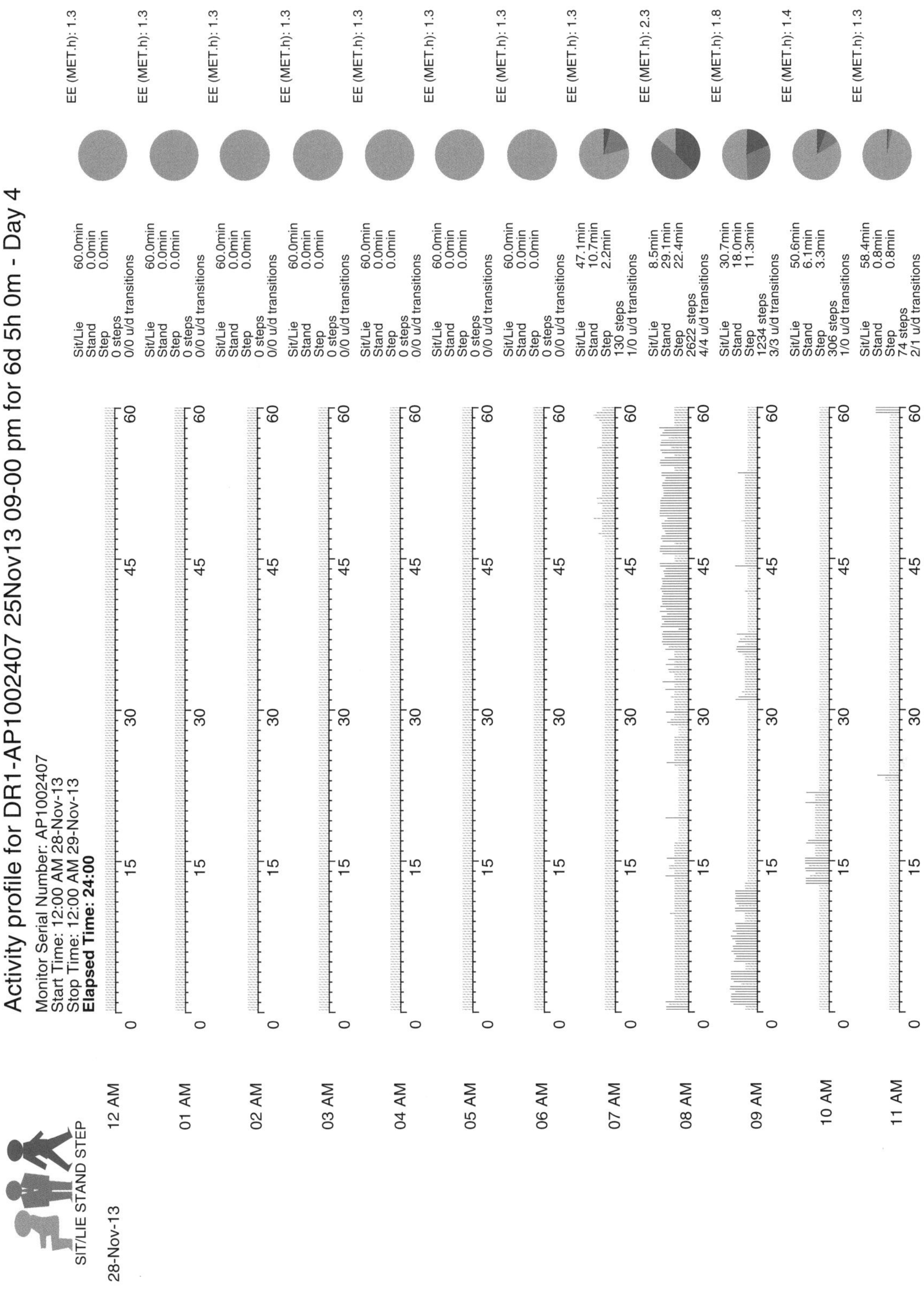

Activity profile for DR1-AP1002407 25Nov13 09-00 pm for 6d 5h 0m - Day 4

Monitor Serial Number: AP1002407
Start Time: 12:00 AM 28-Nov-13
Stop Time: 12:00 AM 29-Nov-13
Elapsed Time: 24:00

Fig. 14.7 An Example 24-Hour Output Collected Using activPAL.

Continued

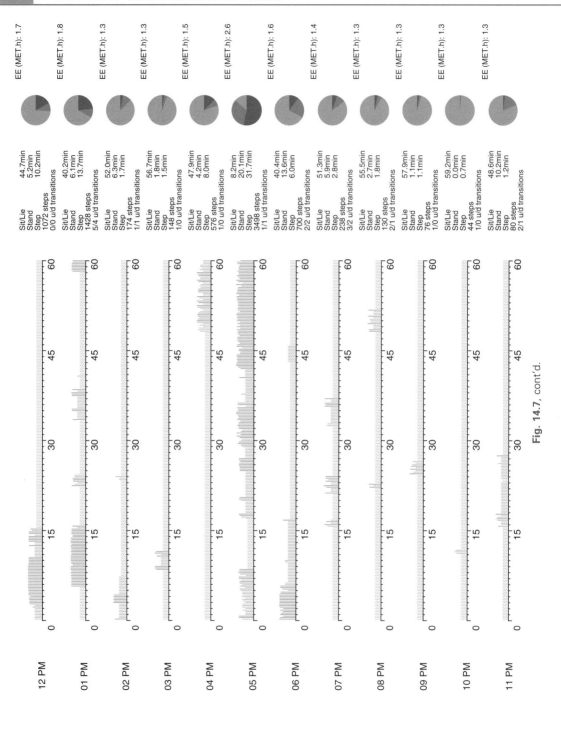

Fig. 14.7, cont'd.

What is the difference in approach? What has the first offspring done that the second offspring, through a conception of empathy, has not? Or is the first offspring inherently lazy?

Yes, the first offspring has broken the sedentary behaviour of the parent. The parent is capable of getting up and making tea. The second offspring has shown empathy but failed to realise the importance of breaking sedentary behaviour. These small behaviour changes could go a long way to improving health and well-being for the elderly parent.

Scenario 2

A patient with a heart condition gets his newspaper delivered every day (yes, this was before online media dominated). You have measured his physical activity using an activity monitor. Your observation is that the volume of stepping is reasonable (approximately 10,000 steps per day), but most of these are accumulated in the lower cadence bands, generally considered to be household tasks. However, there is evidence to suggest that while these would not be considered MVPA, the patient is capable of slow or medium walking. What would be the advice? You could suggest that he is capable of walking and therefore should cancel the delivery and walk to the nearest shop to buy his newspaper. This increases physical activity and probably saves money.

Scenario 3

You are working with a chronic television addict. How do you break the sedentary behaviour associated with this? Easy. Rather than watch television get them to go for a walk. Well, the chances of that happening are probably small. So why not suggest that they should stand up during the breaks between programmes or during the adverts.

Scenario 4

Think back to the activity profile presented previously (Fig. 14.7). How could we affect this? Well, the longest periods

---

> ### ACTIVITY BOX 14.5 Case Study: How Do You Improve a Patient's Physical Activity?
>
> A 49-year-old man with back pain is referred for physiotherapy. He is a little bit overweight (BMI = 26) but does almost no physical activity, perhaps 10 min of walking all day. You have assessed him and started treating his back symptoms with some appropriate exercises. How do you address his lack of physical activity? Do you need more information? Where do you start? List three things you might do to get the ball rolling.
>
> 1.
> 2.
> 3.

---

of sedentary behaviour occur during the working day and in the evening. Potentially suggesting more regular breaks in sedentary behaviour during the working day might help. This could be done via prompts. In the evening, standing up between television programmes or commercial breaks might help. How do we increase their physical activity? You may have observed that after 12 noon there is a period of purposeful walking followed by a period of sitting, and then after 1 pm a period of purposeful walking again, which definitely indicates a lunch break (it is me so I know this). Suggest they go for a standing lunch. Additionally, suggest a longer walk to work; as the Osaka study (Hayashi, 1999) would suggest, moderately increase your route to work.

None of these scenarios are scientifically tested to make a difference. However, if we follow the deductive logic that precedes them in the chapter, hopefully they would make a difference.

▌ SUMMARY

Accruing physical activity is very complex and variable both within and between individuals. We operate differently on a workday to a rest day. We also operate differently and have a different physiological response if we have long-term condition(s). However, understanding the overall pattern of behaviour at an individual level may provide evidence on how to change behaviour.

Are physical activity guidelines important? Yes, they are. Scientifically they provide a basis for both maintaining and improving health. Is reducing sedentary behaviour the most

important aspect of improving or maintaining health? We are required to think innovatively as to how we can combine interventions that both combine a reduction in sedentary behaviour and an increase in physical activity that is scientifically supported and caters to the individual influencers of our patients. Rarely in such scenarios does one size fit all. Changing behaviour patterns is a difficult task; understanding by quantifying them (objective activity monitoring) may go some way to effecting change.

To put some of this into practice try Activity Box 14.5.

SELF-ASSESSMENT QUESTIONS

1. What is 1 metabolic activity (MET) equal to?
   a. Total energy expenditure in 1 day
   b. 1 Moderate exercise time
   c. Resting metabolic rate, equal to sitting quietly
   d. Basic metabolic rate, equal to complete standing
2. Moderate to vigorous physical activity (MVPA) has a MET value of
   a. Anything above 1.5.
   b. Between 3 and 6 METs.
   c. Anything that is not sitting.
   d. Less than 9.
3. You do the ironing in a seated position. The MET value of this is 2.5. You are
   a. Not sedentary.
   b. Sedentary.
   c. Accumulating MVPA.
   d. All of the above.
4. Walking is physical activity because
   a. It is MVPA.
   b. The cadence is above 100.
   c. It is easier than running.
   d. You are moving.
5. Define sedentary behaviour.
   a. Seated or lying with a MET of less than 1.5
   b. A MET value of less than 1.5
   c. Anything that is not MVPA
   d. Standing with a MET of less than 1.5

6. If you exercise for 30 minutes/day, 5 days/week, you should consider this
   a. Job done as it meets the guidelines.
   b. A good reason to take more rest.
   c. A good reason to buy more cakes to replace energy.
   d. Along with your sedentary behaviour.
7. Sedentary behaviour affects
   a. Only older adults.
   b. Only people living with long-term conditions.
   c. Everyone.
   d. People that commute to work.
8. Oxygen uptake is
   a. Impossible to measure.
   b. The difference in oxygen levels between the air we inhale and the air we exhale.
   c. Similar to accelerometry.
   d. Not meaningful.
9. People living with long-term conditions should be advised
   a. To take it easy and get as much sedentary time as possible.
   b. That if they can't walk with a cadence of greater than 100 not to bother walking.
   c. To wait until their condition improves.
   d. To try and stay active within their limits.

ANSWERS TO QUESTIONS POSED IN TEXT

Answer to Activity Box 14.2, Ranked Lowest to Highest in Energy Cost (Metabolic Activity)

1. Sitting on a bus (1.0) and lying on couch watching TV (1.0)
2. Spectating at a sports event (1.5)
3. Watering plants (2.5)
4. Vacuuming (3.5)
5. Country dancing (4.5)
6. Doubles tennis (5.0)
7. Cycling (8.0)
8. Roller blading (12.5)

Some Suggestions for Activity Box 14.5

1. Find out if there are any medical reasons for him not participating (or modifying participation) in physical activity, for example, cardiovascular disease or renal disease. If there are then there may be a need for a medical examination before suggesting moderate/vigorous activity.
2. Find out what activities he has done recently (past few years) and enjoys.
3. Find out his occupation and method of commute.
4. Get a better (objective) measure of current physical activity, for example, diary, physical activity monitor.
5. Educate him on health benefits (including low back pain) from being physically active.
6. Suggest small changes to his daily routine, for example, walking upstairs at work twice a day, or walking kids to school twice a week. This should be done cooperatively.
7. Set clear and achievable goals; for example, doubling the amount of time walking every day within 4 weeks.
8. Set medium- to long-term goals, such as joining an exercise club or cycling to work, which will help sustain behaviour change.
9. Encourage the involvement of family and friends.

REFERENCES

Ainsworth, B.E., Haskell, W.L., Herrmann, S.D., et al., 2011. Compendium of physical activities: a second update of codes and MET values. Med. Sci. Sports Exerc. 43, 1575–1581.

Byrne, N.M., Hills, A.P., Hunter, G.R., Weinsier, R.L., Schutz, Y., 2005. Metabolic equivalent: one size does not fit all. J. Appl. Physiol. 99 (3), 1112–1119. doi:10.1152/japplphysiol.00023 .2004.

Celis-Morales, C., Lyall, D.M., Welsh, P., Anderson, J., Steell, L., Guo, Y., et al., 2017. Association between active commuting (walking and cycling) and incident cardiovascular disease, cancer and mortality: prospective cohort study of 264,337 UK biobank participants. BMJ 357, j1456.

DiClemente, C.C., Velasquez, M.M., 2002. Motivational interviewing and the stages of change. In: Miller, W.R., Rollnick, S. (Eds.), Motivational Interviewing: Preparing People for Change, second ed. Guilford Press, New York, pp. 201–216.

Ekelund, U., Steene-Johannessen, J., Brown, W.J., Fagerland, M.W., Owen, N., Powell, K.E., et al., 2016. Lancet sedentary behaviour working group. Does physical activity attenuate, or even eliminate, the detrimental association of sitting time with mortality? A harmonised meta-analysis of data from more than 1 million men and women. Lancet 388 (10051), 1302–1310.

Graham-Rowe, E., Skippon, S., Gardner, B., Abraham, C., 2011. Can we reduce car use and, if so, how? A review of available evidence. Transport. Res. A-Pol. 45 (5), 401–418. doi:10.1016/j.tra.2011.02.001.

Hagströmer, M., Oja, P., Sjöström, M., 2006. The international physical activity questionnaire (IPAQ): a study of concurrent and construct validity. Public Health Nutr. 9 (6), 755–762. doi:10.1079/PHN2005898.

Hansen, B.H., Kolle, E., Dyrstad, S.M., Holme, I., Anderssen, S.A., 2012. Accelerometer-determined physical activity in adults and older people. Med. Sci. Sports Exerc. 44, 266–272.

Harvey, J.A., Rafferty, D., Martin Chastin, S.F., 2017. Consequences of short interruptions of bouts walking on estimates of compliance to physical activity guidelines. Physiol. Meas. 38 (5), N93–N100. doi:10.1088/1361-6579/aa66c2. [Epub 2017 Mar 14].

Hayashi, T., Tsumura, K., Suematsu, C., Okada, K., Fujii, S., Endo, G., 1999. Walking to work and the risk for hypertension in men: the Osaka health survey. Ann. Intern. Med. 131 (1), 21.

Hirotsu, C., Tufik, S., Andersen, M.L., 2015. Interactions between sleep, stress, and metabolism: from physiological to pathological conditions. Sleep Sci. 8 (3), 143–152.

Lee, I.M., Shiroma, E.J., Lobelo, F., Puska, P., Blair, S.N., Katzmarzyk, P.T., et al., 2012. Effect of physical inactivity on major non-communicable diseases worldwide: an analysis of burden of disease and life expectancy. Lancet 380, 219–229.

Matthews, C.E., Chen, K.Y., Freedson, P.S., et al., 2008. Amount of time spent in sedentary behaviors in the United States, 2003–2004. Am. J. Epidemiol. 167, 875–881.

McArdle, W.D., Katch, F.I., Katch, V.L., 1986. Exercise Physiology. Lea and Lebiger, Philadelphia.

Morency, C., Trépanier, M., Demers, M., 2011. Walking to transit: an unexpected source of physical activity. Transp. Policy 18 (6), 800–806.

Morris, J.N., Heady, J.A., Raffle, P.A., Roberts, C.G., Parks, J.W., 1953. Coronary heart disease and physical activity of work. Lancet 265, 1053–1057.

Owen, N., Healy, G.N., Matthews, C.E., Dunstan, D.W., 2010. Too much sitting: the population health science of sedentary behavior. Exerc. Sport Sci. Rev. 38 (3), 105–113. doi:10.1097/JES.0b013e3181e373a2.

Paul, L., Rafferty, D., Young, S., Miller, L., Mattison, P., McFadyen, A., 2008. The effect of functional electrical stimulation on the physiological cost of gait in people with multiple sclerosis. Mult. Scler. 14, 954–961.

Platts, M.M., Rafferty, D., Paul, L., 2006. Metabolic cost of overground gait in younger stroke patients and healthy controls. Med. Sci. Sports Exerc. 38, 1041–1046.

Rafferty, D., Dolan, C., Granat, M.G., 2016. Attending a workplace: its contribution to volume and intensity of physical activity. Physiol. Meas. 37 (12), 2144–2153.

SBR Network, 2012. Letter to the editor: standardized use of the terms "sedentary" and "sedentary behaviours". Appl. Physiol. Nutr. Metab. 37, 540–542.

Schmid, D., Leitzmann, M.F., 2014. Television viewing and time spent sedentary in relation to cancer risk: a meta-analysis. J. Natl. Cancer Inst. 106 (7), doi:10.1093/jnci/dju098.

Slootmaker, S.M., Schuit, A.J., Chinapaw, M.J., Seidell, J.C., van Mechelen, W., 2009. Disagreement in physical activity assessed by accelerometer and self-report in subgroups of age, gender, education and weight status. Int. J. Behav. Nutr. Phys. Act. 6, 17.

Tudor-Locke, C., Camhi, S.M., Leonardi, C., Johnson, W.D., Katzmarzyk, P.T., Earnest, C.P., et al., 2011. Patterns of adult stepping cadence in the 2005–2006 NHANES. Prev. Med. 53, 178–181.

Wen, C.P., Wai, J.P., Tsai, M.K., et al., 2011. Minimum amount of physical activity for reduced mortality and extended life expectancy: a prospective cohort study. Lancet 378, 1244–1253.

World Health Organisation (WHO). http://www.who.int/topics/physical_activity/en/.

Restoring and Optimising Human Movement

15

Motor Relearning Principles

Madeleine A. Grealy and Andy Kerr

OUTLINE

LEARNING OUTCOMES

After reading this chapter, you will be able to:
1. Describe different theories of skill acquisition
2. Understand how varying the performance of a skill can impact on learning and retention and describe the contextual interference effect
3. Appreciate the role of mental practice in skill learning
4. Describe how manipulating feedback can change skill learning
5. Appreciate how we can motivate people whilst they are learning skills
6. Understand the role of virtual reality in skill acquisition.

PRINCIPLES OF MOTOR LEARNING

The process of learning or relearning a motor skill involves creating and developing a memory representation for the action in our brain. However, the memories we create for movements are not the same as the memories we have for past events; we do not remember every movement we make or routinely recall them; rather we remember how we have learnt to control our bodies in relation to our environment. We have evolved to do this because even seemingly simple skills such as picking up a cup require us to continuously modify and adapt our movement patterns to accommodate for example the size, shape, weight, location and contents of the cup along with our intention to lift, push, pull, shift or rotate it. Studying the complex process of skill learning has been conducted at different levels, from the functional and structural changes that occur in the brain to the changing behaviour patterns that emerge over time as a person develops a coordinated movement pattern. In this chapter we are going to focus on changes in behaviour and how we can influence these by manipulating the learning experience or the environment.

THEORIES OF SKILL LEARNING

Several theories of skill learning have been proposed to map out the complex process of skill learning, and an understanding of how we learn to control our movements allows us to tailor the learning environment to maximise the rate of learning and gain optimal performance levels. Amongst the most commonly cited skill learning theories are the three-stage model proposed by Paul Fitts and Michael Posner and the two-stage model proposed by Ann Gentile. These focus on how adults or young people develop skills; however, other scientists such as Nikolai Bernstein and Janet Starkes have written about how infants and children develop motor skills as their brains and bodies mature.

Three-Stage Model (Fitts and Posner, 1967)

Fitts and Posner (1967) described a three-stage model of skill learning based on their observations of the phases that most people seem to go through when they learn a new motor skill. The first stage is called the **cognitive stage** and during this the learner tries to understand how to do the skill and how to use feedback to modify their actions. During this cognitive stage the learner engages in a process of trial-and-error and typically asks questions or they will talk themselves through the problem-solving process. With practice they begin to understand the nature of the skill and how changes they make impact on the outcome. This can be a tiring stage with error filled practice. The second stage is called the **associative stage** and here the learner begins to understand how the various components of the skill are interrelated and how they are able to modify these. They still make movement errors but they are better able to detect these and solve them without having to rely on a coach or therapist telling them what they did wrong and what to change.

The final stage, the **autonomous stage**, is when the learner can perform the skill almost automatically. They no longer need to focus all their attention on the mechanics of performing the skill and can start to broaden their attention to other aspects of the environment. For example, in a hockey game, rather than having to concentrate on the mechanics of passing and receiving the player can look to see where other players are positioned and start to read the tactics of the game. They can perform the skill consistently without errors and they have learnt how to make subtle changes to the movement pattern to refine it. Unlike in the first stage where a great deal of effortful processing, problem solving, planning and reflection were required, in the final stage these processes seem to occur automatically. In fact it is interesting to note that when the skill becomes autotomised to this level the learner no longer has access to the cognitive processes they experienced in the first stage.

Two-Stage Model (Gentile, 1972)

In a complementary model Gentile proposed two stages of learning. The first stage is similar to the cognitive and associative stages of Fitts and Posner's model where the learner learns how to coordinate their movements in relation to the environment and learns to tune into relevant cues and to use feedback. In the second stage, however, Gentile makes an important distinction in relation to what we need to learn for different types of skill. For skills where the performance environment is relatively stable (sometime referred to as closed skills) Gentile proposed that we need

to learn to fixate. That is we learn how to make the movement patterns as consistent as possible. A good example of this would be a gymnast learning to perform a somersault on a balance beam. They need to repeatedly practise the skill to develop a consistent movement pattern. In contrast, for skills where the environment changes Gentile proposed that the learner must learn how to diversify the skill. That is they need to learn how to adapt the movement to suit the environment. For example, a soccer player learning to pass the ball must learn to kick the ball to different distances and at different angles (Activity Box 15.1).

Lifespan Model (Starkes et al., 2004)

In order to accommodate skill learning in both children and adults Janet Starkes and colleagues extended and expanded on previous theories to create a lifespan model (Fig. 15.1). This model describes four developmental phases but also makes the distinction between two important processes, one being able to perceive and understand (perceptual-cognitive stream) and the other being able to perceive and do (perceptual-motor stream). Starkes et al. noted that performance is the product of both of these processes so, whilst they may develop at different rates, they are inextricably linked so that performance is facilitated or constrained by either process or the interaction between the two.

During the first phase the learner acquires both declarative knowledge (facts and information about the skill) and procedural skills (how to do the skill). By 'trying out' the skill the learner establishes knowledge in the form of 'if I do this then that happens' type statements. As practice continues the number and range of procedural skills increases and the learner starts to refine the coordination pattern (known as constraining the degrees of freedom). Moving on to phase two the learner starts to both condense and elaborate their knowledge. In this phase movements become linked and more efficient and the number of movement options may increase. The learner is also able to create

---

ACTIVITY BOX 15.1

Think back to when you learnt a motor skill as an adult. It might be that you learnt a new sport, or you learnt to drive a car, or played a video game.

- Can you identify the different learning phases you went through?
- Did these map onto the phases describes by Fitts or Gentile?
- Approximately how long did you spend in each phase of learning?
- What were the biggest challenges you faced in terms of learning this skill?

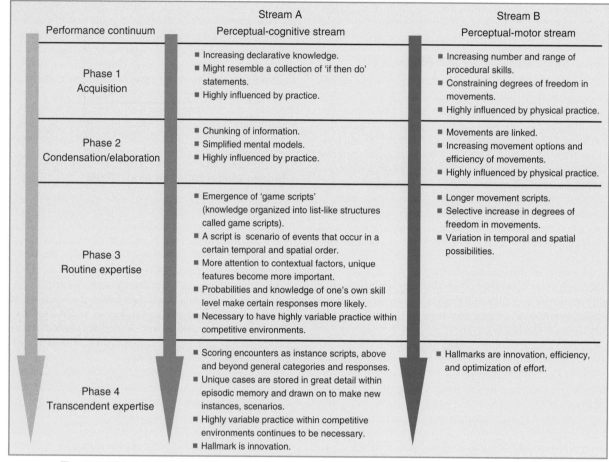

Fig. 15.1 A Model of the Acquisition and Retention of Perceptual Motor Expertise. (Adapted from Starkes, J. L., Cullen, J. D., & MacMahon, C. (2004). A life-span model of skill acquisition and retention of expert perceptual-motor performance. In A. M. Williams & N. J. Hodges (Eds.), *Skill acquisition in sport: research theory and practice* (pp. 259–281). London: Routledge.)

increasingly complex scenarios relating to strategies and decision making and is able to start stringing movements together so they form larger chunks. This is a lengthy phase of skill acquisition and if the person is able to progress beyond it they move into the first of two expert phases, that of the routine expert and transcendent expert.

The routine expert learns to develop and use 'game scripts' and 'movement scripts'. 'Games scripts' relate to aspects such as the game plan or performance strategy whilst the 'movement scripts' relate to movement sequences or patterns of coordinated actions. These 'scripts' are not necessarily verbally articulated; in fact the expert may find it difficult to describe them in words. This is similar to the autonomous phase of learning described by Fitts and Posner where the skill is automated. The majority of experts stay in

this phase but the Lifespan Models also accommodates the minority of people who are able to go beyond this level and demonstrate truly exceptional ability. They referred to this phase as transcendent expertise with the characteristics of maximum efficiency, optimisation of effort and innovation (Activity Box 15.2).

How Much Practice Do We Need?

How much practice do you need to do to learn a new skill, to become an expert or to recover movement after an injury? This frequently asked question has been the matter of considerable debate in the literature over the years. Ericsson et al. (1993) attempted to answer this by studying a group of good and a group of elite violinists. He asked them to estimate how many hours per week they had practised their violin during each year since they had started to learn. The findings showed the top violinists had practised intensely and deliberately for approximately 10,000 hours over a ten-year period. This 10,000 hours 'rule' is now commonly quoted, however, the extent to which it applies to all skills needs to be considered. For example, are some musical instruments more difficult to learn than others and should we expect differences in the rate at which we learn fine motor skills (like violin) and gross motor skills (such as running)? In terms of rehabilitation we also need to consider how much improvement is possible, and what the person's goals are. So whilst 10,000 hours is a good estimate for an elite violinist it is unlikely to be the case for everyone in every situation. Probably the best way to establish how much practice is required is to track how the person's performance changes over time (by plotting a learning curve) so that the rate of change can be determined.

How Should We Practise?

The concepts of variable, random, massed, distributed, part, whole and mental practice. It goes without saying that learning or relearning of a motor skill requires practice, but what is not so obvious is that the rate of learning and the degree of retention can differ depending on how practice sessions are structured and conducted. Changing the degree of variability within the practice session, when rest periods are given, whether the whole or part of the action is practised can all improve skill learning. Some of these manipulations will lead to short-term gains with little retention whilst others lead to slower rates of improvement during practice but better retention in the long term. This section will outline the key concepts of adopting variable or random practice and the contextual interference effect, massed versus distributed practice and practising the whole skill or part of the skill.

Variable and Random Practice

There are several different ways in which variability can be incorporated into practice, but the two that have been studied extensively are varying the conditions under which one particular skill is performed and varying the order in which a number of different skills are practised.

Variation With the Same Skill

A good example of varying the conditions under which one skill is performed is a golfer practising putting. During a session they could choose to practise putting from the same distance and position from the hole, or they could vary this so that each attempt is taken from a different position and distance. The potential advantage arising from including this type of variation when practising a single skill emerged as a prediction of Schmidt's Schema Theory (1975). Schmidt proposed that learning a motor skill involves the generation and elaboration of a Generalised Motor Programme (GMP). The idea of a GMP is that we have a stored representation of the spatial and temporal patterns of muscle activity that are required to perform an action. When the person attempts the action in different contexts the GMP is elaborated, and the accuracy with which the person can then predict the required patterns, when they are faced with performing the skill in a new context, increases. The most popular way to investigate this variable practice hypothesis has been to investigate what happens when one group of participants practise an action in exactly the same way each time and another group practises with variations. Both groups are tested afterwards (post-test task) on their ability to perform a novel variation of the task. Some studies have shown that variable practice enhances performance on the post-test task (e.g. Shoenfelt et al., 2002; Landin et al., 1993); however, there have been some inconsistencies in the findings of studies which suggest other variables need to be taken into account. One of these variables is the person's stage of learning when the practice variation is introduced. During the initial stage of learning, when the learner is still learning the basic movement pattern and the requirements of the task, introducing variation is unlikely to help. Later on, however, it is likely to be of value. Another thing to note is that the types of variations that should be introduced need to reflect how the person will eventually want to use the skill. For example, during the rehabilitation of walking, introducing a number of variations such as different surfaces, doorways, crowded environments etc. is likely to benefit, and when helping someone to relearn how to use their key to open their front door by getting them to practise when it is light and dark, or when it is raining or dry would be helpful.

Varying Between Skills

A practice session that includes a number of different skills performed in a random order is another way in which to introduce variation. Within the sport science literature including this type of variability into practice sessions has been shown to slow the rate of learning for each of the skills, but improve performance on retention or transfer tests. This seemingly contradictory finding is known as the **Contextual Interference** effect.

Shea and Morgan (1979) conducted one of the first studies on contextual interference. They recruited 72 college students and asked them to learn three different movement patterns.

The basic task was to pick up a tennis ball and knock over three out of six wooden barriers and return the tennis ball as quickly as possible. The movement pattern required on any trial was indicated by lights which illuminated which barriers were to be knocked down. Half the students were assigned to a blocked condition where they practised movement pattern A, then B and then C. The other half practised the patterns in a random order never performing the same pattern twice in a row. Half of the participants in each group completed retention trials 10 minutes after the end of the learning phase whilst the other half completed a retention test 10 days later. When the investigators looked at the recorded movement times they found that during the practice phase the average movement time from participants in the random group was slower than the average movement time for those in the blocked practice group (Fig. 15.2). However, 10 days later the pattern reversed with the random practice group outperforming the blocked practice group. Thus, Shea and Morgan demonstrated that blocked practice produced faster performances during learning but this was not maintained, whilst random practise led to slower performances during learning but this was maintained.

Taking this finding out of the laboratory Robert Hanlon studied the effect of random versus blocked practice in stroke patients (Hanlon, 1996). Twenty-four participants with chronic hemiparesis were assigned to one of two practice groups (random or blocked) or a control group. The random practice group completed 10 practice trials per day on an experimental task comprising extending the limb to a cupboard door, opening the door and picking up cup by the handle, transferring the cup up on to a platform and releasing the cup. After each attempt they completed one of three other tasks (pointing, touching objects or touching a location). The blocked practice group just practised the experimental task 10 times per day and the control group did not practise at all. Retention tests were undertaken by all groups 2 and 7 days after the end of practice. When they looked at successful performance on the experimental task, they found that there was no significant difference in success rates between the random and blocked practice groups during practice, but the random practice group performed significantly better on the retention tests than either the blocked or control group. This finding suggests that the contextual interference effect could be used effectively in clinical settings. However, not all studies have been able to show the contextual interference effect. A good example of this is the study by Brydges et al. (2007) who examined possible contextual interference effects in surgeons learning to perform orthopaedic surgical tasks that differed in the degree of complexity. During the learning phase the findings indicated an advantage for practising the easier skills in a block as opposed a random order, but on the novel transfer test 1 week later there was

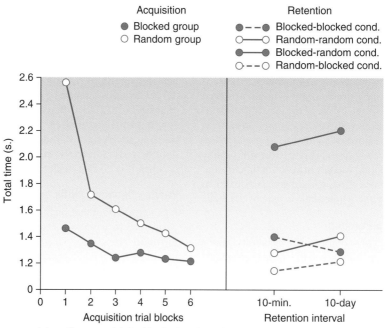

Fig. 15.2 Mean total time (in seconds) for blocked and random groups during the acquisition trial blocks and retention tests. (Adapted from the graph for Shea, J.B., Morgan, R.L., 1979. Contextual interference effects on the acquisition, retention, and transfer of a motor skill. J. Exp. Psychol. Hum. Learn. Mem. 5, 179–187.)

ACTIVITY BOX 15.3

Think about a person who has experienced a stroke and is trying to relearn how to use their arm and hand. What kinds of practice might a physical therapist employ to help them, and when would they introduce these?

no overall advantage for the group who had practised the skills in a random order. One possible reason for this finding is that the tasks did not differ sufficiently, as previous studies have shown that the contextual interference effect is greatest when the skills practised vary in the required patterns of coordination (Activity Box 15.3).

Massed Versus Distributed Practice

Apart from deciding which skills are to be practised during a session the rehabilitation practitioner also needs to decide how much rest to give the person between attempts, and this has been investigated by comparing the effects of massed or distributed practice on the rate of skill learning and skill retention. Massed practice is where the amount of time spent practising during a session is greater than the time spent resting, whilst distributed practice is where the amount of time spent resting is equal to or greater than the time spent practising. However, despite there being a number of studies in this area, there is no consensus view on this as a number of factors need to be considered for each individual. Fatigue, energy demands and complexity of the skill are obvious factors but the amount of cognitive effort required and the time needed to process the outcome and to make changes to the General Motor Programme also need to be accounted for. This is particularly true in rehabilitation where the relearning of an activity can require considerable cognitive effort to translate instructions into actions and to process feedback, so a distributed practice session may be more advantageous in these circumstances. The individual's level of motivation will also dictate the amount of rest needed, and frustration at repeated failures will make it more difficult for the person to process and act on feedback.

Whole Versus Part Practice

The inherent complexity of the skill will dictate whether it is best to practise it as a whole or in parts, but the practitioner must also consider the capabilities of the learner. For example, in a rehabilitation setting a patient with poor working memory or difficulties with sustaining or switching attention may benefit from part practice methods such as segmentation or simplification. Similarly when teaching children it is important to take into account the degree to which they can cope with cognitively demanding tasks and to break

them down accordingly. One way to do this is segmentation, which is where the skill is split into components, usually based on spatial or temporal characteristics. An alternative is simplification, which is where an easier version of the skill is taught, for example by allowing the person to use assistive devices (like a walking frame) or modifying the equipment (like using a large racket to hit a ball). A third technique involves components of a skill which are usually performed simultaneously being practised independently first before being combined.

MENTAL PRACTICE

Mental practice is when a person imagines themselves making a movement, or a series of movements, without actually physical doing them. Mental imagery is a type of mental practice where the person creates some form of visual or kinaesthetic representation of the action. There are two types of mental imagery: internal where the person 'views' the action from the perspective they would have if completing it and external imagery where the person views the action from the external perspective, as if they were watching a recording of themselves.

There have been a lot of studies carried out in the field of sports psychology assessing the use and effectiveness of mental imagery as a form of mental practice for athletes, and the overall consensus is that mental imagery is both a useful and effective technique to promote learning and to help athletes focus their attention and remain calm.

However, the literature on the use of mental imagery and practice in clinical rehabilitation is currently less extensive and more mixed. The majority of the current studies have focused on the use of mental imagery on the rehabilitation of neurological impairments, mostly from the effects of a stroke, and Guerra et al. (2017) published a systematic review of the published clinical trials. They found 32 studies which had assessed the effects of mental imagery on improving activities of daily living, balance, gait/lower limb and upper limb in stroke survivors. Guerra et al. assessed the quality of these studies included in their review, taking into account factors such as whether participants had been randomly allocated to either the intervention group or the control group, whether the participants in the groups were similar at the start of the study and whether a lot of participants had dropped out of the study. This revealed nine high quality studies and when they analysed these studies collectively they found that mental practice did not significantly improve outcomes for balance, activities of daily living, lower limb/gait or upper limb. However, when all 32 studies were included more positive findings emerged. They concluded that whilst the majority of existing studies show benefits for the use of mental imagery there are some

ACTIVITY BOX 15.4

People differ in their ability to form mental images for actions. One way to determine the accuracy of a person's mental imagery is to get them to time how long it takes them to imagine a task and then time them actually doing the task to see whether there is a discrepancy in their mental and physical timings. You can try this for yourself to see what your mental imagery accuracy is like. First, imaging yourself moving a short distance, say from a desk to a door. Get a stopwatch and time yourself mentally doing this. Then time yourself actually moving from the desk to the door. Next increase the distance and see what happens. You will probably find that when the actions are longer than 5 seconds you become less accurate in your mental imagery timing.

conflicting results and that at this time there are not enough high-quality studies on which to base a decision as to the value of using mental imagery in the rehabilitation of stroke (Activity Box 15.4).

FEEDBACK

Feedback about performance comes from two sources, internal and external. Internal feedback comes from our sensations and perceptions and includes **exteroception** (visual, auditory, cutaneous senses), **proprioception** (information from the muscle spindles, tendons, vestibular system) and **exproprioception** (the movement of the body relative to the environment) (see Chapter 9). External feedback is often referred to as augmented feedback and can relate to the outcome of the performance and/or aspects of the movement pattern. Information about the outcome of the performance is known as knowledge of results (KR) whilst information about the movement pattern is called knowledge of performance (KP). Both of these forms of feedback can be given verbally or nonverbally and during or after the performance. The nature and timing of augmented feedback can have a profound effect on motor learning and in the next sections we will explore this more.

GUIDANCE HYPOTHESIS

The influence of augmented feedback on learning has been studied for over 50 years and a review of the early studies was undertaken by Salmoni et al. (1984). Based on their findings they proposed that feedback guides the learner to the optimal performance. However, they noted some interesting findings such as providing augmented feedback after every attempt does not always improve performance. One argument that has been put forward to account for this relates to the early cognitive stage of motor learning when the learner goes through a trial and error process to develop appropriate patterns of coordination. It is proposed that if KR is given too frequently during this phase the learner may become dependent on it rather than using their intrinsic error detection processes to develop an understanding of the skill. There are also considerable variations in the movement patterns during this phase of learning and providing feedback to correct errors after every attempt can result in what is known as maladaptive short-term corrections. This is where the person over-compensates for an error associated with one aspect of their performance and as a result of further feedback the performance can then begin to oscillate. This would suggest that reducing the amount of feedback given could be beneficial but giving too little can leave the learner in state of not knowing what they are doing wrong which can be demotivating.

A number of studies have examined the effect that reducing the amount of feedback has on learning under either constant or variable practice conditions. Overall the findings have been somewhat mixed, with little empirical support for the idea that providing feedback after each attempt reduces the extent to which people use their own error detection and problem-solving strategies. However, there is some support for a reduction in the frequency of feedback resulting in more stability between attempts, which aids learning. This is the case for simple skills but not for more complex skills where there is a high demand on attention and memory. For these skills providing feedback after every attempt is the best approach.

A further point for consideration relates to when feedback is given relative to the end of the attempt. Here the research points to the most benefit occurring when feedback is given 2 to 3 seconds after the performance ends rather than immediately. However, a study by Schmidt and Wulf (1997) also found that giving concurrent feedback during practice can improve performance although when it is withdrawn on a retention or transfer test they noticed clear performance decrements. Feedback can also be given after blocks of trials, or when the performance has improved beyond certain limits, which is known as bandwidth KR. In theory, providing feedback after a number of trials could encourage the learner to engage in more problem solving which would aid learning; however, currently there are not enough experimental studies to demonstrate whether this is the case.

ATTENTIONAL FOCUS

One important way in which feedback affects learning is by drawing the learner's attention to a particular aspect of the skill. The focus of attention induced by the verbal feedback given by a coach or therapist can have a considerable effect on learning. Typically studies have shown that when attention is directed to the person's body movements, known as an internal focus of attention, the rate of learning is reduced compared to conditions where the focus of attention is directed externally, that is, how the movement is made in the environment. It appears that by focusing in on the movement itself can interfere with some of the automatic processes used to control the action. You may have experienced this phenomenon yourself when you walk down stairs. If you walk down looking ahead or towards the bottom of the stairs as you normally would, your feet and legs seem to automatically know how to form the correct movement pattern. If you consciously look down at the feet, though, and then visually guide each foot to the next step you may get the sense of feeling unsteady. This interference effect is noticeable on well learnt automatic skills, but this is not necessarily the case for new skills or the relearning of motor skills.

Spotlight on the Use of Virtual Reality Technology in Skill Acquisition

One way of increasing variability into practice and manipulating the feedback a person gets is to use virtual reality systems. Virtual reality (VR) has been around for some time now. It is already well used to develop skills in pilots and surgeons (among others) but only relatively recently applied to the rehabilitation of movement. The production of low-cost VR systems means this technology is now widely accessible and its use in rehabilitation is predicted to grow, particularly in the area of neurorehabilitation where repetitive movement practice is conversely problematic and essential. Weiss et al. (2006) defined virtual reality as 'interactive simulations created with computer hardware and software to present users with opportunities to engage in environments that appear and feel similar to real world objects and events'. The idea is that it creates an enriched, interactive environment for practising movement. Not only is this regarded as more enjoyable (Lewis and Rosie, 2012) but there is good evidence from animal studies that enriched environments promote recovery of brain functions following a stroke (Janssen et al., 2010).

Clearly a more enjoyable experience will have therapeutic benefits, but there are specific advantages for learning/relearning movement with VR that map onto the principles of motor learning we have outlined in this chapter. Firstly it enables a high volume of practice as the tasks in a VR environment are easily repeated. This practice can also be varied more easily and to a much greater extent than in the real world (depending on the software), so the learner can be more challenged in terms of motor problem solving

and introduced to situations which might be risky in the real world (e.g. crossing a busy road) without the risk of actual harm.

Perhaps the most exciting feature of VR, however, is the ability to manipulate the feedback to the individual. The most common way to provide feedback with VR is visually on the screen, although many systems also include sound, touch, balance (e.g. a moving platform) and even smell (Serrano et al., 2016). As we have already stated there are many parameters to feedback and these can all be tailored to the individual. So, for example, a VR system could exaggerate the visual representation of a patient's movement so that it appears more successful (this idea is discussed later on) or even swap the movement of an unaffected side with the affected side; this is termed discordant feedback and can be surprisingly effective. There are many other variations possible; what works best has not been established and is likely to vary according to the individual and task. The point, however, is that VR can offer more variety in feedback than is possible in the real world. Importantly, there is good evidence to support its use in the recovery of upper limb movement and activities of daily living in stroke survivors and growing evidence of its effectiveness for lower limb activities (Laver et al., 2015).

An important characteristic of effective VR is the feeling of being part of the virtual world. This is called presence and various technologies have tried to achieve this through head-mounted systems and large curved screens. One of the more successful systems for achieving presence is the Computer Assisted Rehabilitation Environment (CAREN) (Motek Medical B.V., The Netherlands), Fig. 15.3. This system

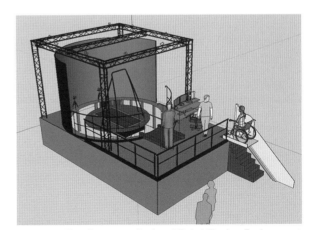

Fig. 15.3 The Computer Assisted Rehabilitation Environment (CAREN) (Motek Medical B.V., The Netherlands) system incorporating 180-degree VR screen, treadmill, safety harness, 6-degree of freedom platform and motion capture cameras.

ACTIVITY BOX 15.5

Rehabilitation with VR is not the same as playing a video game but there are many aspects of video games that can be used to encourage movement. Think about a video game you have played and consider which parts of the game might be used in a rehabilitation setting and which parts could not.

ACTIVITY BOX 15.6

Try to think of a time when you think you learned a movement skill particularly well with the help of a coach/teacher/parent/driving instructor. How did they give you feedback? Was it at the end, or during your performance? Did they get you to think about the movement? Did they encourage you to identify the errors yourself? How did they motivate you to continue learning?

Spend 5 min reflecting on this and the whole area of motor learning and write down five things you might consider when you are next working with a patient to recover a movement.

provides mechanical feedback through a treadmill mounted on a platform that can move in every direction (useful for recreating outdoor walking), a 180-degree curved screen and a surround-sound system. The system also benefits from a motion-capture system and forceplates (see Chapter 12) which can be used to provide very precise feedback on the body's movement (Activity Box 15.5).

Optimal Performance

So far we have focused on how practice conditions and feedback influence motor learning, but equally important are the motivational factors of the learner. In an attempt to draw together what we currently know about motivation Wulf and Lewthwaite (2016) reviewed the literature and proposed the OPTIMAL theory of motor learning. OPTIMAL stands for Optimising Performance Through Intrinsic Motivation and Attention for Learning. Based on an analysis of studies from psychology, neuroscience and sports science, they identified two areas of motivation that appear critical for skill learning, enhanced expectancies and autonomy. Expectations of future success are powerful drivers of behaviour so enhancing them can, not surprisingly, improve learning. Wulf and Lewthwaite point to a number of ways in which expectations can be enhanced. Self-modelling is one such technique. This is where the learner is shown video feedback of their best performances, or the video is edited to show the person performing a skill or combination of skills that they have not yet attained. For example, a video of a gymnast performing two skills separately can be edited to make it look like they are performed in a sequence. This technique, known as feedforward modelling, was studied by Ste-Marie et al. (2011) who found that gymnasts who viewed edited videos of themselves prior to competing scored higher than in competitions when they did not watch videos of themselves.

Another key element, related to enhancing expectations of success, is the perceived difficulty of the task. The person's belief about their ability can be altered in a number of ways. For example, telling a person that people like them typically perform well on a task can be sufficient to improve performance (Wulf et al., 2012) or setting criteria for a successful performance that can be easily reached can provide a subjective experience of success that aids learning. Similarly, if the person believes that their ability level is fixed and cannot change then their motivation for engaging in learning is going to be low, but if they believe their motor abilities are changeable they are more likely to try to improve. Beliefs about abilities can also be influenced by feedback and task instructions, for example, by giving false positive feedback. Telling a person that they are performing above average for people who are similar to them can lead to them improving faster than people who are not told this. Providing feedback after 'good' attempts rather than after 'bad' attempts can also improve motivation and aid learning.

The second motivational factor included in the OPTIMAL model is autonomy, as studies have consistently shown that giving the learner control over some aspects of the practice session can improve skill learning. Autonomy can be introduced in a number of different ways and can provide the person with a sense of control and ownership over their learning. Controlling when feedback is given, access to video, the use of assistive device, the practice schedule and task difficulty have all been shown to be beneficial (Sanli et al., 2013) although more work needs to be done to establish the nature of the motivational benefits that can be gained from these (Activity Box 15.6).

SELF-ASSESSMENT QUESTIONS

1. What are the three stages of motor learning proposed by Fitts and Posner?
2. What does Gentile mean by 'fixate' and 'elaborate'?
3. What is a General Motor Programme?
4. What is the difference between blocked and random practice?
5. What is the Contextual Interference effect?
6. What is mental imagery and mental practice?
7. Why can giving feedback too often be detrimental?
8. Is it better to encourage a learner to focus their attention internally or externally?
9. How can VR systems help in rehabilitation settings?
10. Describe two ways in which the motivation of a learner can be improved.

REFERENCES

Brydges, R., Carnahan, H., Backstein, D., Dubrowski, A., 2007. Application of motor learning principles to complex surgical tasks: searching for the optimal practice schedule. J. Mot. Behav. 39, 40–48.

Ericsson, K.A., Krampe, R.T., Teschromer, C., 1993. The role of deliberate practice in the acquisition of expert performance. Psychol. Rev. 100, 363–406.

Fitts, P.M., Posner, M.I., 1967. Human Performance. Brooks Cole, Belmont, CA.

Gentile, A.M., 1972. A working model of skill acquisition with application to teaching. Quest 17, 3–23.

Guerra, Z.F., Lucchetti, A.L., Lucchetti, G., 2017. Motor imagery training after stroke: a systematic review and meta-analysis of randomized controlled trials. J. Neurol. Phys. Ther. 41, 205–214.

Hanlon, R.E., 1996. Motor learning following unilateral stroke. Arch. Phys. Med. Rehabil. 77, 811–815.

Janssen, H., Bernhardt, J., Collier, J.M., Sena, E.S., McElduff, P., Attia, J., et al., 2010. An enriched environment improves sensorimotor function post-ischemic stroke. Neurorehabil. Neural. Repair 24, 802–813.

Landin, D.K., Hebert, E.P., Fairweather, M., 1993. The effects of variable practice on the performance of a basketball skill. Res. Q. Exerc. Sport. 64, 232–237.

Laver, K., George, S., Thomas, S., Deutsch, J.E., Crotty, M., 2015. Virtual reality for stroke rehabilitation: an abridged version of a Cochrane review. Eur. J. Phys. Rehabil. Med. 51, 497–506.

Lewis, G.N., Rosie, J.A., 2012. Virtual reality games for movement rehabilitation in neurological conditions: how do we meet the needs and expectations of the users? Disabil. Rehabil. 34, 1880–1886.

Salmoni, A.W., Schmidt, R.A., Walter, C.B., 1984. Knowledge of results and motor learning—a review and critical reappraisal. Psychol. Bull. 95, 355–386.

Sanli, E.A., Patterson, J.T., Bray, S.R., Lee, T.D., 2013. Understanding self-controlled motor learning protocols through the self-determination theory. Front. Psychol. 3, 611.

Schmidt, R.A., 1975. A schema theory of discrete motor learning. Psychol. Rev. 86, 225–260.

Schmidt, R.A., Wulf, G., 1997. Continuous concurrent feedback degrades skill learning: implications for training and simulation. Hum. Factors 39, 509–525.

Serrano, B., Banos, R.M., Botella, C., 2016. Virtual reality and stimulation of touch and smell for inducing relaxation: a randomized controlled trial. Comp. Hum. Behav. 55, 1–8.

Shea, J.B., Morgan, R.L., 1979. Contextual interference effects on the acquisition, retention, and transfer of a motor skill. J. Exp. Psychol. Hum. Learn. Mem. 5, 179–187.

Shoenfelt, E.L., Snyder, L.A., Maue, A.E., McDowell, C.P., Woolard, C.D., 2002. Comparison of constant and variable practice conditions on free-throw shooting. Percept. Mot. Skills 94, 1113–1123.

Starkes, J.L., Cullen, J.D., Macmahon, C., 2004. A life-span model of skill acquisition and retention of expert perceptual-motor performance. In: Williams, A.M., Hodges, N.J. (Eds.), Skill Acquisition in Sport: Research Theory and Practice. Routledge, London.

Ste-Marie, D.M., Rymal, A., Vertes, K., Martini, R., 2011. Self-modeling and competitive beam performance enhancement examined within a self-regulation perspective. J. Appl. Sport Psychol. 23, 292–307.

Weiss, P.L., Kizony, R., Feintuch, U., Katz, N., 2006. Virtual reality in neurorehabilitation. Textbook Neural. Rep. Rehabil. 51 (8), 182.

Wulf, G., Chiviacowsky, S., Lewthwaite, R., 2012. Altering mindset can enhance motor learning in older adults. Psychol. Aging 27, 14–21.

Wulf, G., Lewthwaite, R., 2016. Optimizing performance through intrinsic motivation and attention for learning: the OPTIMAL theory of motor learning. Psychon. Bull. Rev. 23, 1382–1414.

Ergonomics: The Influence of the Environment on Human Movement

Philippa Coales

OUTLINE

LEARNING OUTCOMES

After reading this chapter, you will be able to:

1. Describe a systems approach to human activity.
2. Explain the effects of the physical environment on human movement.
3. Give examples of the way the design of a task affects human movement.
4. Recognise the impact of technology on human movement.
5. Consider the impact of organisational design and psychosocial environment on human movement.
6. Discuss the influence of anthropometrics on human movement.

INTRODUCTION

Reading this book, you will have become aware of the many factors that influence human movement. Many of these have been involved with the anatomical and physiological processes within the body as well as the human's psychological situation, and could be termed *intrinsic factors*. Factors *extrinsic* to the individual can also have an impact on movement; these can be described as environmental, task and organisational factors. In this chapter we shall discuss what these factors are and how they influence human movement.

WHAT IS THE ENVIRONMENT?

The dictionary definition of the environment is 'the surrounding objects or circumstances in which a person, animal or plant lives or operates' (Oxford English Dictionary, 2018).

In this day and age, the term *environment* has taken on a rather different connotation, and you are most likely to hear the word used in relation to climate change, rain forest destruction, sustainability and other factors relating to the natural world and the impact of human activity on its condition.

However, if we consider the environment in relation to human movement we need to understand which environmental factors may have an impact on it. If we go back to the original dictionary definition, we can break it down into two parts: surrounding objects and surrounding circumstances (Activity Box 16.1).

In Activity Box 16.1, you may have mentioned things like clothing, a computer mouse/keyboard, a desk, carpets, chairs, doors, tables. If you were outside you might have said pavements, walls, bins and street furniture (such as lampposts). All these objects could be considered as surrounding objects capable of changing your movements. Factors such as the weather, level of lighting, temperature and noise can be considered as physical circumstances surrounding a person. These are simple physical factors; however, there is a further dimension that could best be categorised under the division of surrounding circumstances which needs to be considered for a more complete picture. This factor concerns the psychosocial circumstances or situation of an individual, rather than the physical. An example of this may be the impact on a person who is required to work in an open-plan office environment when they prefer to work in a single office environment. This, in addition to the physical environment factors encountered, may have a detrimental psychosocial impact on the individual.

WHY DO WE NEED TO CONSIDER THE ENVIRONMENT?

Human movement can be affected, either positively or negatively, by the environment within which the movement takes place. Consider an athlete who runs the 100 m wearing training shoes. She is unlikely to achieve as good a time wearing these shoes as she would if she wore specifically designed spiked running shoes. During athletic competitions wind speed is always measured as it is recognised as having an impact, either positively or negatively, on performance times. If our runner was running into a headwind, her speed would be reduced, as some of her force would be needed to overcome the additional obstacle of the wind. On the contrary, if she had a tailwind her performance would be enhanced and movement assisted by the wind (Chapter 5). Let us also consider other surrounding circumstances, such as what is motivating the athlete to run. Is she there because she really wants to be, or is she there just because her brother is also a runner and so her parents bring her along as well? Motivation is a key factor in sports training and performance (Keegan et al., 2010).

Thinking about one activity such as running 100 m, it is clear that it can be impacted on by many aspects of the environment, surrounding objects, surrounding physical circumstances and surrounding psychosocial circumstances, all of which have an influence on the human movement performance. For a full and clear understanding of the achievement of human movement it is important to consider the environment in which any movement occurs.

It is clear that movement can be affected by numerous aspects of the environment in which the movement takes place, and it would be helpful to have a strategy by which the environmental impact on the movement could be considered logically and systematically.

A SYSTEMATIC APPROACH

Considering the environmental impacts on movement is very desirable to ensure all influences on movement are addressed. Professionals involved in analysing human movement—including physiotherapists, bioengineers, architects, occupational therapists and ergonomists (can you think of any more), as well as others involved in specific aspects of human movement, such as sports coaches and trainers—aim to maximise a person's safety, comfort and productivity. A logical, thorough analytical process using a system approach can attain the best outcome. This approach considers all the parts that may impact on an individual's ability to perform their movement objective.

A *system* is any interaction that a human may have, in any aspect of their life, that involves cognitive thought; initiation of movement and/or activity; interaction with physical, human and psychosocial influences; and a desired outcome (Arnold et al., 1998). This is similar to our definitions of the balance and motor system (see Chapters 8 and 9). In all these definitions there is the idea of things working together where there is an input (e.g. need to do a task, make a movement), communication/integration of this input and formation of a movement plan (cognitive processes) and then an output (execution of the movement task), with the sequence often repeating. This chapter is more concerned with the way humans interact, through movement and postures, with the systems that surround us.

An example of a system would be a person loading a dishwasher. The individual identifies (vision) that the dishwasher needs loading (input); after a bit of quick motor planning (cognitive processes), initiates the activity to load it including any adjustments to plates, cups, dishwasher etc. (more motor planning), closes the door and starts the machine, achieving the goal. What movements were used to achieve this may be influenced by the position of the dishwasher, the size and weight of the plates, the psychological state of the individual (see the discussion of the balance model below) and of course the individual's own motor capacity.

Another example of a system would be a woman working at a conveyor belt in a factory; she is required to load components that are in front of her into boxes that come along the belt. In this case, she initiates the repeated movements;

interacts with the components, boxes and conveyor belt, and possibly her colleague working on the opposite side of the belt; and achieves the desired pile of filled boxes. How this is achieved may depend on the height of the individual in relation to the conveyor belt, the duration that the activity has to be done for, and possibly the relationship the individual has with her colleagues (see the discussion of the balance model below) and employer.

The system approach can be applied in all aspects of life—for example having a shower, playing a game of badminton, sitting in a lecture, eating a meal, watching the television and putting on a coat—and in that way all aspects of a person's life can be considered as an interaction with a system (Activity Box 16.2; Case Study 16.1).

You can see from the above case studies that there are some core systems that are common to both people and are mostly to do with basic self-care, such as washing, eating and dressing. While they may be a common activity, the way in which they are carried out will differ between them because of factors that are intrinsic and extrinsic, such as environmental factors.

In addition to the differences in performing similar activities, there are differences in the actual type and number of systems in which each individual is involved. Jenny has many more systems within which she interacts, and these are of a more active nature, requiring movement, strength and flexibility. It is also clear that Jenny has more interactions with other people in her systems, whereas Agnes spends much of her time alone. This interaction with others, or lack of it, may have an impact on each individual's psychological factor. Isolation may demotivate Agnes and reduce her desire to move. Jenny's attitude towards schoolwork will impact on whether she runs to the bus stop or walks dragging her feet, and whether it is raining or not may impact on whether she is able to go outside to play at break time.

Having completed Activity Box 16.2 and looked at the case studies, you will be beginning to understand how many and varied are the activities and systems within which human movement may occur. In the next section we will look specifically at how the environment influences these systems, and therefore our movement.

ACTIVITY BOX 16.2   Your Daily Systems

Spend 5 minutes making a list of some of the systems in which you have been involved with in the last hour: making coffee? using a personal computer? mobile phone? using a toilet?

THE ENVIRONMENT'S IMPACT ON MOVEMENT SYSTEMS

As we have already seen, there are many components in the environment that affect a person's movement, which include their immediate physical surroundings, their immediate surrounding circumstances and their surrounding psychosocial situation.

Some of the obvious influences the environment has on movement include clothing (may restrict joint movement) and a mismatch between their physical stature and the objects/machines they are using (e.g. if you are small or in a wheelchair it is hard to turn a doorknob). Some aspects of a person's surrounding circumstances include temperature, which may make movement difficult if at extremes of physical comfort; light levels, which can either enhance or detract

CASE STUDY COMPARISON 16.1

Let us consider Agnes, who, at 85, spends most of her time in the house on her own. She is self-caring and able to do small domestic jobs around the house to assist the family. She uses the bathroom along the landing from her bedroom. In the morning, Agnes is able to get herself out of bed (system 1), get to the bathroom and wash herself (system 2) and return to her bedroom and dress herself (system 3). Once downstairs (system 4), she can prepare her breakfast (system 5), eat it and wash up (systems 6 and 7). Having eaten her breakfast, she tends to wrap herself in a light blanket and sit in her armchair in the sitting room to read (system 8) and watch a bit of TV (system 9). Although she is able to stand up from sitting, she tends not to get up until it is time for lunch (system 10), as it is warmer to stay sitting and wrapped in the blanket. She is able to make herself a sandwich (system 11) and cup of tea (system 12).

Agnes's granddaughter, Jenny, is 9 years old and is able to mirror her grandmother in the morning's activities as systems 1–6 are all completed, though the age difference may mean they are executed in a different fashion (see Chapter 10 for more information on ageing and child development). Jenny then collects her school bag and walks to the bus stop (system 7); travels to school by bus (system 8); attends classes, in which she works as part of a group (system 9); and moves between classrooms, which can be on different floors (system 10), to attend a science class in a laboratory (system 11). At lunchtime, Jenny eats her packed lunch (system 12), chats with her friends (system 13) and plays outside with a skipping rope (system 14).

from easy or safe movement; noise, which may alter ways in which movement is achieved; and the duration of the activity, which may alter movement patterns because of fatigue.

As you can see, there are many aspects of the environment that need to be considered when thinking in relation to human movement, and it is important to address them all to achieve the best quality of movement possible.

Therefore a broad systematic approach is needed to consider all the environmental factors. A useful model, based on balance theory, is shown in Fig. 16.1. This model focuses on the individual while considering the impact of various factors on that individual, giving a considered, balanced, approach. As you can see, the multiple factors are grouped together into five areas: the individual, technology, task design, task environment and organisational design. This framework is very helpful when used in conjunction with a system approach to movement, as described above, as it can be applied to any identified system and allows logical and thorough consideration of factors that may impact on human movement.

Using this balance model the individual is the most important factor, and it allows factors that impact on the individual to be considered. In this case, the task can be considered to be any system in which the individual is actively involved, be it work, school or leisure, and numerous aspects of environmental factors are able to be considered. By analysing these impacts, some ideas about the individual's personal situation can be identified.

Let us consider each component of the balance system and see how it impacts on human movement using different members of a family as examples.

THE BALANCE THEORY MODEL

The Task Environment

This factor in the model considers the environmental surrounding circumstances (e.g. light, temperature, noise and vibration), as well as the immediate physical surrounding environmental objects (e.g. space, furniture and flooring). As an example, let us consider the posture adopted and the speed of walking that someone may achieve when walking in the rain and wind when compared with walking in sunny and dry conditions. A crouched or hunched posture, with a rushing speedy walk, may be apparent in the rain (to minimise how wet you get) as opposed to an upright relaxed and slow walk in the sun (to maximise warmth and pleasure). The surface over which the person is walking may also alter gait if it is uneven cobbles compared with smooth tarmac, as less speed and greater care in foot placing will be required. Consider someone who works in a noisy environment that requires them to struggle to hear their colleague speak, their posture may be altered, with hunched shoulders and an awkward head/neck position to facilitate hearing their colleague (Activity Box 16.3; Case Study 16.2).

The case study above identifies how some of the physical environmental factors can impact on Agnes's movement, unfortunately mostly in a negatively way, reducing her movement, mobility and safety. Physical factors can also impact on movement in a positive way, for example a swimmer who wears a specially designed swimsuit is able to improve her technique and speed because of less movement restriction and reduced drag (Activity Box 16.4).

The Task Design

It is always desirable to fit the task to the person rather than attempt to fit the person to the task (Parker and Wall, 1998),

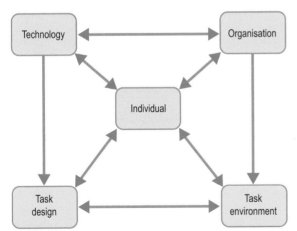

Fig. 16.1 A System Model Based on Balance Theory. (From Smith, M.J, Sainfort, P.C, 1989. A balance theory of job design for stress reduction. Int. J. Ind. Ergon. 4 (Part 1), 67–79.)

ACTIVITY BOX 16.3

Look around yourself in your immediate environment and identify all the factors (not just the objects you did in Activity Box 16.1) that may influence your movement.

ACTIVITY BOX 16.4

Return to the list you made in Activity Box 16.3 and consider how the environmental factors might influence your own movement and the perhaps the movement of others with different movement abilities.

Think about one aspect of your life (e.g. work, university or leisure) and consider how the physical environment impacts either positively or negatively on your movement, including your motivation to move.

CASE STUDY 16.2

Let us consider some of the systems in which Agnes was involved in (see Case Study 16.1), and consider how the task environment may have had an impact. Agnes is 85 and spends most of her time in the house on her own. She is self-caring and able to do small domestic jobs around the house to assist the family. In her bedroom, there is a single bed, a chest of drawers, a wardrobe, a bookcase on which she displays her ornaments, an armchair and two favourite floor rugs, which she brought from her own home, on the floor. This cluttered room is likely to reduce Agnes's movement, as she has to shuffle around the limited floor space and step over the rug edges (trip hazard). Many older people have reduced balance (Muir et al., 2010, and see Chapters 8 and 10) and she may feel safer using the furniture as support when she moves around the room. While this may give her an added feeling of security, it is likely to increase her risk of falling as she reaches forwards for support and moves her centre of gravity too far out of her base of support for recovery. She uses the bathroom along the landing from her bedroom. The landing has a central light, the switch for which is at the far end of the landing from her bedroom. Although Agnes is more able to walk freely along the length of the landing than in her own room, it is poorly lit until she reaches the far end and is able to switch the light on. Older people require

adequate lighting to assist in balance (Figueiro et al., 2012) and the dimness of the landing increases the potential for falling.

Once downstairs, which Agnes is able to negotiate with the use of two banister rails, there is a much less cluttered environment and she is able to move around more freely and safely. However, as she is the only person in the house during most of the day; she is reluctant to put the heating on due to the cost and so the house is quite cool during the daytime, until the rest of the family return home. Having eaten her breakfast, she tends to wrap herself in a light blanket and sit in her armchair in the sitting room to read and watch the TV. The chair was recently bought for her to assist herself rising from sitting, as she had previously been finding it more difficult to rise unassisted from the lower three-piece suite (see Chapter 17 for a case study on the sit-to-stand movement). Although she is now able to stand up from sitting more easily, she tends not to get up until it is time for lunch, as it is warmer to stay sitting and wrapped in the blanket. Her mobility is constrained by the lack of warmth, and the lack of mobility further reduces her temperature, setting up a vicious circle of being sedentary and cold, whereas if the heating was on during the day the warmth would encourage more general movement and mobility.

and there are various issues that need to be considered when designing or redesigning any task or system.

One aspect that can really impact on how individuals interact in a system within which they must operate is how their body stature relates to the objects that they use within that system. This is termed *anthropometrics* and relates to the dimensions of people in terms of height, limb length, forward reach distance, overhead reach distance, length of thigh, chest circumference etc. These dimensions are probably the most basic consideration for ensuring that a person is comfortable and safe in an environment, and it is therefore unfortunate that most objects, systems and activities are designed around the nominal average male person or average female person, who unfortunately do not truly exist (Pheasant and Haselgrave, 2006). This means that frequently people are moving and interacting with objects and the environment in which there is a size relationship mismatch, which may cause restriction of movement or altered posture, or cause someone to overstretch to achieve their goal. For example, a person of 155-cm height has much more difficulty reaching a product from the top shelf of a supermarket than a person of 185-cm height. Equally, these two people will find sitting postures and comfort levels

ACTIVITY BOX 16.5

Take some basic anthropometric measurements of two people with different physical statures (e.g. upper limb length, lower limb length, upper limb reach forwards and upwards, and trunk length). Take an average of these measurements and see how far from the average each person is. Consider how these deviations from the average may affect a person when sitting at a desk, cycling a bike, using a laptop, driving a car and vacuuming the carpet.

very different when they sit in a similar armchair (Activity Box 16.5).

Other factors that need to be considered in designing a task are the frequency an activity is performed, the number of repetitions of the activity that are performed, and the load of the activity. Consider the person working at a supermarket checkout, who repeatedly reaches for and grasps the items on the conveyor belt then drags or lifts the items and pushes them along the belt after checking them. The position of the person in relation to the belt, the size and weight of each item, and the number of items moved will

CASE STUDY 16.3

Chris is 19 years old; he is home from university and working at a temporary job in a factory to raise money to travel. He works an 8-hour shift with two half-hour breaks during this time, packing items into boxes from a conveyor belt. He is required to lift the items from the belt and pack them into a box that is on another belt at right angles to, and lower than, the first belt. This necessitates him reaching forwards to different positions, as the items are not regularly spaced on the conveyor belt, rotating and flexing his trunk to pack them into the box, and once the box is full he steps through 90 degrees and pushes the filled box along the second conveyor line. The speed at which he does these activities is dictated by the conveyor belt speed, and he is unable to regulate this to his own comfort. He has to wear protective clothing for his own safety, but the weight and bulk of this restricts his mobility. Although others work on the belt, the noise prohibits conversation (see The Task Environment section). By the end of each shift, he is fatigued physically, bored and demotivated mentally.

ACTIVITY BOX 16.6 Enhancing the Working Environment

Consider the case study above and make a list of some simple modifications that could be made to the above work design that would enhance the working environment. Think how you could alter the movements, the load, the duration etc.

ACTIVITY BOX 16.7 Design of the Task Impacting on Movement

Think about some activities that you routinely do, at work, at home or for leisure, and consider how the design of the task impacts on your movement.

Can you think of any ways in which the task could be adapted to make it:

- *Safer or easier* for you?
- *Easy* for a much taller or shorter person, e.g. adjusting dimensions?
- *Possible* for a person with impaired mobility or a wheelchair user to complete?

all affect the way in which the activity will be performed. Add to this the anthropometric variation and it is possible to see that a 'simple' activity can be highly influenced by other factors (Case Study 16.3).

It is quite clear that this is not a good work design for any individual, and there is the potential for both physical and mental harm as well as a reduction in productivity (e.g. accidents, damaged goods). This case study may seem fairly exaggerated, but there are numerous people who regularly work in this type of environment, which will impact on their movement and potentially cause musculoskeletal and/or mental health harm (Activity Boxes 16.6 and 16.7).

Technology

In this day and age technology saturates our daily life, and you may wonder how it may impact on human movement. For this, we need to think about what is meant by technology. The most obvious answer seems to be the plethora of electronic gadgets such as mobile phones, computers and automated systems in shops but technology includes a much broader spectrum. Cars, mechanical lifting equipment, kitchen appliances, walking sticks, household appliances, and public transport, the list goes on. The word technology has been adapted from the Greek word for craft in art and skill (*techne*) and covers, processes, techniques, skills and methods used to accomplish an objective such as the manufacture of goods or provision of a service. A stick may

be considered a technology when used by a chimp to lever out some delicious ants. The definition by Bain (1937) is probably the most apt as it covers both the hardware (tools etc.) and the knowledge/skills:

> "*technology includes all tools, machines, utensils, weapons, instruments, housing, clothing, communicating and transporting devices and the skills by which we produce and use them*"

In many cases, the purpose of technology is to reduce human movement, which can have a positive outcome for the individual; for example the use of a mechanical earth mover requires the driver to sit and operate instruments in the cab instead of using a spade and bending, twisting and lifting to shovel the soil himself. Reduction of movement is not always positive though, as in the case of the water engineer who previously physically inspected the water treatment facilities by walking around them and looking but who now sits and watches the computer screen as the facilities are monitored remotely. This causes him back pain from long periods of static sitting postures and boredom from watching the screens, leading to loss of concentration and general demotivation for the work that had previously been an outdoors physical job that he enjoyed. The impact of technology on physical activity is explored further in Chapter 14.

As you will see from Case Study 16.4, some of the technologies available in life today have a positive effect on

CASE STUDY 16.4

Liz is a very busy individual as, in addition to doing the majority of household duties for the family, she works part-time as an administrator in a building company. In many of her household roles, technology assists her to achieve all of her goals and includes assistive devices such as a washing machine, dishwasher and vacuum cleaner. Each of these machines reduces the effort involved in managing a large family while also working outside the home. While aiding Liz, they also have an impact on the types of movements she needs to be able to achieve; for example either good spinal flexibility or full range of knee flexion is needed to be able to load the washing machine and dishwasher. If, however, she hangs washing on an outside line instead of using a tumble drier she will need to be able to reach above her head. These types of technologies direct the type of movement necessary but also reduce the physical effort required for the activity, therefore enabling individuals with less movement and strength to continue to carry out the chore and maintain independence.

Liz uses a car to get to work instead of walking, which reduces her overall daily physical activity which, if not compensated for elsewhere in her lifestyle, could impact on her general health and fitness levels. Once at work, her main role is entering data into a computer. This type of activity requires specialised movement, in which the body remains in static postures for long periods of time, and small-range repetitive finger movements, not usually used in any other type of activity, are used. Long periods of static postures are not desirable for the human body and the repetitive nature of the keyboard work needs to be assessed in light of the information from the section on task design.

ACTIVITY BOX 16.8   Technology in Leisure

Spend 5 minutes making a list of what technologies are involved in your leisure time. Consider whether these technologies increase or decrease your physical activity.

ACTIVITY BOX 16.9   Your Organisations

Make a list of all the organisations within which you currently operate.

chess within a club organisation and Liz works within a business company organisation. Every individual will operate within a number of organisations at any one time depending on their family situation, education, work and leisure activities (Activity Box 16.9).

You may wonder why considering the wider organisational environment is valuable. Within any organisation, policies and procedures, whether they are formal (as in the case of a school or company) or informal (as in the case of most families), will impact on what each individual within that organisation is able to do. For example, in Jenny's school the policy is that the subject teachers stay in the same room and the pupils move to the room for the subject, which means that Jenny regularly gets up and walks along corridors and up and down stairs. The company for which Liz works recognises the potential risk of long periods of keyboard work, and the staff are encouraged to take regular breaks to move and to do different aspects of their job, for example filing, in sequences to avoid long static periods. While it is clear that the approach of the organisation will have an impact on the movement an individual is able to do, it has a more far-reaching effect which may impact on the psychological situation for the individual. In this example, Liz is aware that her company is concerned about her well-being, which makes her feel valued and motivated. This has benefits not only for Liz but also for the company, as a well-motivated workforce is more productive. In most cases it is the organisation that determines the rules of our activity, what we can and can't do; sometimes this can be to the benefit of the individual but the rules are made primarily for the organisation's efficiency and effectiveness and not for the individual.

From Case Study 16.5, you should be able to see that the organisation within which movement systems occur can have a profound impact on the movement that an individual person may achieve or perform. In this case, a policy that was implemented to encourage workers has led to John carrying out heavy physical activity despite the availability of assistive devices to help him (Activity Box 16.10).

human movement and allow individuals to achieve their goals, but sometimes the technology has a limiting effect on human movement, the reduction of which may cause health and fitness problems (Activity Box 16.8).

The Organisation

Up until now, we have considered how task design, the task environment and technology may impact on a human's movement within a system approach. Now the aspect of the organisation within which the system operates will be considered.

What is meant by the organisation is any larger environment within which systems operate. In the context of our case-study family, Jenny's science lesson in the laboratory is within an educational organisation, Agnes's activities of daily living are within the family organisation, Dan plays

CASE STUDY 16.5

John works as a van driver for a furniture delivery company. The van he drives is new and has a good seat, steering wheel and pedal position, and he therefore has a good posture and is comfortable while driving. Each day, he receives a list of his deliveries for that day, identifies the items in the warehouse, and loads them onto his van in an order that will allow him to make the deliveries using the shortest possible route. To assist him, he has a two-wheeled trolley, the van has a hydraulic tail lift and an inbuilt satellite navigation system. He then drives round the computer-optimised route, unloading the items at each address and taking them into the house or flat.

John's company has provided him with an assistive moving device, the trolley, a hydraulic tail lift and a satellite navigation system, all of which have an impact on reducing the physical workload that John has to perform and reducing activities such as bending and lifting and making him more efficient. It also has a policy of having unfixed hours, which means that once John has made all of the deliveries for that day, he finishes work, whether that be early or late in the day. This flexible type of working helps to motivate John, and it encourages him to work fast so that he can finish earlier. There is no benefit to the company of John finishing early as he has fulfilled his work quota for that day, but it benefits John, who likes to get home early so he can spend time with his mother, Agnes. This desire to finish early means that John works fast and avoids using the trolley and tail lift, as they slow him down. He therefore, unnecessarily, increases his physical workload and his movements by physically lifting and moving the furniture without assistance.

ACTIVITY BOX 16.10

Think about an organisation within which you are currently functioning, whether at home, studying, at work or for leisure. Think about the aspects of that organisation that may impact on your physical activity and identify if these are positive or negative impacts.

It is interesting to identify how some innocuous, or even historical, situations actually impact on human movement without us being aware. In some cases, the organisation can be manipulated by altering the use of technology (e.g. John's assistive devices in Case Study 16.5) to alter a person's movement. The ability to adjust the rules operating within an organisation, in the same way as you may adjust a task design, may need careful negotiating skills but may ultimately allow safer human movement.

The Individual

Using the balance theory approach to human movement (see Fig. 16.1), the main component is the individual. How the other components impact on that individual is important, as we have seen, but individuals have their own characteristics, which will have an impact on their movement and will impact on the other components.

We have already mentioned human anthropometrics in the section on task design and looked at how body stature and physique may impact on the movement it can achieve. We identified that each individual's unique anthropometrics (e.g. height, chest girth and overhead reach) will impact on how similar activities are carried out and whether or not an individual is actually able to achieve the goal.

Let's look at someone shopping in a supermarket whose height is 155 cm; they are able to reach objects on lower- and middle-height shelves but unable to reach objects on the top shelf and so will require assistance. As we know, the majority of systems are designed for the 'average' person, which may cause considerable difficulty for those at extremes of this norm. Take, for example, a man of 190 cm who is trying to buy a new car that is comfortable for him to drive. It is very difficult, as many of his anthropometric measurements limit his ability to achieve a comfortable position. For example, his lower leg length means it is difficult to comfortably reach the pedals, while his foot size may make safe use of the pedals impossible. His thigh length means that he has to sit with his hips flexed to more than 110 degrees, and it is difficult for him to get his knees under the steering wheel, while his trunk length means that his head is rubbing on the ceiling. Someone who is at the shorter end of the scale may have difficulty actually reaching the pedals and/or the steering wheel and may not be able to see adequately over the steering wheel without the strategic placement of a cushion.

Car manufacturers design features such as adjustable seat height, steering wheel position and seat position, which mean that the majority can achieve comfort, but there will always be the extremes who are not so easily accommodated. If a person is too far from the norm to achieve the goal of a movement system, they may require adaptation of the systems to enable them to achieve the goals without further outside assistance (Activity Box 16.11).

In addition to anthropometrics, other personal characteristics may influence how a person moves. For example, a person's strength may allow them to achieve an activity or movement that a weaker person may achieve differently or even not at all. Let us go back to John's work, in which

CASE STUDY 16.6

John and Liz are keen gardeners. They enjoy working together in their flower and vegetable garden and are out in the garden in all weathers (the weather may have an impact on their movement, as already discussed in the section on the task environment above). Their enthusiasm for their hobby means that, whatever the weather, they are happy to be gardening, ensuring repetitive activity that will help maintain smooth, coordinated and efficient movement. John is 180 cm and heavily built, while Liz is 155 cm with a petite physique. Over the years that they have created and managed their garden, they have realised that each is better suited to some of the regular jobs than others and they work to their individual strengths. John digs and fertilises the vegetable garden, as he is strong enough to achieve good soil turnover and is able to lift and manoeuvre the fertiliser bags. Liz works in the greenhouse bringing on the seedlings, as John finds the height of the greenhouse shelving forces him to bend his back and he becomes uncomfortable. Although the height of the shelving is appropriate for Liz, she is not strong enough to lift the bags of potting compost, so John decants the big bags into several smaller bags so that she can lift them. When planting time comes, it is Liz's job to plant out the young plants into furrows that John has created. During the growing season, the garden is kept tidy by Liz using a hoe regularly to keep the weeds under control. Although she is weaker than John, he is hampered in this job as his height in relation to the length of the hoe handle means he is uncomfortable working in a flexed posture. The lawn is kept neat by John doing the actual mowing and Liz trimming the edges, so each does activities suited to their individual characteristics so they are safe and effective. Their different characteristics come in very useful when it is time for pruning, as their different statures mean that they can each reach areas that the other cannot and they complement each other's activities.

he moves furniture from a warehouse on to a van and from the van into people's homes. We already know that to speed the process up, and get home early, he avoids using the devices in situ to help him, the trolley and the hydraulic lift, and physically lifts and carries the items. He is able to do this as he is muscularly strong enough to do so, whereas a work colleague with less strength may not be able to or, in trying to, may harm themselves (Activity Box 16.12).

Another characteristic of an individual that could influence how movement is performed or achieved is the individual's present or previous health. Agnes, who at 85, may have arthritis in her hips and knees decides to climb the stairs one step at a time and use the banisters on both sides to reduce joint loading, while 15-year-old Dan may run up the stairs taking two steps at a time and not use the banister at all. Long-term conditions may influence movement; for example someone with chronic low back pain may walk in a more flexed posture and at a slower speed, while a person with chronic bronchitis may have a hunched upper body posture that may limit shoulder and neck movements. Acute illness or injury may also impact on movement in a variety of ways from the person who is acutely ill and bed-bound temporarily to someone who must use aids to achieve movement, such as the individual with a fractured ankle who needs to use crutches to walk.

However, it is not only an individual's physical health that may impact on movement quality and quantity. Someone suffering from depression may limit their movement in all aspects, and when they do move it may be achieved slowly and possibly in a flexed posture. An individual's psychological profile and personal motivation may influence the quality of their movement. For example, Jenny, who at 9 years old is very enthusiastic about school, rushes along the pavement running and skipping to get the bus; however, Dan, at 15 years old, is bored with school and disinterested in it so walks along the pavement with his head down, shoulders drooped and dragging his feet.

As can be seen from Case Study 16.6, a person's individual characteristics mean that they are more suited to some activities than to others. It is clear that both John and Liz could achieve each of the jobs in the garden, but they have divided the activities to allow each to achieve them using easily achieved and safe movement, for one to achieve a job the other does may require exertion and potential harm.

SUMMARY

In this chapter, we have introduced the idea that human movement can be considered in relation to movement systems and how environmental factors, which may influence this movement, can be logically addressed using a balance theory model. This model applies factors such as task environment, task design, the influence of technology, and the organisation within which the movement system occurs to the individual person doing the movement, and considers how each factor, separately and collectively, may influence movement achieved. Additionally, it considers individuals' unique personal characteristics and how they may influence the movement achieved. This approach allows both physical and psychosocial aspects of each factor to be applied to the movement system.

It is hoped that, after reading this chapter and completing the activities, you will have a much clearer understanding of how physical and psychosocial environmental factors influence human movement. The following self-assessment questions are designed to help you retain this understanding. Once you have completed them please return to the learning outcomes stated at the beginning and make sure you feel confident you have achieved them, if not then you know what to do.

SELF-ASSESSMENT QUESTIONS

1. Name the five elements of the framework/model based on balance theory.
2. Name five environmental factors that could affect movement.
3. What do we mean by anthropometrics?
4. Is the following statement true or false?
   Technology means the physical tools we use to achieve our objectives.
5. Name three technologies used by a physiotherapist.
6. How might a recently torn ankle ligament alter the way you walk downstairs?
7. Using the Balance Theory model, reflect on a work or leisure system of activity in which either you or an associate/friend/colleague are engaged regularly. Consider the impact of the influences of all the factors in the model on how the system or activity is achieved. If detrimental impacts are identified create a plan which, if implemented, would improve the system of activity to optimise human movement for health, safety and the wellbeing of the person.

REFERENCES

Arnold, J., Cooper, C.L., Robertson, I.T., 1998. Work Psychology. Understanding Human Behaviour in the Workplace, third ed. Prentice Hall, Harlow.

Bain, R., 1937. Technology and state government. Am. Sociol. Rev. 2 (6), 860–874.

Figueiro, M.G., Gras, L.Z., Rea, M.S., Plitnick, B., Rea, M.S., 2012. Lighting for improving balance in older adults with and without risk for falls. Age. Ageing 41 (3), 392.

Keegan, R., Spray, C., Harwood, C., Lavallee, D., 2010. The motivational atmosphere in youth sport: coach, parent, and peer influences on motivation in specializing sport participants. J. Appl. Sport Psychol. 22 (1), 87–105.

Muir, S.W., Berg, K., Chesworth, B., Klar, N., Speechley, M., 2010. Quantifying the magnitude of risk for balance impairment on falls in community-dwelling older adults: a systematic review and meta-analysis. J. Clin. Epidemiol. 63 (4), 389–406.

Oxford English Dictionary. Oxford English Dictionary. http://www.askoxford.com (Accessed 17 January 2018.)

Parker, S., Wall, T., 1998. Job and Work Design. Sage Publications, London.

Pheasant, S., Haselgrave, C.M., 2006. Bodyspace: Anthropometry, Ergonomics and the Design of Work. Taylor & Francis, London.

17

Case Studies in Human Movement

Seda Bilaloglu, Roy Bowers, Bruce Carse, Megan Caughey, Konstantinos Kaliarntas, Andy Kerr, Andrew Murphy, Preeti Raghavan, Jennifer Stone and Alvin Tang

OUTLINE

LEARNING OUTCOMES

After reading this chapter, you will be able to:

1. Apply knowledge of human movement (biomechanics, anatomy, physiology and motor control) to the understanding of clinical problems and sports techniques.
2. Apply principles of measurement to movement problems.

3. Recognise the value that movement analysis can have in identifying movement impairment and recovery of movement function.
4. Gain greater insights on the effect of interventions (surgical and conservative) for the recovery of functional movement.

INTRODUCTION

In this final chapter we will apply your newly gained understanding of human movement (biomechanics, anatomy, physiology and motor control) to the kind of movement problems you might see during your professional work. This will cover lower limb movements such as gait; upper limb movements such as a reach to grasp; and a sports technique, when we look at rowing. In these case studies you will be introduced to some clinical conditions, such as stroke and cerebral palsy. We will only provide a short background to these conditions so that you can follow the movement problem presented. You are advised to look at disease-specific books to gain the required depth of knowledge of the conditions. The chapter is composed of six case studies written by experts in their area, and the data they present are all real data collected from their movement labs and clinics. Of course, there are many different movement problems that we have not covered here and, while there will be more examples made available to you through the evolve website, the idea is that you build a general understanding of movement analysis so that you can apply this knowledge to your own movement problems.

CASE STUDY ONE: GAIT OF A CHILD WITH CEREBRAL PALSY BEFORE AND AFTER CORRECTIVE SURGERY*

Background

Walking is the most frequently used type of gait and provides independence and the ability to perform many important activities of daily living, facilitating many occupations and social activities. The average person takes between 5000 and 15,000 steps per day (Kirtley, 2006). It is a highly complex biomechanical activity; however, the majority of it takes place subconsciously and therefore we do not require a detailed understanding in order to complete the task.

A person's gait pattern can be adversely affected by a large number of conditions including: cerebral palsy, stroke, multiple sclerosis, Parkinson's disease and common musculoskeletal injuries. Gait requires joints to be flexible, muscles to be sufficiently strong, skeletal alignment to be correct, and an intact motor control of the entire musculoskeletal system.

A normal healthy gait pattern can be quite variable. You may have noticed that you can identify particular people from a distance by their style of gait, so within what is considered 'normal range' there is a surprising amount of variation. Clinical gait analysis is used when a person's gait

abnormalities are such that they have a detrimental effect on their quality of life and their ability to participate fully, usually through causing them pain, increased trips and falls, or high levels of fatigue. It provides detailed information on the person's walking pattern, which can help a multidisciplinary health care team to decide on an appropriate intervention. It can also be used to assess the efficacy of the intervention to ensure it has provided the desired improvement to the person's walking pattern with a before-after comparison.

The Movement

The kinematics of the normal gait cycle can be broken down into eight distinct phases as described by Perry and Burnfield (1992); these are described in Table 17.1.

When the body contacts the ground, it exerts a force on the ground, and the ground exerts an equal and opposite force to the body (see Chapter 4 for reminder of Newton's laws of motion). The force that the ground applies to the body is called the ground reaction force (GRF). The GRF is a vector that can be split into three components: anterior-posterior (Fx), mediolateral (Fy) and vertical (Fz). The magnitude and alignment of the GRF vector relative to the joint centres determine how our body segments, and ultimately our centre of mass (CoM), move as we walk. While the GRF is measured in newtons, using the person's body mass it is converted into percentage body weight (BW) so it is comparable across different people.

Case Study

The data presented below were collected during a clinical gait analysis with an 8-year-old boy with diplegic cerebral palsy, 1.21 m in height and weighing 22.6 kg. His main complaints were that he was getting very tired when walking at school and found it difficult to keep up with his friends. He also complained that he frequently tripped and fell due to his feet turning inwards when he was walking. A recent fall had resulted in a visit to the accident and emergency department.

His clinical examination, which assessed his lower limb joint ranges of motion, muscle strength and spasticity, and skeletal alignment, identified the impairments detailed in Table 17.2.

He regularly used ankle-foot orthoses (Fig. 17.9), and also took oral Baclofen to reduce the spasticity in his muscles. He had previously had serial casting to stretch his calf muscles, but this only provided a short-term benefit.

Retro-reflective markers were placed on various anatomical landmarks in accordance with the conventional gait model (Davis et al., 1991). These markers were then tracked by a 10-camera Vicon system (sampling rate 100 Hz) in conjunction with two force platforms as the child walked barefoot up and down the gait laboratory. The marker and force platform data allowed the calculation of three-dimensional

*Bruce Carse

TABLE 17.1   The Phases of the Normal Gait Cycle as Described by Perry and Burnfield (1992).

	Phase	Description
1	Initial contact	The hip is flexed, the knee extended and the ankle is dorsiflexed to neutral. Floor contact is made with the heel.
2	Loading response	Body weight is transferred onto the leading limb. Using the heel as a rocker, the knee is flexed for shock absorption. A brief period of ankle plantar flexion interrupts the heel impact, but the heel rocker is preserved until the end of the phase.
3	Midstance	In the first half of a single leg stance, the limb advances over the stationary foot by ankle dorsiflexion while the knee and hip extend. The opposite limb is advancing through its midswing phase.
4	Terminal stance	During the second half of single leg stance, the heel rises and the limb advances over the forefoot rocker. The knee completes its extension and then begins a new arc of flexion. Increased hip extension and heel rise put the limb in a more trailing position. The other limb is completing terminal swing.
5	Preswing	Terminal double limb support is initiated by floor contact of the other limb. The reference limb responds to the initial weight transfer with increased ankle plantar flexion, knee flexion and a reduction of hip extension. The opposite limb is in loading response.
6	Initial swing	Increased knee flexion lifts the foot for toe clearance, and hip flexion advances the other limb. Ankle dorsiflexion is incomplete. The other limb is in early midstance
7	Midswing	Advancement of the limb anterior to the body weight line is gained by further hip flexion. The knee is allowed to extend in response to gravity while the ankle continues dorsiflexing to neutral. The other limb is in late midstance.
8	Terminal swing	Limb advancement is completed by knee extension. The hip drops slightly (to a 20-degree flexion) and the ankle remains dorsiflexed to neutral. The other limb is in terminal stance.

TABLE 17.2   Description of Patient Impairments Observed During the Clinical Examination.

	Impairment Description
Range of Motion	
1	Increased internal hip rotation bilaterally
2	Decreased external hip rotation bilaterally
3	Reduced range of hip extension bilaterally
Muscle Spasticity	
4	Tibialis posterior spasticity bilaterally
5	Bilateral gastrocnemius spasticity
Skeletal Measures	
6	High femoral anteversion bilaterally
7	Internal foot-thigh angles bilaterally
8	Bilateral forefoot adduction

(3D) joint angles as well as ground reaction forces, joint moments and joint powers. The child completed the gait assessment barefoot, and the average of 10 gait cycles per limb were used for the analysis.

An 'impairment-focussed interpretation' of the data was conducted (Baker, 2013) and after the multidisciplinary team discussion, it was decided that the main surgical intervention would be to conduct bilateral femoral derotation osteotomies. This was supplemented by physiotherapy, botulinum toxin injections to his gastrocnemii, new ankle-foot orthoses and continued use of oral Baclofen. A repeat gait assessment using the same equipment and test conditions was conducted 12 months after surgery.

Results

Kinematic Data

The overall improvement in his 3D gait kinematics was shown by the Gait Profile Score (Baker et al., 2009) changing from 16.9 to 7 degrees, which indicated that his walking pattern was much closer to normal. Using just the video footage, an Edinburgh Visual Gait Score (Read et al., 2003) was also used both pre- and postsurgery and his scores improved from 9 (right 4, left 5) to 3 (right 1, left 2). The specific kinematic improvements achieved are shown in the kinematic graphs in Fig. 17.1, and are explained fully below.

- Corrected his internal hip rotation angles [c], so his knees faced straight forwards when he was walking instead of being rotated internally
- Improved his internal foot progression angles [g], so they were less internal and made him less likely to trip and fall
- Eliminated the bilateral gastrocnemius spasticity in stance [e], so he no longer 'bounced' up on his toes during midstance
- Achievement of bilateral ankle dorsiflexion in swing [f], which also reduced the likelihood of tripping and falling as his feet cleared the ground better during swing
- Increased knee flexion in swing [d], which also helped both feet to achieve ground clearance
- Improved anterior pelvic tilt [a] and reduced his pelvic retraction [b]

His walking speed also reduced from 1.5 to 1.1 m/s, which was considered to be an improvement as it implied a more controlled gait pattern.

Kinetic Data

The most striking changes in his GRF profiles, shown in Fig. 17.2, were that the vertical GRF during loading response changed from excessive (i.e. >200% BW) to a normal magnitude of 110% to 120% BW [j]. During the same phase of the gait cycle, his posterior GRF also changed from excessive (40% BW) to normal (20% BW) [h]. The abnormal peak in his anterior GRF [i], caused by spasticity in his gastrocnemii prematurely plantar flexing his ankles in midstance, was also successfully eliminated.

As with his walking speed, these changes in his GRF suggest that the package of interventions allowed him to walk with more control than previously. As the vertical CoM accelerations and decelerations were no longer so severe postsurgery, he walked with increased efficiency.

CASE STUDY TWO: SPINAL BIOMECHANICS CASE STUDY—SPINAL RESPONSES DURING WALKING AND LOW BACK PAIN*

Introduction

Walking is an important function for an independent and normal life. However, there are numerus conditions that affect normal walking and others where symptoms can be aggravated by walking. Low back pain (LBP), is a complex

*Konstantinos Kaliarntas

condition that usually involves biological, social and psychological factors (Dunn and Croft, 2004). About 85% of LBP cases are classified as nonspecific, because definitive radiographic diagnosis cannot be established (Dillingham, 1995), and up to 85% of all people will be affected by LBP at some point in their life (Dunn and Croft, 2004). In the past, LBP management practice included recommendations for bed rest and reduced activity. Current guidelines suggest that people who are affected by LBP should be encouraged to stay active and consider exercise as a management option (National Institute of Health & Care Excellence, 2016). Also, there is evidence suggesting that physical activity and exercise may reduce pain and improve physical function and quality of life (Geneen et al., 2017). (See Chapter 14 for more details on physical activity.) However, how much exercise or activity should a person with LBP safely undertake? Can physical activity potentially aggravate pain? What happens in the spine when we perform a very simple physical activity such as walking?

In this case study we will consider a different aspect of gait from the previous case study. In this case study we will look at the way the spine moves, especially how it changes length as we walk.

As Bruce stated in the previous case study, the average person takes up to 10,000 steps per day (McCormack et al., 2006) but this is highly dependent on their physical fitness, gender, age, occupation, comorbidities and multiple other factors. But if it is true, it means there are about 10,000 heel strikes performed every day, on average, and therefore 10,000 compressive loads applied to the spine. So, it is worth looking first at what happens during walking and then discuss the effects on the spine.

Analysing Walking

To analyse walking we usually break it down into gait cycles. A gait cycle usually starts with the heel contact of one foot (0%) and ends with another heel contact of the same (ipsilateral) foot (100%). In healthy people at 50% of the gait cycle, we have the heel contact of the opposite (contralateral) foot. During the gait cycle, we can observe two main periods (1) when the foot is on the floor (stance phase); and (2) when the leg is swinging forwards (swing phase). In healthy walking the stance phase accounts for about 60% and the swing phase for the remaining 40% of the gait cycle. The stance phase of the gait cycle is further subdivided into three subphases of equal duration: early, middle and late (Baker, 2013) (Fig. 17.3). Please note the differences in terminology with the previous case study. As is usual in life there are always different views and this includes gait analysis, so it is good to be aware of these differences in terminology. By definition, since the foot is coming into contact with the ground with some velocity,

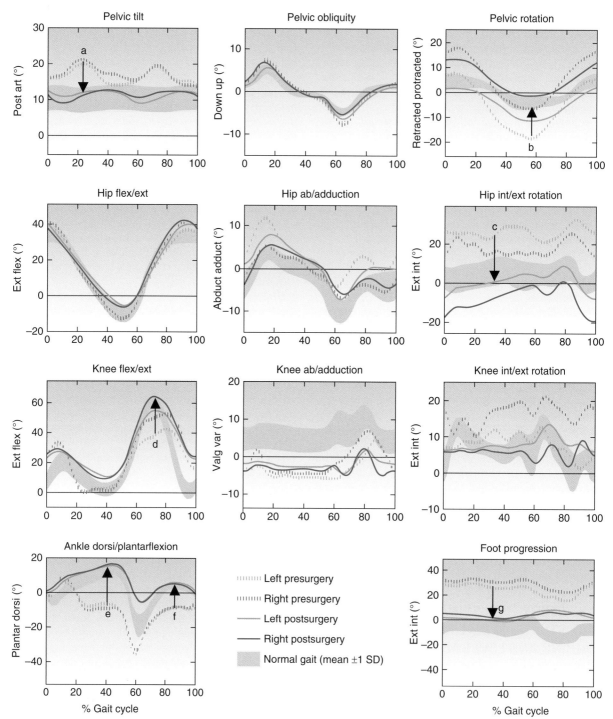

Fig. 17.1 Kinematic Gait Graphs Showing a Pre- and Postsurgery Comparison. Key kinematic improvements are indicated by the letters *a* to *g*.

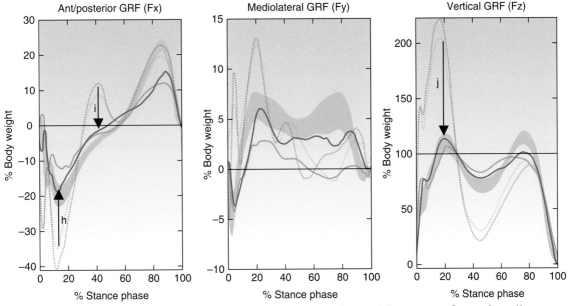

Fig. 17.2 Ground Reaction Force *(GRF)* Graphs Showing a Pre- and Postsurgery Comparison. Key kinematic improvements are indicated by letters *h* to *j*.

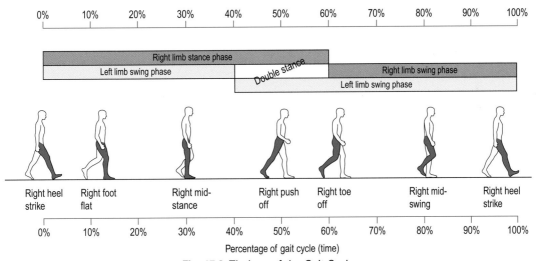

Fig. 17.3 Timings of the Gait Cycle.

there will be forces involved, and if you consider Newton's third law of motion (see Chapter 4) you will remember that for every action there is an opposite and equal reaction. These forces are called external forces and are the result of the body's interaction with the environment; as Bruce mentioned in case study 1, we call these forces the GRF, which are separated into anteroposterior, mediolateral and

vertical. In this case study we will focus on the vertical GRF, which has, by far, the highest magnitude. At a self-selected walking speed, the vertical GRF during early stance will exceed BW by 10% to 20% (Fig. 17.4).

At the start of early stance, initial contact (usually heel strike) occurs and we can observe a rapid increase of force, which usually exceeds BW. This force development typically

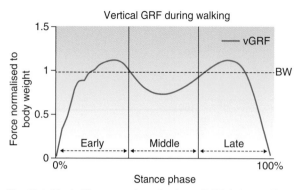

Fig. 17.4 *Vertical line,* ground reaction force *(GRF)* during walking. *Horizontal line,* body weight *(BW)*. vGRF, Vertical ground reaction force.

ACTIVITY BOX 17.1   Shock Absorption at Heel Strike

While you are walking at your usual walking speed, try striking the ground without allowing the hip to flex, the knee to flex or the ankle to plantarflex (i.e. keep the leg straight when it hits the ground). What did you feel? Do you think this could irritate a sore back or perhaps even lead to other injuries?

---

happens very fast and produces transient shocks and vibrations that propagate up the body. Shock and vibration resulting from heel impact during walking have an occurrence frequency between 1 and 2 Hz (i.e. one to two times per second) and may well aggravate LBP. At heel strike, the hip is in flexion, the knee is more or less fully extended and the foot is dorsiflexed, or in a neutral position. Just after ground contact the knee goes into flexion and the heel into plantarflexion. This is a very useful mechanism, which increases the time that the force acts (impulse–momentum relationship, see Chapter 4) and hence reduces the potentially harmful impact of GRFs. The steeper the force slope, the higher the rate of force development, and therefore the higher the impact of force in the body during early stance (Activity Box 17.1).

Case Study

In this case study, the participant was a 45-year-old man with chronic (>12 weeks) LBP. He was 1.82 m in height with a body mass of 77 kg.

The participant walked on a treadmill at a self-selected walking speed (0.86 m/s) for 30 minutes during two different conditions: (1) normal walking, and (2) supported walking (40% of his BW was lifted with an upper body harness).

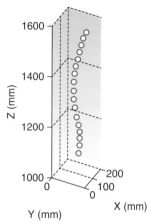

Fig. 17.5 Reflective markers placed on each spinous process (T1 to L5).

Seventeen retro-reflective markers were attached on each spinal process from thoracic 1st to lumbar 5th (Fig. 17.5).

A six-camera VICON motion capture system was used to capture 3D dynamic positional data (100 Hz) for 10-second intervals every 5 minutes. In this way it was possible to measure the length of the spine as he walked (Fig. 17.6). Using Fourier analysis, which is a mathematical technique to break up a signal into its frequency components (a bit like using a prism to break white light up into the different components, red, orange, yellow etc.), we are able to explore the frequency and power of the transient shocks caused by the heel strikes on the lumbar spine (Fig. 17.7). We also measured the pain levels of the patient by using visual analogue scales every 5 minutes during the 30 minutes of treadmill walking (see Fig. 17.8).

In Fig. 17.6 we can clearly see the lumbar length variation during walking and observe the characteristic peaks, which are the heel strikes during normal walking. The magnitude of this length variation is slightly smaller during supported walking and slightly out of phase with the heel strikes during normal walking. In this figure we can also see that there are approximately two heel strikes per second. Now, if we have a look at the power spectral density (PSD), which is the power of the signal at different frequencies (see Fig. 17.7), we can observe predominant peaks at 1 and 1.5 Hz (clearly associated with the heel strikes, particularly in normal walking), which are substantially attenuated (reduced) during supported walking. For this particular person, this reduction of lumbar spinal length variation and peak vibration activity is followed by a reduction in pain levels during the 40% BW supported walking condition (Fig. 17.8), whereas a similar reduction is not observed in the normal walking condition. Due to the complexity and the biopsychosocial

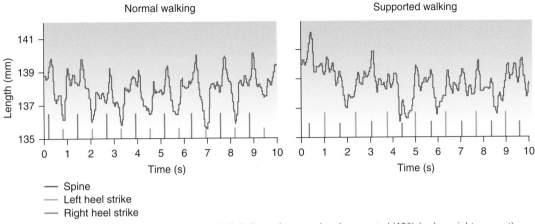

Fig. 17.6 Length of the lumbar spine (L1 to L5) during gait, normal and supported (40% body weight support).

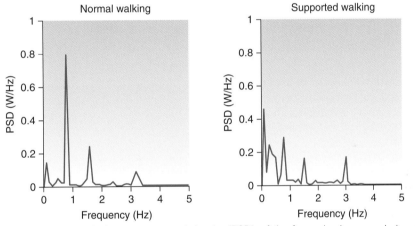

Fig. 17.7 Frequency analysis, power spectral density (PSD), of the force shock waves during gait.

nature of LBP in most patients, it is usually difficult to manage LBP by simply reducing the mechanical loading of the spine. However, by modifying movement patterns (e.g. a more cushioned heel strike) and controlling exercise parameters (i.e. intensity, duration), we can harness the beneficial effects of exercise while potentially reducing the negative experience of frequent pain aggravations from the GRF at heel strike.

What would you advise this gentleman to do in order to avoid pain aggravation if he wants to exercise by walking?

1. Wear shock absorbing shoes.
2. Control the duration of walking or exercise.
3. Control the intensity of physical activity or exercise.
4. All the above.

CASE STUDY THREE: USING AN ANKLE-FOOT ORTHOSIS TO CORRECT HEMIPLEGIC GAIT IN STROKE PATIENTS*

Introduction

In this final case study on gait we will consider the use of an orthosis to support walking in people with a hemiplegia (weakness down one side of the body) following a stroke. An orthosis is literally something that corrects or straightens (as in orthodontics, which aims to straighten the teeth). An

*Roy Bowers

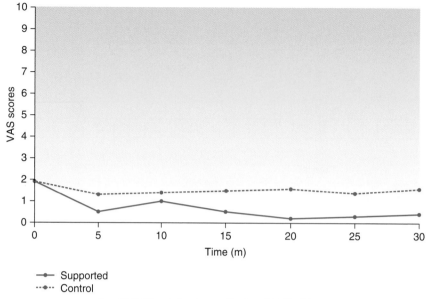

Fig. 17.8 Visual Analogue Scales *(VAS)* of Pain.

orthosis is an 'an externally applied device used to modify the structural and functional characteristics of the neuro-muscular and skeletal systems' (ISO, 1989a). These types of orthoses are typically designed and applied by trained orthotists (ISO, 1989a).

The ankle-foot orthosis (AFO) is an orthosis that covers the ankle joint and part (or all) of the foot. It can be made from different materials, but thermoplastic (polypropylene) is the most commonly used material (ISO, 1989b). Many mobility problems can be improved through the use of a suitable AFO, and you may have already come across one (see Fig. 17.9).

Background

Stroke has been defined by the World Health Organisation as 'a clinical syndrome (a collection of symptoms and signs) of focal (or global) disturbance of cerebral function, lasting more than 24 hours or leading to death, with no apparent cause other than that of vascular origin'. Strokes are caused by a disruption of the blood supply to part of the brain. This may result from either a blockage of a blood vessel (ischaemic stroke) or the rupture of a blood vessel (haemor-rhagic stroke). Most strokes are ischaemic in origin. Of those who survive a stroke, about 40% will remain dependent upon other people for their daily activities. The after-effects of a stroke often include speech deficits, depression, neu-ropsychological disorders, functional difficulties and, most commonly of all, mobility problems. It is the leading cause

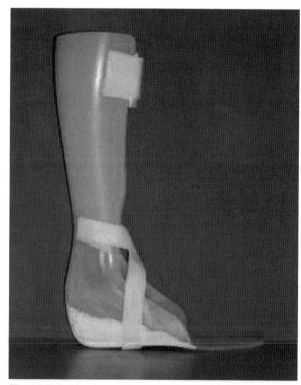

Fig. 17.9 Solid polypropylene ankle-foot orthosis, with wedge to accommodate an existing plantarflexion contracture.

of disability among adults in the developed world, and keeps rehabilitation services around the globe very busy. One of the often-stated priorities (patients and therapists) for rehabilitation is the recovery of independent walking.

Walking After Stroke

Gait following stroke has been characterised as slow and stiff, with poorly coordinated movements and a high energy demand. Step length and cadence are adversely affected (Lehmann et al 1987).

In addition to the foot dropping during the swing phase (due mainly to weakness in the ankle dorsiflexors, or over-activity in the plantarflexors), posing an obvious trip hazard, many stroke patients face substantial challenges during the stance phase of gait. In many cases the foot adopts an equino-varus posture (ankle is plantarflexed and inverted), which leads to initial contact being made with the outside of the forefoot. Knee hyperextension in mid to late stance is common, and tibial progression is impeded by the foot position. Hip extension is typically compromised or even absent.

Orthotic Intervention

Many AFOs can prevent the foot falling into plantarflexion during the swing phase (drop foot), thereby reducing the risk of tripping. In addition, if they are adequately stiff, some can prevent plantarflexion of the foot during the stance phase. Many prefabricated AFOs are insufficiently stiff to resist plantarflexion during the stance phase (caused by spasticity in the plantarflexor muscles), and therefore they fail to address the substantial stance phase gait problems faced by the patient. In these cases, custom made, solid AFOs are indicated.

Solid AFOs prevent all motion at the foot and ankle (see Fig. 17.9). They are indicated when there is high tone or spasticity in the plantarflexors, a gastrocnemius contracture, substantial mediolateral instability of the foot and/or a need for the AFO to influence the knee or hip (NHS Quality Improvement Scotland, 2009). The stiffness of a solid AFO is influenced by material choice and thickness, and the location of the trimlines (edges), which should be anterior to the midline of the malleoli. Reinforcements (e.g. carbon fibre inserts) can be incorporated at the ankle section of a solid AFO to further increase stiffness (see Chapter 5 to revise stiffness of materials).

Case Study

The following case study considers the case of a 69-year-old man who sustained a left side basal ganglia haemorrhage. Despite having been cared for in a specialist stroke unit for the 3 months since his stroke, he presented at a local orthotic clinic with a contracture (shortening) in his gastrocnemius

muscle. The maximum amount of dorsiflexion achievable, with his knee fully extended, was 5 degrees of plantarflexion. Tone in the lower limb was assessed as grade three on the Modified Ashworth Scale (this means there was a considerable increase in muscle tone and passive movement was difficult). He was only just able to transfer between chairs with assistance and was predicted by the staff in the stroke unit to become wheelchair dependent. He was referred to the orthotics clinic for assessment for an ankle-foot orthosis to make it easier for him to transfer to and from his wheelchair. His gait was analysed using the Codamotion 3D Motion Analysis System (Codamotion, Rothley, UK), with the PRO-VEC 5 Plus Video Vector System (MIE medical Research Ltd, Leeds, UK).

One useful stage of his gait cycle to look at is the middle of stance phase, the point at which the swinging foot is in line with the standing foot (see point three, Table 17.1). Fig. 17.10 shows this point in the gait cycle when this patient walks with shoes only. What do you think of the alignment of his:

1. Ankle?
2. Knee?
3. Hip?

You can see that his ankle is more plantarflexed than it should be, and is actually considerably more plantarflexed than the 5 degrees we might have expected based on the physical examination. This is due to the increase in tone in the calf muscles, which forces the foot into further equinus when walking, and holds the tibia in a reclined orientation (leaning back). This plantarflexed position of the foot means that the GRF, indicated by the black arrow, is too far forward at the metatarsal heads rather than at the midfoot. The knee

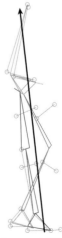

Fig. 17.10 Midstance Alignment With Shoes Only. The figure shows a reconstruction from the motion capture data with the stance side in orange and the swing side in grey.

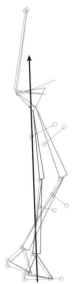

Fig. 17.11 Midstance Alignment With Solid Ankle-Foot Orthosis.

function of an AFO, and may even be a necessary prerequisite to successful AFO fitting.

CASE STUDY FOUR: THE SIT-TO-STAND MOVEMENT*

Background

The sit-to-stand (StS) movement is clearly important for everyday life. Think about the number of times you carry out this movement at home, work or school. Or what about watching a football game or attending a religious ceremony? In fact, healthy people, on average, perform the movement 60 times a day (Dall and Kerr, 2010). Although routine, it is nevertheless one of the hardest movements to perform. You need enough power in your lower limb extensor muscles (mainly gluteus maximus, hamstrings and quadriceps) to quickly lift all that body mass around 0.5 m, and, at the same time, move it forward around 0.4 m. Once you have left the stable environment of the chair there is the additional challenge of keeping yourself balanced, which means controlling the upward and forward thrust. For these reasons, many people struggle to perform the movement independently and safely, and may fail or fall during the attempt. The well-described effects of ageing on muscle strength, joint flexibility and balance can impair an individual's ability to perform this movement (Bohannon, 2012) as does any condition that affects lower limb muscle strength, movement control and balance, for example, hemiplegia following a stroke (Pollock et al., 2014) and Parkinson's disease (Inkster and Eng, 2004). Try Activity Box 17.2 to consider the wider implications of not being able to stand up from sitting on your own.

The Movement

Let's have a more detailed look at the StS movement. Like gait, we can break it down into distinct phases. There have been many different proposals for doing this but perhaps the most logical and easiest thing to do is

is hyperextended. This is caused by the anterior placement of the GRF relative to the knee joint centre. The hip is in flexion with some anterior leaning of the trunk. The presence of an external hip flexion moment makes it difficult for the patient to achieve hip extension and causes the hip to remain in flexion.

Now look at the same stage of the gait cycle (Fig. 17.11) when the patient wears a solid ankle-foot orthosis (like the one in Fig. 17.9). The gait data were collected on the same day (in case you were wondering). We can see that the ankle alignment is now controlled by the AFO, and the tibia is held in slight forward inclination as would be the case at this stage in normal gait. Notice how the GRF has been relocated to the midfoot, rather than being at the forefoot when walking in shoes only, Fig. 17.10. The GRF is now slightly posterior to the knee joint, rather than excessively anterior, and knee hyperextension has been eliminated. At the hip, the GRF now passes posterior to the joint, rather than being anterior as previously noted when walking without the AFO. This GRF alignment facilitates extension of the hip and a more normal alignment of the pelvis and trunk.

It is important to remember that the use of an AFO should be seen as part of an integrated package of care. For example, an appropriate AFO may be beneficial during physiotherapy sessions by reducing the biomechanical challenge facing the patient during gait reeducation and providing the brain with 'normal' sensations (i.e. joint position) when walking. In the same way, the use of pharmacological interventions to moderate the effects of increased tone can enhance the

*Andy Kerr

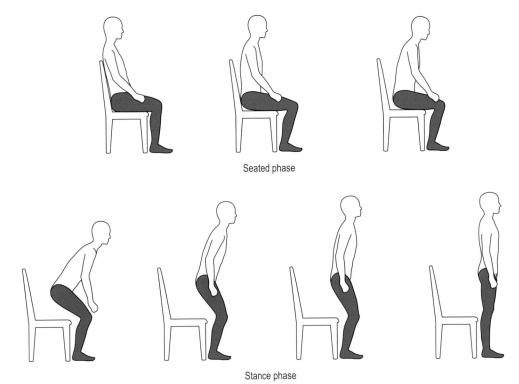

Seated phase

Stance phase

Fig. 17.12 The Pattern of Movement When Rising From a Chair.

ACTIVITY BOX 17.3 **Bending Forward in the Sit-to-Stand Movement**

While you are sitting there reading this, why don't you try standing up without bending forward first and then try bending forward very slowly.

Hopefully this should confirm the importance of this phase to you.

to divide it into two phases with distinct challenges, see Fig. 17.12.

Phase 1: The seated phase (sometimes called pre seat-off) is all about bringing the body forward, mainly through hip and trunk flexion, but can also include the arms. Typically, this is done pretty quickly (~0.2 m/s) to generate enough forward momentum for the body to travel forward to its new position (Activity Box 17.3).

Phase 2: The rising phase is all about lifting all that mass vertically. This is achieved through hip and knee extension, and the forces involved are considerable. If we briefly revisit Newton's first law of motion, *a body will remain at rest unless acted on by an unbalanced force*, then we know that

to move upwards we have to produce a force that exceeds the downward force of gravity acting on our mass. In fact, most studies record forces between 1.1 and 1.2 × BW. This force is produced by the combined actions of the knee and hip extensors with some assistance from the arms, either by swinging them upwards or pressing down on the armrests. For most people producing this magnitude of force is not a problem, but for the elderly this may be equivalent to their maximum power capacity. For this reason a StS movement has been likened to a maximal vertical jump for older adults. Now perhaps you can understand why older people sometimes struggle a bit to get off the sofa (Table 17.3).

Case Study

The following graphs were produced by a 68-year-old woman weighing 72 kg, who was 1.7 m in height and had a stroke 8 days previously, which resulted in a hemiplegia on her left side.

She was asked to stand up from a plinth that was adjusted to the height of her knee. Retro-reflective markers were placed on various anatomical landmarks in accordance with the standard model of gait; these markers were tracked by a 12-camera motion capture system (sampling rate was

TABLE 17.3 Reference Data of Unimpaired Subjects Performing the Sit-to-Stand Movement From a Starting Position of Hips and Knees at 90 Degrees.

	Joint Movement	Duration	Forward Velocity	Vertical Velocity	Vertical Force
Phase one	Trunk flexes forward 20–30 degrees (pelvis, spine and hips). Knees may move a little in preparation.	0.75 s	Increases to around 0.2 m/s	Slight downward velocity. Around 0.06 m/s	May slightly decrease if the feet are lifted up. This is speed dependent.
Phase two	Trunk returns to neutral (0 degrees). Knees extend from around 90 degrees to almost straight.	0.75 s	Decreases to zero	Rapid increase up to 0.5 m/s	Peaks shortly after seat-off and increases to > BW 1.2

100 Hz). This allowed us to calculate the 3D movement of multiple joints during the movement, as well as calculate the instantaneous position of the CoM. (See Chapter 3 for a reminder of what the CoM is.)

Let's have a look at the overall performance by plotting the forward and vertical CoM velocity. (We can ignore side-to-side velocity at the moment, although this may be important for some individuals.)

During phase 1 (before seat-off) there are three clear 'bounces' in the velocity (Fig. 17.13A) and force signals (see Fig. 17.13B). This is not an uncommon observation among people with balance problems; it's actually a smart move if you are worried about controlling your balance once you are standing. If you generate too much forward velocity while seated, you will have to control all that momentum (mass and velocity) while perched on a relatively small base of support in standing. Therefore, a bit of trial and error until you get the minimal momentum required to stand up is probably a sensible approach to reducing the risk of a fall. The final, successful, attempt is different in two ways: first, there is a larger initial backwards movement (−ve velocity) with a much sharper increase in velocity (or acceleration, remember change in velocity is acceleration). Secondly, and perhaps the most important characteristic of this successful attempt, is the continued upward velocity, which peaks well after the horizontal peaks (compared to previous attempts). This has been described as the momentum transfer phase, with the forward velocity reducing while the vertical velocity continues to increase.

If we look at the vertical force (B) we can see that the combined force (left and right) does not exceed BW (9.81 × body mass, marked with a horizontal line in the figure) until the final attempt, and then it only just makes it (~1.1 × BW). The unaffected side is mainly responsible for the magnitude

ACTIVITY BOX 17.4 Treatment strategy

What would you work on to improve this gentleman's sit-to-stand performance?
1. Extensor strength and power on the affected side
2. Faster forward movement while seated
3. Perhaps you would simply practice the whole movement.
4. All the above

of this force with the hemiplegic side only contributing around 40% of the push. Now try Activity Box 17.4.

CASE STUDY FIVE: UPPER LIMB IMPAIRMENT AFTER STROKE*

Introduction

As has already been said in Case Study Three, stroke is the leading cause of adult disability in the developed world. Approximately 86% of stroke survivors have persistent deficits in their arm and hand many months and years after their stroke. Therapeutic efforts to address poststroke hemiparesis in the upper limb requires a thorough understanding of the type of impairment involved, and the ensuing functional limitation. In this case study, we aim to show that motion analysis can aid in understanding which upper limb movements are impaired, how they contribute to the functional

*Seda Bilaloglu, Jennifer Stone, Alvin Tang, Megan Caughey, and Preeti Raghavan

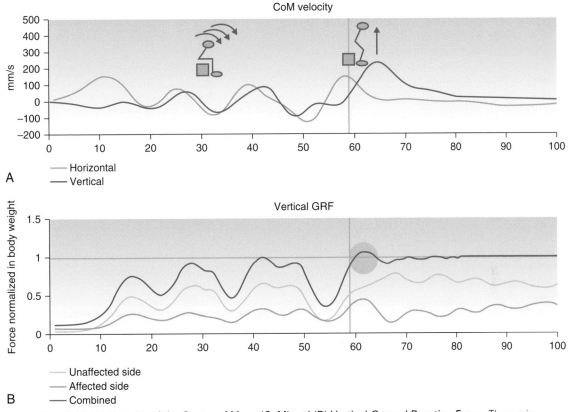

Fig. 17.13 (A) Velocity of the Centre of Mass *(CoM)* and (B) Vertical Ground Reaction Force. The x-axis has been normalised to 100% of the whole cycle (i.e. movement initiation until standing achieved). *Vertical line* = time of seat-off. The y-axis units are mm/s (A) and N/Kg (B). *GRF* is the Ground reaction force.

deficit in an individual and what things might be useful to focus on during therapy.

Medical History and Evaluation of Motor Impairment and Functional Limitation

The patient we describe here is a 57-year-old right-hand-dominant male who presented with left-sided hemiparesis resulting from a right middle cerebral artery stroke. At the time of evaluation, he was 17 months poststroke. Following his stroke, he had received both physical therapy and occupational therapy for 1.5 hours a day, 5 days a week for a period of 4 weeks.

His upper extremity motor impairment was assessed using the upper extremity component of the Fugl-Meyer Scale (FMS; Fugl-Meyer et al., 1975). He scored a total of 14/66 on the FMS, which was further broken down into the upper extremity component, and the wrist and hand component (Table 17.4). Note that the patient scored poorly on both components, which suggests that he had a severe

deficit in the entire upper limb. However, the scores don't provide information on exactly what movements to target to reduce impairment. The patient's functional ability was assessed using the Wolf Motor Function Test (WMFT; Wolf et al., 2001). Table 17.5 shows the time taken to perform selected tasks in the WMFT battery. The time limit was 120 s, and a score of 120, for example for elbow extension, suggests that the patient was unable to complete the task in the given time frame. However, the patient was able to reach and retrieve quite easily. The time on the WMFT provides an indication of what the patient has difficulty accomplishing but does not indicate exactly how to improve the functional deficit. Motion analysis is therefore indicated to fill the gap in understanding what movements are impaired and how to target the treatment to reduce the functional deficit.

Motion Analysis

Active range of motion at the shoulder, elbow, forearm and wrist joints (Norkin et al., 1995) were measured using the Motion Monitor 3D electromagnetic motion sensor system (The Motion Monitor, Innsport, Chicago, IL). The system utilises the Ascension 800 sensors (Ascension Technology Corp., Shelburne, VT), sampled at 120 Hz with a static resolution of 0.5 mm for position and 0.1 degree for angular orientation, and an accuracy of 1.4 mm root mean square (RMS) for position and 0.5 degrees RMS for angular orientation.

The patient was instructed to perform the following movements actively: shoulder abduction, shoulder flexion and extension, elbow flexion and extension, forearm pronation and supination and wrist flexion and extension. The start position for each movement was fixed as follows: the shoulder and elbow movements shared the same start position with the subject sitting with their torso straight and arms down by their sides and elbows extended; for the forearm and wrist movements, the participants started with the elbows flexed to 90 degrees and the forearm in neutral (i.e. thumb facing the ceiling). The patient was instructed to move actively to the maximum possible range (peak) and return to the start position. The onset and offset of the movements were defined as the amplitude of the movement at 5% of peak angular velocity. Active range of motion was also assessed in a 41-year-old male, with no contributory past medical history, as a reference (healthy control).

Fig. 17.14 shows a still image and the skeletal model of the patient performing shoulder abduction. Note the degree of

TABLE 17.4 Upper Extremity Motor Impairment.

	FUGL-MEYER (FMA) SCORE	
	Patient Score	Maximum Score
Upper Extremity		
1. Reflexes	4	4
2. Flexor synergy	1	12
3. Extensor synergy	4	6
4. Movement combining synergistics	1	6
5. Movement out of synergy	0	6
6. Normal reflex activity	0	2
Total Upper Extremity Score	10	36
Wrist and Hand		
7. Wrist	2	10
8. Hand	2	14
9. Coordination/speed	0	6
Total Wrist and Hand Score	4	30
Total FMA Upper Extremity Score	14	66

TABLE 17.5 Upper Limb Functional Ability.

WOLF MOTOR FUNCTION TEST	
Task	**Time (s)**
Forearm to table	2
Forearm to box	3
Elbow extension	120
Elbow extension w. weight	120
Hand on table	3
Hand on box	2
Hand on box w. weight	4
Reach and retrieve	3
Fold towel	19
Lift basket	5

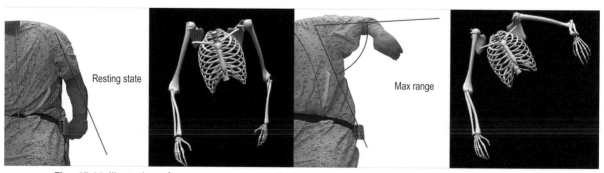

Resting state   Max range

Fig. 17.14 Illustration of compensatory trunk flexion when the patient attempts to perform shoulder abduction.

TABLE 17.6   Upper Limb Active Joint Range of Motion on Motion Analysis.

Joint Movement	Patient ROM (degrees) Values (Onset to Peak)	Control ROM (degrees) (Onset to Peak)	Normal ROM (degrees) (Onset to Peak)
Shoulder flexion	12.63	168.3	0–180
Shoulder extension	9.91	12.35	0–60
Shoulder abduction	34.48	146.2	0–180
Elbow extension	94.21	125.1	0–180
Elbow flexion	88.97	83.31	0–150
Pronation	46.39	58.25	0–80
Supination	14.92	12.77	0–80
Wrist extension	14.33	58.15	0–70
Wrist flexion	11.46	82.71	0–80

ROM, Range of motion.

lateral trunk flexion to the opposite side to facilitate shoulder abduction. The trunk flexion is a compensatory movement that also needs to be quantified to monitor progress in range of motion with treatment. It is shown here as a reminder that compensatory movements must be checked when interpreting range of motion data (Table 17.6).

Shoulder Flexion/Extension/Abduction

The patient showed markedly decreased shoulder flexion and abduction and velocity (Fig. 17.15). Shoulder extension was noticeably less affected.

Elbow Flexion/Extension

The patient also showed decreased range of motion at the elbow joint during extension, but not flexion compared to the control. However, note that the elbow extension, while limited, was not severe (Fig. 17.16).

Forearm Supination/Pronation

The patient showed a fairly intact range of motion during pronation and supination compared to the control (Fig. 17.17).

Wrist Flexion/Extension

The patient showed a decreased range of motion and velocity at the wrist joint during both flexion and extension (Fig. 17.18).

Summary

Motion analysis data on this patient revealed that the key movements impaired were shoulder abduction (performed using compensatory trunk flexion), shoulder flexion, elbow extension, and wrist flexion and extension. Movements that were relatively preserved were shoulder extension, elbow flexion, and pronation and supination. This information can aid in the formulation of therapeutic strategies to both reduce impairment and enable function.

To reduce motor impairment, one may need to ask what is contributing to the lack of range of motion. Weakness or paresis, sensory loss, spasticity and abnormal motor synergy may all contribute to the abnormal movement patterns (Raghavan et al., 2015). Medications and targeted therapeutic exercises can then be used to reduce spasticity and to increase strength in the muscles to restore range of motion, which should secondarily lead to a reduction in motor impairment.

Immediate improvement in function may be enabled by focusing on joints that have preserved range of motion. Tasks can be organised or modified to use these preserved joints. For example, the patient is likely to be unable to perform the elbow extension task on the WMFT because it also required shoulder flexion in which he was severely impaired. However, once shoulder flexion was taken out of the equation (e.g. in the reach and retrieve task) he had little difficulty.

Thus, motion analysis is useful to help understand why a patient's movements are impaired and what can be done to restore movement and function. Besides joint range of motion, the velocity, acceleration (to measure smoothness) and muscle activity can contribute to further understanding the deficits and selecting the appropriate therapeutic strategies for rehabilitation.

Based on this information do you think motion analysis will become commonplace in the rehabilitation gyms of the future?

The optical tracking systems included in many of these case studies are expensive. Do you know of any lower cost solutions? (Have a look again at Chapter 12.)

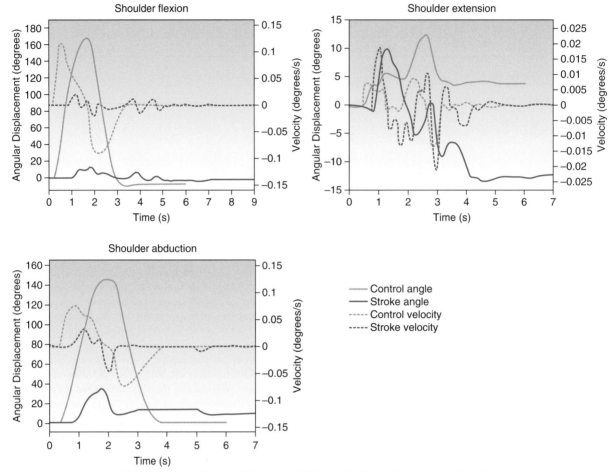

Fig. 17.15 Shoulder Range of Motion and Velocity in the Patient and Healthy Control.

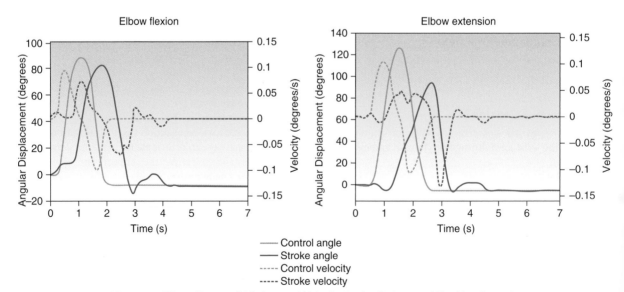

Fig. 17.16 Elbow Range of Motion and Velocity in the Patient and Healthy Control.

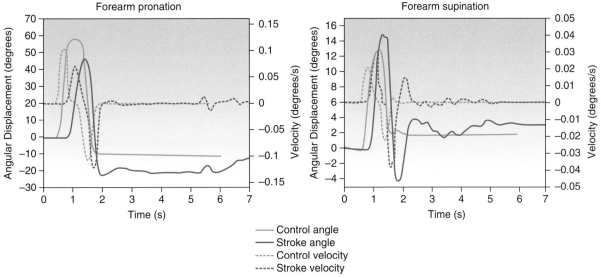

Fig. 17.17 Forearm Range of Motion and Velocity in the Patient and Healthy Control.

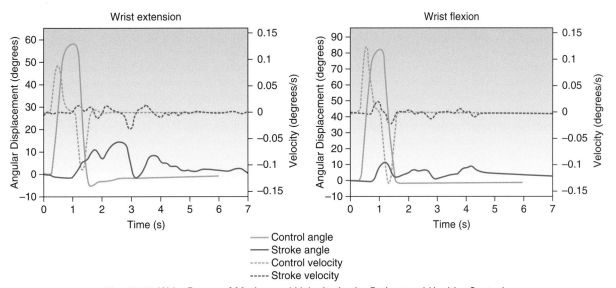

Fig. 17.18 Wrist Range of Motion and Velocity in the Patient and Healthy Control.

CASE STUDY SIX: THE ROWING STROKE*

Background

To achieve success at the highest level of sport would be considered by many to be one of the most challenging goals that a person can set themselves. At the elite level, the

demands and pressures on athletes are many and varied; however, their personal objectives and final aim will almost always be conversely singular: to win. In the United Kingdom elite rowers are supported by multi- and interdisciplinary teams of specialists, including sports psychologists, nutritionists, physiologists, biomechanists, various coaching experts, as well as sports therapists, physiotherapists, medical professionals and more. Each of these disciplines have a role to play in supporting the athletes they work with, and must

*Andrew Murphy

attempt to work together to affect the performance gains which are the difference between success and failure at the pinnacle of sporting competition.

Put very simply, the goal of competitive rowing is to travel a set distance as quickly as possible. This may be generalised in mechanical terms as a need to maximise the average forward velocity of the boat over the total race distance, and this is achieved by the rower using their muscles to generate force and power and controlling their movement patterns in order to efficiently transfer this output to the boat via the oars. Nolte (2011) offered that there are two main mechanisms by which one may improve their rowing performance: (1) rowers can produce more energy, and (2) rowers can use their energy more efficiently: it is probably fair to say that the roles of the sports biomechanist would fall into the second of these categories. There is a huge amount of past and current research that demonstrates the necessity of optimising biomechanics-related performance variables, such as peak power output and stroke length. There is also a growing body of literature that attempts to consider the movement strategies that rowers use in order to achieve these major determinants of rowing performance (Baudouin and Hawkins, 2004; Bourdin et al., 2017; Buckeridge et al., 2015a, 2016; Cerne et al., 2013; Hofmijster et al., 2008; Soper and Hume, 2004).

Inextricably linked with performance in sport is injury and injury risk; if one is unable to compete or train due to injury then it naturally follows that performance will suffer. Several authors have reported on the relatively high incidence of injury in elite international rowers; all agree that some of the most common sites for chronic and acute injuries are the lumber spine, chest and ribs, forearm and wrist, and the knee; and some have attempted to identify movement behaviour that may be related to injury risk, for example increasing levels of flexion and twisting through the lumbopelvic region (Hickey et al., 1997; Rumball et al., 2005; Smoljanovic et al., 2015; Wilson et al., 2010).

With all of this in mind (and much more that is beyond the scope of these few pages) it is hopefully clear that gaining an understanding of exactly how rowers move is an important goal.

The Movement

Precise aspects of rowing technique can vary considerably between individual athletes, and indeed it should be recognised that if one considers parameters such as size, strength and ability, this variation is expected and thus individual athletes will achieve maximum efficiency in slightly different ways. That being said, the fundamental movement (the rowing 'stroke') can be well defined as consisting of two major phases: the 'drive', and the 'recovery' (Fig. 17.19). The drive is the work phase, and it is during this period that the rower must generate force and power in order to ultimately propel the boat through the water; the drive begins with the rower in a position known as the 'catch', and ends with them reaching the 'finish'. The recovery phase is the return of the rower from the finish position to the instant before the catch of the subsequent stroke. At all times the rower should attempt to keep their back long and straight, maintain relaxed shoulders as far as possible and consider the major pivot point of the torso rocking movement to be the hips, not within the spine.

At the catch, the athlete's lower limbs are in full flexion with shins vertical, combined with full extension of the upper limbs. The majority of force and power generated during the rowing stroke should come from the legs, and peak propulsive forces should be generated within the first half of the drive phase. The rowing stroke requires a significant whole-body effort and many muscles are involved; some of the major muscles that should be working at the catch and/or throughout (or at specific points) during the drive phase include (but are not limited to) quadriceps, gastrocnemius, soleus, hamstrings, gluteal, erector spinae, rectus abdominus, rhomboids, deltoids, trapezius, pectoralis major, biceps brachii, triceps brachii and wrist extensors and flexors (marked in dark and light orange in Fig 17.19). Only a small proportion of the power needed to row effectively will be generated by the upper body. To avoid expending energy unnecessarily, athletes should consider trying to keep their arms, hands and upper body as relaxed as possible; they should also avoid gripping too hard or pulling with the arms too early in the stroke. This can be a difficult concept to grasp, and significant training is needed to master the skill.

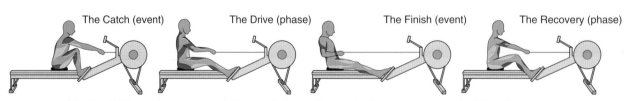

The Catch (event)   The Drive (phase)   The Finish (event)   The Recovery (phase)

Fig. 17.19 The major events and phases of the rowing stroke illustrated using a land-based ergometer set-up.

Once the athlete has reached the finish position, the recovery phase begins. The hands should lead the recovery by moving down and away from the torso; this is followed by a smooth 'rockover' of the upper body by rotating about the hips while keeping the legs and back straight (switching on the glutes helps with this). As the hands progress further sternwards the knees are allowed to 'break', bringing the lower limbs gradually back into a flexed pose in preparation for the next stroke try Activity Box 17.5.

It is worth noting that various rowing associations have produced general guidance and recommendations to assist athletes and coaches with a better understanding what the 'perfect' stroke looks like (British Rowing, 2018).

Case Study

The following is based on data collected from an elite British rower. In order to maintain anonymity and to protect confidential data, there are some limits to the information and interpretation provided. The athlete is male and was in preparation for an Olympic competition at the time of his assessment. Testing was carried out in a laboratory setting using a bespoke instrumented ergometer, an electromagnetic-based motion capture system, and according to an incremental Step test—one where exercise intensity is systematically increased over the duration of the protocol. Full details of the methods have been previously published elsewhere (McGregor et al., 2005, 2007, 2016; Murphy, 2009; Murphy et al., 2010, 2011a, 2011b).

Fig. 17.20 provides selected kinematic data of the athlete's performance at Step 3 and Step 6 of the incremental protocol. Step 3 would be considered low-intensity exercise for this elite individual: below the onset of blood lactate accumulation, heart rate 65% to 75% of maximum, rating of perceived exertion = 2 to 4. Step 6 would be considered high-intensity exercise: above the onset of blood lactate accumulation and metabolic acidosis, heart rate 87% to 95% of maximum, rating of perceived exertion = 9.

All vertical axes units are degrees of rotation. The dark orange lines show Step 6 (high-intensity exercise) and orange lines show Step 3 (low-intensity exercise) for a complete representative stroke (0% to 100% on the horizontal axes). The timings for peak handle force production (15% and 19%) and the finish (35% and 43%) are indicated by the oversized tick marks.

During Step 3 and Step 6, the athlete rowed at 21 and 32 strokes per minute respectively, utilised a drive/recovery duration ratio of 1.0:1.8 and 1.0:1.3, produced peak tensile forces on the ergometer handle of 12.1 N/kg and 12.5 N/kg, achieved a stroke length of 1.60 m and 1.56 m, completed 792 J and 805 J of work, and generated 3.9 W/kg and 5.9 W/kg of power.

Fig. 17.20 shows that at both low and high exercise intensities the athlete raised his heel away from the foot stretcher creating an angle between fore- and hindfoot at the catch of the stroke. This pose was accompanied by an approximately neutral ankle position, deep knee and hip flexion, 15 to 20 degrees of anterior pelvic tilt and 4 to 7 degrees of flexion at the lumbopelvic junction. This body position will have allowed the athlete to achieve good stroke length 'at the front' of the stroke without the need for significant thoracic flexion or shoulder protraction (Activity Box 17.6).

After the catch, the rower in this case manages to limit active intersegmental lumbopelvic rotation to within ±2 degrees change during rapid force generation, and regardless of exercise intensity. First, this control provides some protection against acute injury to the lower back, and it could be argued also against potential long-term overuse injury; and second, this pattern of movement assists in efficiently transferring the forces and power being generated by the legs through the kinetic chain to the arms, and ultimately

---

ACTIVITY BOX 17.5 Activating Abdominal Muscles

While you are sitting reading this: sit up straight in your chair, relax your shoulders, extend your knees a little (you can move your feet forward), try to keep your feet flat on the floor and your back in contact with the backrest. Now lean forward. Did you bend forwards through your trunk, flexing your spine? If yes, get back in your starting position, now squeeze your glutes and lean forward. When you squeezed your glutes some of your abdominal muscles probably switched on too, so when you leaned forward you rotated about the hips this time. Play around with any variations that you can think of and try to be aware of what is going on in your glutes, abdominals and hip extensors.

ACTIVITY BOX 17.6 Anterior Pelvic Tilt

Consider for a moment the flexibility and control needed in order to achieve anterior pelvic tilt while in a seated posture, with your feet only a few centimetres below the buttocks, and in combination with deep hip and knee flexion. Do you think that you could do this? Do you think that you could do it approximately 200 times during a 6- to 8-min race, or 4000 times every day during training as elite rowers do? Easy eh?!

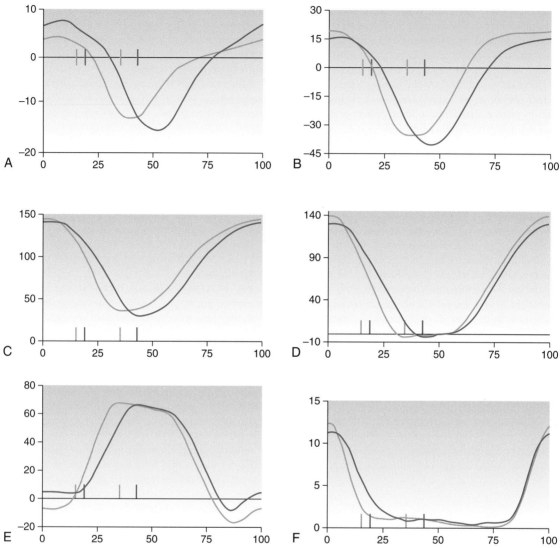

Fig. 17.20 Selected Kinematic Data Illustrating the Performance of an Elite Male Rower. (A) Intersegmental lumbopelvic flexion (+ve) extension (–ve), (B) anterior (+ve) posterior (–ve) pelvic tilt, (C) hip flexion, (D) knee flexion (+ve), (E) ankle dorsi (–ve) plantar (+ve) flexion and (F) interfore/hindfoot sagittal plane angle.

out into the ergometer handle or oars, which will be beneficial to ergometer performance and boat speed. Much (though probably not all) coaching philosophy and research would argue that it is important to minimise lumbopelvic flexion at the catch (Buckeridge et al., 2015b; Wilson et al., 2013). Possibly even more important, though, for both efficient transmission of power as well as reducing injury risk, is the concept of 'holding what you have'. The idea that whatever posture an athlete can or does achieve through the lower

back at the catch, they must hold it during the first half of the drive phase. It would be hard to argue that by any measure Sir Steve Redgrave is one of the most successful Olympians of all time, yet he did not have a bolt upright flat back while in the drive phase. However, he was strong and skilled enough to be able to ensure that the joints in his back did not move after he had 'collected the boat' at the catch.

Fig. 17.20 is an illustration, and real-world example, of the rowing stroke described in the previous section. As expected during the drive phase of both low- and high-intensity exercise, the athlete exhibits rapid extension of the lower limbs through a wide range of motion at the hips and knees, combined with plantarflexion of the ankles, and effort to 'get the heels down' quickly. There is a clear rocking motion of the pelvis about the hips (compare the gradient of the lines for pelvic tilt and hip and knee flexion early in the recovery phase). There are also some differences between the graph traces for each exercise intensity—in joint ranges of motion, absolute angles, and the timing of rotations between low and high intensity efforts. For example, total range of motion of intersegmental rotation at the lumbopelvic junction increases from 17 degrees to 23 degrees (an increase of 35%). Such changes in kinematics are not uncommon, even at the elite level, and are not particularly surprising when one considers the substantial effects that factors such as fatigue can render. However, it should be an aim of any sports biomechanist to develop the means by which the athletes' movement patterns may be measured and monitored carefully so that they will be better armed to work with their colleagues and athletes in the pursuit of performance gains, injury prevention and optimisation of rehabilitation strategies (Activity Box 17.7).

Hopefully this short introduction to the rowing stroke will have been found to be interesting. It is far from a complete guide to rowing well, safely or efficiently, but if it has highlighted the importance of monitoring athletes' movement behaviour then it has served its purpose. The hard work and dedication of staff and students at the Imperial College London, as well as staff and athletes within British Rowing, contributed to this case study and are gladly acknowledged.

ACTIVITY BOX 17.7 Speed and Complexity

In this case study, the rower was working at 21 (Step 3) and 32 (Step 6) strokes per minute; that equates to an average of 2.9 and 1.9 seconds per stroke—a decrease of 34% in real time. Take a moment to think about virtually any complex movement (getting out of a bathtub, reaching for a jar at the back of a high cupboard, rising to stand after sitting on the floor). Do you think that generally speaking it would be easier or harder to perform such a complex movement involving the coordination of every body part if you had one-third less time to do it? What about if you were extremely fatigued too? What if you had to do it 200 times in a row without stopping?

SELF-ASSESSMENT QUESTIONS

1. What is the magnitude of a normal vertical GRF during the loading response phase?
2. What scoring tool could you use to measure a patient's gait pattern if you only had digital video footage of them walking?
3. When should you refer a patient for clinical gait analysis?
4. What vibration frequencies are associated with walking?
5. What do you think the effect of increasing walking speed would be on
   a. The force magnitude during the early stance phase?
   b. The duration of the whole stance phase?
   c. The peak vibration activity in the lumbar spine?
6. Is knee hyperextension inevitable after a stroke, or might early use of an AFO prevent this?
7. Do you think a prefabricated (off the shelf) AFO could achieve the kind of stance phase control seen above?
8. Is there a role for AFOs during the early rehabilitation of stroke?
9. What magnitude of force does the body need to exceed in order to stand up from sitting?
10. Which joints perform the most movement during phase 1 of the sit-to-stand movement?
11. What do you think the effect of raising the chair height might have on
    a. The force required to stand up?
    b. The knee movement?
12. What do you think might be the effect of increasing the speed of the sit-to-stand movement on
    a. Joint angle range?
    b. The forces applied to the ground?
13. Why do you think some older people use arm rests when standing up? What impairment might this strategy address?
14. How might an individual with hemiplegia compensate for a loss of shoulder range of motion post stroke?
15. Which upper limb movements appeared to be more affected in the upper limb hemiplegia case study?

16. In the upper limb hemiplegia case study why do you think pronation and supination were less severely affected than other movements?

17. Can you name five muscles or groups of muscles that are important to the rowing stroke?

18. Can you suggest any specific acute or chronic injuries that a rower might experience if they do not utilise safe movements of the lumbopelvic region of their back?

19. Do you think that the risk of lumbar injury has been more closely linked with rowing on ergometers, or on the water? Why?

REFERENCES

Baker, R., 2013. Measuring Walking: A Handbook of Clinical Gait Analysis. Mac Keith Press, London.

Baker, R., McGinley, J.L., Schwartz, M.H., Beynon, S., Rozumalski, A., Graham, H.K., et al., 2009. The gait profile score and movement analysis profile. Gait Posture 30, 265–269.

Baudouin, A., Hawkins, D., 2004. Investigation of biomechanical factors affecting rowing performance. J. Biomech. 37 (7), 969–976.

NHS Quality Improvement Scotland (Funder), 2009. Best Practice Statement: Use of Ankle–Foot Orthoses Following Stroke. Edinburgh.

Bohannon, R.W., 2012. Measurement of sit-to-stand among older adults. Topics Geriat. Rehabil 28 (1), 11–16.

Bourdin, M., Lacour, J.R., Imbert, C., Messonnier, L.A., 2017. Factors of rowing ergometer performance in high-level female rowers. Int. J. Sports Med. 38 (13), 1023–1028.

British, Rowing., 2018. British rowing—the perfect stroke. Available at https://www.britishrowing.org/upload/files/CoachingTraining/PerfectStrokePoster.pdf. (Accessed 31.January.2018.)

Buckeridge, E.M., Bull, A.M.J., McGregor, A.H., 2015a. Biomechanical determinants of elite rowing technique and performance. Scand. J. Med. Sci. Sports 25 (2), e176–e183.

Buckeridge, E.M., Bull, A.M.J., McGregor, A.H., 2015b. Incremental training intensities increases loads on the lower back of elite female rowers. J. Sports Sci. 34 (16), 369–378.

Buckeridge, E.M., Weinert-Aplin, R.A., Bull, A.M.J., McGregor, A.H., 2016. Influence of foot-stretcher height on rowing technique and performance. Sports Biomech. 15 (4), 513–526.

Cerne, T., Kamnik, R., Vesnicer, B., Zganec-Gros, J., Munih, M., 2013. Differences between elite, junior and non-rowers in kinematic and kinetic parameters during ergometer rowing. Human Mov. Sci. 32 (4), 691–707.

Dall, P.M., Kerr, A., 2010. Frequency of the sit to stand task: an observational study of free-living adults. Appl. Ergon. 41 (1), 58–61.

Davis, R.B., Õunpuu, S., Tyburski, D., Gage, J.R., 1991. A gait analysis data collection and reduction technique. Hum. Mov. Sci. 10 (5), 575–587.

Dillingham, T., 1995. Evaluation and management of low backpain: an overview. State Art. Rev. 9 (3), 559–574.

Dunn, K.M., Croft, P.R., 2004. Epidemiology and natural history of LBP. Eura Medicophys. 40 (1), 9–13.

Fugl-Meyer, A.R., Jääskö Leyman, L., Olsson, S., Steglind, S., 1975. The post-stroke hemiplegic patient. 1. A method for evaluation of physical performance. Scand. J. Rehabil. Med. 7, 13–31.

Geneen, L.J., Moore, A.R., Clarke, C., Martin, D., Colvin, L.A., Smith, B.H., 2017. Physical activity and exercise for chronic pain in adults: an overview of Cochrane Reviews. Cochrane Database Syst. Rev. (4), CD011279, doi:10.1002/14651858. CD011279.pub3.

Hickey, G., Fricker, P.A., McDonald, W.A., 1997. Injuries to elite rowers over a 10-yr period. Med. Sci. Sports Exerc. 29 (12), 1567–1572.

Hofmijster, M.J., van Soest, A.J., Koning, J.J., 2008. Rowing skill affects power loss on a modified rowing ergometer. Med. Sci. Sports Exerc. 40 (6), 1101–1110.

Inkster, L.M., Eng, J.J., 2004. Postural control during a sit-to-stand task in individuals with mild Parkinson's disease. Exp. Brain Res. 154 (1), 33–38.

International Organization for Standardization (ISO), 1989a. General Terms for External Limb Prostheses and External Orthoses. ISO 8549-1: Prosthetics and Orthotics—Vocabulary. International Organization for Standardization, Geneva, Switzerland.

International Organization for Standardization (ISO), 1989b. Terms Relating to External Orthoses. ISO 8549-3: Prosthetics and Orthotics—Vocabulary. International Organization for Standardization, Geneva, Switzerland.

Kirtley, C., 2006. Clinical Gait Analysis—Theory and Practice. Elsevier Churchill Livingstone, London.

Lehmann, J.F., Price, R., Condon, S.M., DeLateur, B.J., 1987. Gait abnormalities in hemiplegia: their correction by ankle-foot orthoses. Arch. Phys. Med. Rehabil. 68, 763–771.

McCormack, G., Giles-Corti, B., Milligan, R., 2006. Demographic and individual correlates of achieving 10000 steps/day: use of pedometers in a population based study. Health Promot. J. Austr. 17 (1), 43–47.

McGregor, A.H., Buckeridge, E.M., Murphy, A.J., Bull, A.M.J., 2016. Communicating and using biomechanical measures through visual cues to optimise safe and effective rowing. Proc. Instit. Mech. Eng. Part P. J. Sports Eng. Technol. 230 (4), 246–252.

McGregor, A.H., Patankar, Z.S., Bull, A.M.J., 2005. Spinal kinematics in elite oarswomen during a routine physiological 'step test'. Med. Sci. Sports Exerc. 37 (6), 1014–1020.

McGregor, A.H., Patankar, Z.S., Bull, A.M.J., 2007. Longitudinal changes in the spinal kinematics of oarswomen during step testing. J. Sports Sci. Med. 6 (1), 29–35.

Murphy, A.J., 2009. Elite Rowing: Technique and Performance. PhD Thesis. Imperial College London.

Murphy, A.J., Bull, A.M.J., McGregor, A.H., 2011a. Optimizing and validating and electromagnetic tracker in a human performance laboratory. Proc. Instit. Mech. Eng. Part H. J. Eng. Med. 225 (4), 343–351.

Murphy, A.J., Bull, A.M.J., McGregor, A.H., 2011b. Predicting the lumbosacral joint centre location from palpable anatomical landmarks. Proc. Inst. Mech. Eng. Part H. J. Eng. Med. 225 (11), 1078–1083.

Murphy, A.J., Chee, S.T.H., Bull, A.M.J., McGregor, A.H., 2010. The calibration and application of a force-measuring apparatus on the seat of a rowing ergometer. Proc. Instit. Mech. Eng. Part P. J. Sports Eng. Technol. 224 (1), 109–116.

National Institute of Health & Care Excellence, 2016. Low back pain and sciatica in over 16s: assessment and management. https://www.nice.org.uk/guidance/ng59/chapter/Recommendations. (Accessed 30.January.2018.)

Nolte, V. (Ed.), 2011. Rowing Faster, second ed. Human Kinetics, Champaign, IL.

Norkin, C.C., White, D.J., 1995. Measurement of Joint Motion: A Guide to Goniometry. FA Davis Co, Philadelphia.

Perry, J., Burnfield, J., 1992. Gait Analysis: Normal and Pathological Function, second ed. Slack Incorporated, Thorofare, NJ.

Pollock, A., Gray, C., Culham, E., Durward, B.R., Langhorne, P., 2014. Interventions for improving sit-to-stand ability following stroke. Cochrane Database Syst. Rev. (5), CD007232.

Raghavan, P., 2015. Upper limb motor impairment post stroke. Phys. Med. Rehabil. Clin. North Am. 26 (4), 599–610. doi:10.1016/j.pmr.2015.06.008.

Read, H.S., Hazlewood, M.E., Hillman, S.J., Prescott, R.J., Robb, J.E., 2003. Edinburgh visual gait score for use in cerebral palsy. J. Pediatr. Orthop. 23, 296–301.

Rumball, J.S., Lebrun, C.M., Di Ciacca, S.R., Orlando, K., 2005. Rowing injuries. Sports Med. 35 (6), 537–555.

Smoljanovic, T., Bohacek, I., Hannafin, J.A., Terborg, O., Hren, D., Pecina, M., et al., 2015. Acute and chronic injuries among senior international rowers: a cross-sectional study. Int. Orthop. 39 (8), 1623–1630.

Soper, C., Hume, P.A., 2004. Towards an ideal rowing technique for performance: the contributions from biomechanics. Sports Med. 34 (12), 825–848.

Wilson, F., Gissane, C., Gormley, J., Simms, C., 2010. A 12-month prospective cohort study on injury in international rowers. Br. J. Sports Med. 44 (3), 207–214.

Wilson, F., Gissane, C., Gormley, J., Simms, C., 2013. Sagittal plane motion of the lumber spine during ergometer and single skull rowing. Sports Biomech. 12 (2), 132–142.

Wolf, S.L., Catlin, P.A., Ellis, M., Archer, A.L., Morgan, B., 2001. Assessing Wolf motor function test as outcome measure for research in patients after stroke. Stroke 32, 1635–1639.

APPENDIX

CHAPTER 2: SELF-ASSESSMENT ANSWERS

1. A mechanical force is a push or a pull caused through physical contact.
2. a, c and e are vectors
3. Magnitude, point application, direction and angle of application
4. It is false. Although used interchangeably in everyday life, these are different in physics; speed is a scalar quantity (i.e. magnitude only), whereas velocity is a vector so requires both magnitude and direction.
5. Muscles cause joints to rotate because:
   The muscle is attached at a distance from the joint centre (centre of rotation), (b).
6. If the biceps brachii muscle pulls on the radius with 50 N of force (acting perpendicularly) at a distance of 5 cm from the elbow joint centre it will create a turning of 2.5 Nm, (c).
7. If a pulling force (such as a muscle) is applied at an angle, the overall force is broken down/resolved into horizontal and vertical components, (c).
8. Examples of a force couple (muscular or otherwise) include:
   Two hands being used to turn a steering wheel
   Rectus abdominus and hamstrings to posteriorly tilt the pelvis.
9. The two types of force transducer commonly used in forceplates are strain gauges and piezoelectric crystals.
10. A moment of force is a force that causes rotation.

CHAPTER 3: SELF-ASSESSMENT ANSWERS

1. This is false. The strength of gravity results from the amount of mass. The amount of mass a planet has will determine its gravitational force. The moon, for example, has much less mass than Earth (approximately 1/80th) so its gravitation pull is much less (approximately 16% of earth's or 1.62 m/s^2 compared to 9.81 m/s/s on earth).
2. Weight is a force, calculated as mass × gravity (acceleration). Therefore if you had a mass of 75 kg and lived on Earth (gravity = 9.81), your weight would be 735.75 kg (75 × 9.81), (b).

3. Yes it can. The CoM is an abstract point representing the averaged position of all the mass. Think about a ring doughnut (I do a lot); its CoM will be located in the hole in the middle.
4. A stable body will move momentarily to a new position but then return to its original state, (a).
5. Force is measured in newtons (N). Named after Sir Isaac Newton, (b).
6. The rear stabiliser wheels on a wheelchair prevent the chair tipping back, (d).
7. A clown might carry an umbrella for any, or all, those reasons, but from a biomechanical perspective it provides an additional counterbalancing moment, (b).
8. The ankle dorsiflexors (a) perform this function. Lifting the feet up shifts the CoP backwards to create a stabilising moment. Older people who fall have been observed to have greater weakness in this muscle group compared to plantarflexors. The activity also has to be quick.
9. Of course the 'ideal' standing posture will do all of these things; the answer is therefore a, b, c and d.
10. The body maintains stability during these instances of instability by maintaining momentum to a new stable position, (b). Think of the body's position just after the trailing leg leaves the ground when walking; if it wasn't moving forward the body will fall as the CoM is well behind the only point of contact on the ground (the forward foot).

CHAPTER 4: SELF-ASSESSMENT ANSWERS

1. Inertia simply means a reluctance to move and is directly related to the mass of an object.
2. Momentum is mass × velocity (a)
3. Momentum is in fact a vector quantity, so this is true.
4. In a balanced (not accelerating) rotating body the centripetal and centrifugal forces are equal, so the answer is b.
5. Impulse is force × time, (a).
6. Newton's third law of motion is usually stated as 'For every action there is an equal and opposite reaction', (a).

7. Sliding friction is calculated as F = μ (coefficient of friction) × N (weight of object), answer is therefore (a).

8. Work is force × displacement, (d).

9. A lever consists of four parts: a rigid beam, a pivot, an effort and a load, (d).

10. A type 2 lever has the effort and load on the same side as the fulcrum with the effort furthest away (think of a wheelbarrow), (c).

11. The most common type of lever in the body is type 3, (c).

12. Power is work divided by time, (b).

13. Mechanical potential energy due to gravity (also known as gravitational potential energy) is calculated as mass (of body) × gravity × height above ground, (c).

14. This is false. Energy can neither be created nor destroyed. This is the first law of thermodynamics also known as the law of energy conservation.

15. You have a choice of:
    a. Pelvic rotation.
    b. Pelvic tilt/obliquity.
    c. Knee flexion during mid-stance.
    d. Ankle DF at heel strike and PF during terminal stance (heel off).
    e. Knee flexion during loading response (early stance).
    f. Lateral movement of the pelvis (weight shift).

16. The determinants of gait are a really useful way to analyse walking but there isn't hard evidence to support the idea that they directly reduce CoM displacement when walking, with the exception of except heel raise (see Kerrigan et al., 2000).

CHAPTER 5: SELF-ASSESSMENT ANSWERS

1. Briefly, stress is the force applied to a material per unit area (i.e. stress is force/area). Strain is the amount of deformation a material will undergo when stressed (usually as a ratio between new length and original length).

2. Tensile strain is the amount of elongation a material undergoes when stressed. You measure the original length (before stress is applied) and then when the stress is applied, the strain is the ratio between the two (new length when stressed/original length); also, it can be expressed as a percentage.

3. Young's modulus is the ratio between stress and strain, so the answer is (b), stress divided by strain.

4. This statement is true, a material with high viscosity has a high resistance to flow.

5. Shear stress is stress applied parallel to the surface, (d).

6. If a material returns to its original size and properties after a stress is removed, the material has been taken into its elastic range (b).

7. Type 1 collagen is the most abundant in the body, found in tendons, skin, artery walls and bone, (a).

8. Collagen gives tendon its strength, (b).

9. If a material has isotropic properties it means its properties (stiffness, strength, etc.) are the same, irrespective of the direction that stress is applied.

10. The middle layer of skin called the dermis, (a).

11. The two types of bone are compact (on the outside) and cancellous (on the inside), which is also called spongy bone.

12. Tendon fibres have a wavy pattern called a crimp, (b).

13. The collagen in tendons and ligaments are arranged densely and in the same direction, (b).

14. Elastic fibres are made of elastin, (c).

15. Wolff's law states that bone adapts to the forces they experience, (a).

16. The three factors that make immobilisation worse are a prolonged period of immobilisation, inflammation and age, (a), (b) and (c).

17. This statement is true; stress relaxation is where there is a gradual decrease in tension within the stretched muscle when it is held at a constant length.

18. Connective tissue consists of three basic ingredients, fibres (collagen and elastin), cells (fibroblasts, macrophages and neutrophils) and ground substance, (d).

19. Density is mass/volume, (c).

20. 4% of the body would float, (a).

21. Hydrostatic pressure is density × gravity × height (depth), (c).

22. Pascal's law states that a pressure change in a **contained** fluid or gas is transmitted evenly throughout the gas/fluid, (a).

23. The movement of a gas or a fluid where the layers slide on top of each is called laminar flow, (d).

24. The FET technique is all about increasing the velocity of the expired air. This will cause turbulent (as well as fast) air flow next to the airway wall, helping to dislodge any mucus adhering to it.

25. Bernoulli's principle is all about creating pressure differences with increased speed of the fluid (water). The sculling motion of the hand helps to lift the body by creating a pressure difference between the top part of the hand and the lower part.

CHAPTER 6: SELF-ASSESSMENT ANSWERS

1. The two proteins are actin and myosin.
2. The thick filament consists of myosin, (d).
3. The molecule that releases myosin from its attachment to actin is ATP (adenosine triphosphate).
4. The basic functional unit of the muscle is called the sarcomere.
5. Bundles of fibres makes up a fascicle, (b).
6. Strength is equivalent to force. Usually strength means the maximal force that can be generated during a muscle contraction; for example, the largest weight that can be lifted. This is different from power, which is the rate of muscle work (force applied over stated distance, i.e. work/time). Power then is really a measure of how quickly a muscle can perform its work.
7. An isometric contraction is a contraction that does not result in joint movement, that is, the muscle does not change its length. An isotonic muscle contraction, on the other hand, is where there is a change in length as the muscle contracts.
8. An eccentric contraction is when the muscle length increases while tension is generated (e.g. lowering a weight [slowly] in your hand by extending your elbow – eccentric contraction in biceps brachii). A concentric contraction where the muscle length shortens (e.g. lifting a weight in your hand by flexing your elbow – concentric contraction in biceps brachii).
9. An eccentric contraction performs negative work over time, that is, it absorbs power.
10. This is false. A type 1 fibre is slow twitch, but this means it resists fatiguing due to its use of aerobic energy pathways, which are more sustainable.
11. A muscle produces its maximal force during an isometric contraction in its middle range, (b).
12. This is not true. A muscle's ability to produce force does indeed vary according to speed of contraction. During a concentric contraction the faster the muscle shortens the less strength it can generate. This logically means that a zero-contraction speed (i.e. an isometric contraction) creates the highest forces.
13. A female muscle fibre is exactly the same as a male muscle fibre, (c).
14. A grade 3 on the Oxford Muscle Grade Scale is full range of movement against gravity, (a).
15. A 10RM is the resistance/weight that can be lifted 10 consecutive times (safely and with good performance), (b).
16. Using your movement analysis and the FITT principles as a guide, design a programme for an individual who wants to improve his strength so that he can climb the stairs. This individual has undergone significant atrophy due to forced inactivity due to illness. Therefore they have limited muscle strength (Oxford Muscle Grading Scale 3) through their whole lower limb.
    a. The main muscles involved in lifting your body up each step are the knee and hip extensors (gluteus maximus [glut max] and quadriceps [quads] particularly) but there are other muscles that help with balance, foot clearance, posture, etc.
    b. To lift you up each step the glut max and quads muscles are performing concentric contractions. It is impossible to know exactly what the speed of contraction will be exactly, but the important thing to bear in mind is that there is some speed of movement; it is not an isometric contraction so training needs to target muscle power.
    c. No it is quite different. In terms of the key muscles (quads and glut max) these will be working eccentrically during stair descent.
    d. The main physiological adaptation that you want to occur is an improvement in muscle power (perhaps also endurance if there are a lot of steps).
    e. Training needs to be specific to the task, so performing repetitive step-ups is most likely to improve stair climbing. This could be supplemented with other movements that require concentric quads and glut max, such as sit to stand or even cycling in recumbent static bikes (although you should try to match the speed of movement with what might be expected during stair ascent).
    f. These would depend to some extent on the individual but you would need to do these at least two to three times a week (frequency), using body weight as the size of resistance (intensity), high repetitions (think about the number of stairs at home) with low number sets (time) and focus on exercises that are similar to stair climbing (similar joint movement and muscle activity) (type). Probably best of all is simply to practice stair climbing (with supervision).

CHAPTER 7: SELF-ASSESSMENT ANSWERS

1. Fibrous joints (synarthroses) have no movement at all, (a).

2. The synovial fluid does two of these things; it both nourishes the cartilage and reduces friction, (a and b).
3. This is true.
4. Abduction and adduction movements occur in the frontal plane about a sagittal axis, (c).
5. The knee is a hinge joint, (d).
6. A joint's close-packed position is the position of maximum congruency between the surfaces, (b).
7. Rub is not (usually) a joint accessory movement, (c).
8. The apposition of soft tissue is one of the normal constraints to joint movement, (b).
9. Manual passive movements are indicated when a patient is unable to actively perform the movement themselves, (a).
10. Contractures are an adaptive shortening of the muscle, (b).

CHAPTER 8: SELF-ASSESSMENT ANSWERS

1. The two functions that evolution has bestowed on the modern human's foot are rigidity for propulsion (b) and an ability to adapt to varying surfaces, (c).
2. The thoracic spine is curved convexly, (a).
3. The line of gravity does not always lie within the base of support (BoS), this is incorrect, (d).
4. In the sagittal plane the LoG 'ideally' passes through the mastoid process, the shoulder (or just in front), the hip joint (or just behind), the knee joint (or just in front) and just in front of the ankle joint, (c).
5. The pelvis tilts posteriorly, (a), when you sit down (from standing) on a standard chair.
6. The swayback standing posture demands the least energy, (a).
7. Sitting creates the most pressure between the lumbar intervertebral discs, (c).
8. The ankle strategy is where the ankle dorsiflexors and plantarflexors control the forward and backward sway of the body (in the sagittal plane), much like an upside-down pendulum.
9. You could test balance in a number of ways, with and without technology, for example:
   a. Timing a one-legged stand.
   b. Berg Balance Scale.
   c. Romberg test.
   d. Centre of pressure sway recorded from a forceplate.
   e. Centre of mass movement recorded from a body worn sensor (e.g. an inertial sensor).
10. Three things associated with ageing that effect balance could include:
   a. Increased body sway.
   b. Decline in sensory systems (e.g. vestibular system).

c. Loss of strength.
   d. Decreased nerve conduction velocity.
   e. Reduced ability to dual task, such as talking and walking.
11. Feedback is the information we receive from our sensory systems that can be used to adjust a movement. Feedforward is essentially movement preparation; it involves preplanned anticipatory movements that do not require any information from the sensory system.
12. If you experienced a very large push from behind you would probably use the stepping strategy, (c), to maintain stability.
13. The three main sensory inputs used to control balance are:
   a. Vision.
   b. Proprioception (body position awareness).
   c. Head position and acceleration (vestibular system).
14. Technologies that could be used in balance training include:
   a. Balance platforms for measuring centre of pressure location.
   b. Body worn inertial sensors (e.g. your smartphone).
   c. Wobble boards.

CHAPTER 9: SELF-ASSESSMENT ANSWERS

1. The transmission of information between neurons occurs at the synapse, (b).
2. The resting potential across a neuron membrane is approximately −70mV. This is created by the relative (inside and outside the membrane wall) concentration of both sodium (Na^+) and potassium (K^+) ions, (a & b).
3. Axon size, (a), and presence of a myelin sheath, (d), both increase the speed of signal propagation.
4. A muscle spindle detects both the length and rate of change of the length of a muscle, (b & d).
5. Soma means it is about the body (soma means body). Somatosensory means sensations arising from the body, as opposed to the traditional sensations from the sensors in the head (taste, smell, sight and sound) eyes and nose. Therefore somatosensory includes proprioception (body position sense) as well as touch and arguably temperature).
   For the purposes of a body schema it would be proprioception.
6. Stimulation of the stretch reflex leads to a reflexive contraction of the muscle being stretched, (a).
7. Opening of sodium ion (Na^+) channels at the postsynaptic membrane will lead to depolarisation

and therefore excitation of the postsynaptic neuron, (a).

8. The degrees of freedom principle refers to the large number of potential solutions to a movement task, (b).

9. This is true. Feedforward movements do not require feedback.

10. This is false. Although specific motor programmes may not actually be changeable, the output from them, in terms of motor unit action potentials (i.e. instructions to the muscles) can be changed by altering their excitability and combining with other motor programmes.

11. This is false. Central pattern generators, when fired, may be able to set a rhythmic pattern of leg muscle activity that is roughly equivalent to that seen in a walking pattern. However, they are not sophisticated enough to control indoor walking, which is still pretty complex with lots of stops/starts and changes in direction

12. Which of the following statements would you agree with:

I would agree with the second statement (b). Rehabilitation of functional movements should incorporate variability in movement practice to encourage involvement of the feedback system. Practice variability is critical if you want to create real motor learning (the person has to actively think about how they are moving) and will put the person in a better position for returning to everyday life where there are constant variations in posture and movement.

CHAPTER 10: SELF-ASSESSMENT ANSWERS

1. The arm and leg on the left side (side head is turned to) both extend (elbow extends, shoulder may abduct, knee extends and ankle may plantarflex). In contrast, the arm and leg on the right both flex (mainly at elbow and knee) – a bit like an 'on guard' fencing pose. I have also heard it called the ice cream reflex because no matter which hand you hold it in you can't get an ice cream in your mouth (British humour).

2. An infant will start pulling themselves up into standing at around 5 months (even earlier in some cases), but it probably won't be maintained until around 7 months.

3. According to Bandura, the child learns movement by watching others and then imitates it.

4. Reward is considered the primary motivation for movement. Initially this reward is sensory (touch/

sound/vision/taste), but as the child matures the reward involves more complex constructs like achievement and pride, which (according to Bandura) lay the foundation for feelings of self-esteem/worth.

5. Movement, of course, begins long before birth. As early as 7 weeks the foetus can begin to move their trunk with seemingly purposeless twitching movements. By 10 weeks the head and jaw may be moving individually and even hand-to-face movement can be observed.

6. The benefits of physical activity are global. Psychological, social, cognitive and physical gains have all been reported. Specifically, there is evidence for:
   a. **Cognitive domain:** Improved cognitive functioning and reduced risk of dementia.
   b. **Psychosocial domain:** Reduced depression and anxiety, increased social interaction and less social isolation.
   c. **Physical domain:** Age-related cardiovascular changes can be reversed; a reduced risk of hypertension and diabetes (type 2); and increased muscle strength and mass.

7. At the level of body structure, aging causes the following changes to the musculoskeletal system:

   Decreased muscle mass (particularly type 2a and b [fast twitch]), reduced tendon elasticity, reduced ligament strength, loss of bone mineral density, reduced chondrocyte numbers.

   These changes lead to the following loss in function:

   Decreased muscle strength, reduced motor control, increased risk of tendon/cartilage and ligament injury (and longer repair times) and an increased propensity for osteoporosis.

8. Older adults are recommended to engage in physical activity for 150 minutes of moderate, or 75 minutes of vigorous, intensity aerobic activity every week (or a mixture of both). Each physical activity session should last at least 10 minutes. Strengthening exercises, specifically, for the major muscle groups, are recommended at least twice a week and, if they are at risk of falling, they should perform balance exercise at least three times a week.

9. Intrinsic factors include age, gender (higher risk for females), previous history of falls, gait and balance problems, reduced muscle strength (and power) and polypharmacy (i.e. ≥ four medications). Extrinsic factors include things like environmental hazards (e.g. slippery rugs, uneven surfaces), footwear, and

assistive devices (e.g. walking frames) being used incorrectly.

10. As you can imagine, an exercise programme is usually required that includes strengthening, balance, flexibility and endurance. This has been shown not only to reduce the number of falls but also to improve balance confidence, which is probably just as important.

CHAPTER 11: SELF-ASSESSMENT ANSWERS

1. There are nine variables.
   a. Time
   b. Linear displacement
   c. Linear velocity
   d. Linear acceleration
   e. Angular displacement
   f. Angular velocity
   g. Angular acceleration
   h. Force
   i. Moment of force
2. While the mass of an object is unchanging, the moment of inertia depends on how this mass is distributed in relation to its rotation point, which might be changeable, for example, moving the bob at the end of a pendulum or bending the knee up while standing to bring the leg mass closer to the hip, thereby reducing the moment of inertia.
3. To reduce muscle work we reduce the moment of inertia of our moving limbs by bringing the mass closer to the rotation point. In running we bend our arms to make it easier to flex and extend them quickly; we 'shorten' our leg during the swing phase of gait to make it easier to bring it forward.
4. An object will spin if a force is applied with a line of action that is located a distance from its centre of mass, that is, a moment of force is applied.
5. Your lower leg (knee to foot) rotates and translates as you walk. During stance it rotates initially about the heel and then about the ankle (dorsiflexion) before reversing into plantarflexion initially around the ankle and the around the toes. During the swing phase it rotates about the knee through initial flexion to full(ish) extension at terminal swing. However, the knee is translating forward, and hence its movement is a combination of rotation and translation.
6. Velocity is the rate of change of displacement.
7. Acceleration is the rate of change of velocity.
8. Yes. Acceleration is the rate of change of a velocity. Velocity is a vector, which means it has both magnitude and direction, so if direction changes (while speed (magnitude) remains constant) then you will be accelerating (e.g. running around a bend). A force is required to accelerate; in this case the force is directed to the centre of the bend and changes the direction of the velocity, if not its magnitude.
9. Yes, momentum is the product of the mass of an object and its velocity and change in momentum is equal to the product of a force and time (impulse). So if you apply an additional push to a moving object over some time you will increase its velocity and hence increase its momentum.
10. No, the first law of thermodynamics states that total energy remains constant. It can only be transformed from one state to another, for example, from potential energy (ball resting on top of a hill) to kinetic (ball rolling down the hill).

CHAPTER 12: SELF-ASSESSMENT ANSWERS

1. The nine variables are (1) time, (2) linear displacement, (3) linear velocity, (4) linear acceleration, (5) angular displacement, (6) angular velocity, (7) angular acceleration, (8) force and (9) moment of force.
2. A full biomechanical motion analysis will capture (or predict) all nine parameters of human motion (see above) in three dimensions. Movement assessment systems, on the other hand, will measure one or more of the variables in one or more dimension.
3. Stereo-photogrammetry is the process of combining multiple synchronised cameras to get more than one (mono-photogrammetry) point of view.
4. Most motion capture systems use infra-red light.
5. Single marker systems are time consuming (fixing multiple markers to the skin or wearing a special suit).
6. A cluster is a rigid plate with, typically, four individual markers permanently fixed to it.
7. Disadvantages of visual motion analysis include:
   a. It is dependent on the skill of the observer.
   b. There is no permanent record for future comparison/analysis.
   c. Forces and moments cannot be observed.
   d. Velocities and accelerations can only be estimated.
   e. The human visual system (including brain processing) is not quick enough to pick up fast-moving events/functions.

8. Electrogoniometers (electric goniometers) record angular displacement as a changing electrical voltage so they can provide joint angle data.
9. EMG provides an understanding of the muscle activity that creates the movement.
10. An inertial measurement unit (IMU) is a single unit that combines a three-dimensional accelerometer, a three-dimensional gyroscope (which gives angular velocity) and a three-dimensional magnetometer (a three-dimensional compass).

CHAPTER 13: SELF-ASSESSMENT ANSWERS

1. A body function is a physiological or psychological function of a specific body system. This could include mental functions, voice and speech functions and neuromusculoskeletal functions, such as elbow flexion or ankle hip rotation.
2. Pain is a body function; it is listed under chapter two of the ICF.
3. For the participation domain of the ICF (thinking about mobility specifically) you might consider asking about things like:
    Their recreation/hobbies, their social life, the clubs they are involved in etc. It's all to do with an individual's involvement in society, and life in general.
4. The four main classifications of mobility in the activity part of the ICF model are:
   a. Changing and maintaining body position.
   b. Walking and moving.
   c. Carrying, moving and handling objects.
   d. Moving around using transportation.
5. Walking is mainly considered as an activity and has several sub-categories such as walking around obstacles (d4503) and walking indoors (d4600). Gait pattern, on the other hand, is listed as a body function (b770), but this is really in the context of gait analysis. (See https://wwrichard .net/2013/05/31/what-the-icf/ for a discussion on this.)
6. Of course, health professionals need a broad understanding of the impact a disease/injury/ condition can have on a patient's life. This is to ensure the right things (for the patient) are targeted, and the impact of any intervention can be tested against the things that really matter to the patient. Improving ankle joint flexibility may not be important but returning to a social club might be.
7. If you measured motor control in a stroke you would be measuring in the body structure domain of

mobility, specifically this would be b760 (http:// www.icfillustration.com/icfil_eng/b/b75.html).
8. If you measured sit-to-stand ability (e.g. the five times sit-to-stand test) in someone recovering from a total hip arthroplasty you would be measuring in the body activity domains of mobility, specifically category d4104, which deals with moving in and out of a sitting position (http://www.icfillustration.com/ icfil_eng/d/d410.html.)
9. If you measured return to work in someone recovering from cardiac surgery you would be measuring in the participation domain of mobility (http://www.icfillustration.com/icfil_eng/d/d84 .html).

CHAPTER 14: SELF-ASSESSMENT ANSWERS

1. 1 (one) MET is equal to the resting metabolic rate, while sitting quietly, (c).
2. MVPA has a MET equivalent value between 3 and 6, (b).
3. Ironing in a seated position (MET value ~2.5) is categorised as light physical activity so you are not sedentary, but also not accumulating MVPA, so (a).
4. Walking is physical activity because you are moving, (d).
5. Sedentary behaviour is currently defined as being seated or lying down, with a MET value less than 1.5, (a).
6. If you exercise for 30 minutes per day 5 days per week, that is very good, but you still need to consider your behaviour for the rest of the time, (d).
7. Of course sedentary behaviour affects everyone, (c).
8. Oxygen uptake is the difference in oxygen levels between the air we inhale and the air we exhale, (b).
9. People living with long-term conditions should be advised to try and stay active within their limits, (d).

CHAPTER 15: SELF-ASSESSMENT ANSWERS

1. The three stages of motor learning proposed by Fitts and Posner are:
   a. Cognitive.
   b. Associative.
   c. Autonomous.
2. Fixate means to make the movement patterns stable, consistent, for skills taking place in stable, predictable environments. For skills in a changing environment,

elaborate means the need to diversify, to adapt to the changing environment.

3. A General Motor Programme (GMP) is a stored representation of the spatial and temporal patterns of the muscle activity required to perform a specific action.

4. Blocked practice is where the individual carries out a pre-organised set of single movements, for example 10 reaching movements, whereas random practice combines the practice of several different movements presented in a random order, for example reaching, manipulating a small object, gripping a mug etc. In a sports context, for example soccer, you might practice heading the ball, kicking the ball, trapping the ball etc. rather than repetitive kicking.

5. Contextual interference is when the rate of motor learning slows down when practice includes a variety of movements/skills (random as opposed to blocked practice). In an apparent contradiction this leads to better skill retention and transference to other similar skills.

6. Mental practice is simply when a person imagines they are performing the movement without actually moving. Mental imagery is a type of mental practice where the person creates some form of visual or kinaesthetic representation of the action; this could be them watching themselves perform the movement from another person's (e.g. therapist or coach) perspective or from their own perspective.

7. Giving feedback too often during skill acquisition can mean the learner becomes dependent on this extrinsic feedback rather than develop their own intrinsic systems for error correction.

8. The evidence suggests that it is better to focus attention externally, that is, how the movement is made in the environment rather than internally, where the focus is on the muscle activity, joint movement etc.

9. How can VR systems help in rehabilitation settings?
   a. They can enable high repetition as tasks can be easily repeated.
   b. A great deal of variation can be easily included.
   c. They offer a huge range of feedback options to suit an individual's needs.
   d. They may be more motivating, but this will depend on individuals as well as the software being used.

10. A learner's motivation is complex (and can be fragile in clinical environments) but there are ways to improve it. Enhancing expectancies of future success (for example showing videos of their best performances) is where you basically try to make the learner think they will, eventually, master the skill. Autonomy is where the learner takes ownership of some aspects of the training, for example the type and timing of feedback.

CHAPTER 16: SELF-ASSESSMENT ANSWERS

1. The five elements included in the model of human movement using balance theory are:
   a. Organisation.
   b. Task environment.
   c. Task design.
   d. Technology.
   e. The individual.

2. Environmental factors that could affect movement include:
   a. Light.
   b. Noise.
   c. Temperature.
   d. Weather.
   e. Space.
   f. Furniture.
   g. Surfaces.
   h. Objects (clutter).
   i. That's it.

3. Anthropometrics are the measurements taken from the human body; this could be anything from the circumference of the head to mass of a limb.

4. It is almost true, but this definition is just not extensive enough as technology doesn't just mean the actual physical tools—it also includes the skills, techniques and processes involved in pursuing our objectives.

5. A physiotherapist could use any number of physical and procedural technologies including…
   a. A computer.
   b. A video recorder.
   c. A pen/pencil.
   d. A tape measure.
   e. A decision-making flow diagram or guideline.
   f. A walking stick.
   g. An electrical stimulator.
   h. A phone.
   i. A spinal mobilisation technique.

6. With a recently torn ankle ligament you might walk downstairs with the use of crutches or a stick and/or use the bannister. You might also move more slowly and one step at a time. You might also wear a protective boot, strapping or splint.

7. There are too many possibilities to write down but the exercise, if done conscientiously, should help reduce any risk and improve the efficiency of the activity.

CHAPTER 17: SELF-ASSESSMENT ANSWERS

1. The magnitude of a normal vertical GRF during the loading response phase of gait is typically between 110% and 120% of body weight.
2. Standardised scoring tools such as the Edinburgh GAIT score and the Rancho Los Amigos Observational Gait Analysis tool can be used with video footage.
3. This is a clinical judgement (in collaboration with patient/family) with considerations for pain, mobility, rate of deterioration, quality of life and the potential to improve (surgery, orthotics and/or rehabilitation).
4. Vibration frequencies are typically around 1 to 2 Hz (one to two times per second); that is, step frequency.
5. Increasing walking speed would
   a. Increase the force magnitude during early stance phase.
   b. Shorten the duration of the stance phase, in particular the period when both feet are in stance (double support) would diminish as velocity increased until the individual was running. (See Kirtley et al., 1985. J. Biomed. Eng. 7 (4), 282–288.)
6. Knee hyperextension is a common, though definitely not inevitable, gait abnormality after a stroke. If the hemiplegia (muscle weakness) means that knee control is impaired and the knee begins to hyperextend during early to midstance, an AFO could be useful to control these external moments and maintain a good knee posture.
7. Off-the-shelf AFOs tend to be less stiff due to the materials used and their thickness. This means their ability to counteract the potentially very large moments experienced at the knee and hip during gait are not as good as custom-made AFOs. The weight of the patient may also be a factor in this.
8. During the early stages of gait rehabilitation it is important to both practice the movement (or parts of the movement) as much as possible and for the brain to receive sensory (mainly proprioceptive) signals from a 'normally' positioned lower limb. This will help to prevent the adoption of abnormal patterns and to promote good positioning. By holding the lower limb in a 'correct' position, the AFO can help with both these things. It will also

reduce the chances of adaptive shortening in the muscles.
9. The body needs to exceed body weight by around 10% to 20% in order to stand up from sitting.
10. During sit to stand the hip joints move the most during phase 1, around 25 degrees.
11. Raising the chair height will:
    a. Reduce the force required to stand up (less lifting distance required) but it still needs to exceed body weight.
    b. Reduce the amount of knee movement as it will start in a less flexed position.
12. Increasing the speed of the sit-to-stand movement will:
    a. Increase hip/trunk flexion during stage 1 and ankle dorsiflexion during stage 2. Also, there will be more arm movement.
    b. Increase the forces applied to the ground. The need to accelerate the body more will require larger forces.
13. Older people use arm rests to stand up to compensate for an inability to generate the required force from their lower limbs. This might be caused not only by muscle weakness (quadriceps) but also by joint pain. Using the arms will reduce the forces experienced across the knee joint.
14. A loss of shoulder range of motion in people with hemiplegia is common. When carrying out activities of daily living, a good range of shoulder range is often needed (think of reaching for the tomato ketchup on the table). To compensate for this movement loss the individual can use their trunk; for example, to compensate for a loss of flexion they could lean forward; to compensate for a loss of abduction they might lean their trunk to the side (side flexion).
15. The movements mainly affected were shoulder flexion and abduction, elbow extension, wrist flexion/extension.
16. All movements are not affected equally poststroke. It is possible that control of pronation and supination were easier movements for this patient because the muscle strength was sufficient to overcome the smaller gravitational moments, and/or there was less muscle stiffness and spasticity, which can increase resistance to movement and lead to a decrease in range of motion.
17. There are many muscles involved, including:
    a. Quadriceps.
    b. Gastrocnemius.
    c. Hamstrings.
    d. Gluteus maximus.

e. Erector spinae.
f. Rectus abdominus.
g. Rhomboids.
h. Deltoids.
i. Trapezius.
j. Pectoralis major.
k. Biceps brachii.
l. Triceps brachii.
m. Wrist extensors.
n. Finger flexors.

18. Controlling lumbopelvic rotation when rowing should reduce the risk of an acute back injury by maintaining the lumbar posture, particularly during the drive. It will also reduce the risk of overuse injuries to the lower back/lumbar spine.

19. Rowers spend much more time training on rowing ergometers raising the risk of lower back overuse injuries. The increased competitive environment on the water may raise the risk of a traumatic injury. Subtle differences (e.g. different moments of inertia of the oars) between the ergometer and the actual boat may also be a factor. Colder weather may also raise the injury risk but the evidence for this is largely anecdotal.

INDEX

Page numbers followed by "*f*" indicate figures, "*t*" indicate tables, and "*b*" indicate boxes.